Medical Care of the Elderly:
A Practical Approach

THE COLLAMORE PRESS
D.C. Heath and Company
Lexington, Massachusetts
Toronto

MEDICAL CARE OF THE ELDERLY: A PRACTICAL APPROACH

Edited by JACK D. McCUE, M.D.

Chief, Internal Medical Teaching Program
The Moses H. Cone Memorial Hospital
Greensboro, North Carolina
Associate Professor of Medicine
University of North Carolina
Chapel Hill

Every effort has been made to ensure that drug dosage schedules and indications are correct at time of publication. Since ongoing medical research
can change standards of usage, and also because of human and typographical
error, it is recommended that readers check the *PDR* or package insert before
prescription or administration of the drugs mentioned in this book.

Contents

Contributing Authors

Jack D. McCue, M.D.
University of North Carolina at Chapel Hill
The Moses H. Cone Memorial Hospital
Greensboro, North Carolina

Raouf F. Badawi, M.D.
The Moses H. Cone Memorial Hospital
Greensboro, North Carolina

Terry L. Bazzarre, PH.D.
University of North Carolina at Greensboro

Paul Beck, M.D.
University of North Carolina at Chapel Hill

W. Paul Biggers, M.D.
University of North Carolina at Chapel Hill

Dan Blazer, M.D., PH.D.
Duke University
Durham, North Carolina

J. Patterson Browder, M.D.
University of North Carolina at Chapel Hill

Thomas A. Cable, M.D.
University of North Carolina at Chapel Hill
The Moses H. Cone Memorial Hospital
Greensboro, North Carolina

James R. Carter, M.D.
Case Western Reserve University
Cleveland, Ohio

Bryan R. Davis, M.D.
Case Western Reserve University
Cleveland, Ohio

Seymour Eisenberg, M.D.
University of Texas Southwestern Medical School
Dallas

Robert H. Fletcher, M.D.
University of North Carolina at Chapel Hill

J. Dermot Frengley, M.D., CH.B., M.R.C.P.
Case Western Reserve University
Cleveland, Ohio

Peter Gal, PHARM.D.
The Moses H. Cone Memorial Hospital
Greensboro, North Carolina

Vincent J. Giuliano, M.D.
University of Virginia School of Medicine
Charlottesville

M. Andrew Greganti, M.D.
University of North Carolina at Chapel Hill

Colin D. Hall, M.D.
University of North Carolina at Chapel Hill

Alan Halperin, M.D.
University of North Carolina at Chapel Hill

William B. Herring, M.D.
University of North Carolina at Chapel Hill
The Moses H. Cone Memorial Hospital
Greensboro, North Carolina

Wishwa N. Kapoor, M.D.
University of Pittsburgh
Pittsburgh, Pennsylvania

Michael Karpf, M.D.
University of Pittsburgh
Pittsburgh, Pennsylvania

Peter P. Lamy, PH.D.
University of Maryland
Baltimore

Timothy W. Lane, M.D.
University of North Carolina at Chapel Hill
The Moses H. Cone Memorial Hospital
Greensboro, North Carolina

Peter M. Levitin, M.D.
The Moses H. Cone Memorial Hospital
Greensboro, North Carolina

William R. Marshall, PH.D.
The Moses H. Cone Memorial Hospital
Greensboro, North Carolina

C. Thomas Nuzum, M.D.
University of North Carolina at Chapel Hill

Karen S. Oles, PHARM.D.
Bowman Gray School of Medicine
Winston-Salem, North Carolina
University of North Carolina at Chapel Hill

C. Stewart Rogers, M.D.
University of North Carolina at Chapel Hill
The Moses H. Cone Memorial Hospital
Greensboro, North Carolina

R. Balfour Sartor, M.D.
University of North Carolina at Chapel Hill

Robert E. Sevier, M.D.
The Moses H. Cone Memorial Hospital
Greensboro, North Carolina

Sigmund I. Tannenbaum, M.D.
The Moses H. Cone Memorial Hospital
Greensboro, North Carolina

Clinton D. Young, M.D.
The Moses H. Cone Memorial Hospital
Greensboro, North Carolina

Foreword

I attended the symposium organized by Dr. Jack McCue to cover in a systematic way the knowledge about aging that is useful to the primary care physician. The presentations were excellent; making them available in paperback form and expanding the content of the symposium to include even more important issues is a real service to the practicing community.

All physicians except pediatricians care for elderly persons. They know that all cellular functions will be decreased when an elderly patient is tested under stress and that elderly persons may die from illnesses that cause little trouble in younger people. Since we all care for the elderly, what is this fuss about geriatrics?

Those elderly persons who have an adequate income and are able to balance their checkbook, shop, cook, maintain their own living quarters, and engage in sexual activities are easily fitted into most medical practices. Eventually, though, the patient either dies or becomes unable to maintain independent living. Caring for a large number of dependent elderly patients then requires that the physician build up a more extensive support team than is present in the average practice. He must have data to answer a number of questions about each elderly patient: What are the patient's financial resources? What type of support system can the family supply? Are the living quarters well lighted and arranged to prevent falls? What are the fire hazards? Is there a button to press to call for help? Can the patient drive? How far away is the grocery store? Can the patient remember? How will incontinence be handled? How many medicines are being given and what is the cost? Is more than one doctor prescribing? What home health services are available? Are there day care centers? How available and how expensive are visiting nurses? Are there any homemaker services?

The medical history will take longer to elicit, and the physical examination may best be done over several visits. The dangers of hospitals must always be kept in mind. During an elderly patient's convalescence in a hospital, more attention should be paid by health care personnel to activities such as dressing, walking, eating at the table, bathing, and bowels than to the measurement of respiratory rate, pulse rate, and blood pressure.

The physician must know the availability of resources for rehabilitation and take an active role in seeing that all useful measures are carried out. He needs to know something about hearing aids, cataracts, and retinal degeneration. He needs to prepare the person with retinal degeneration to function after sight is gone.

Dependent as the physician is on the talents and skills of others, he will need to spend time each day in their education. The attitudes of attendants are frequently more important than the scientific skills of the physician.

The care of a large number of dependent elderly patients requires the physician to rearrange his time and support system to meet the needs of this population. The material in this book will be useful to any practitioner who treats independently living elderly persons. It will be even more useful to those of us who are involved in a major way with the care of the dependent elderly.

Eugene A. Stead, Jr., M.D.
Professor Emeritus of Medicine
Duke University

Preface

How can we communicate to primary care practitioners the essential knowledge of geriatric medicine? This is a question often asked by caring geriatrics specialists who witness well-meaning physicians making decisions that are philosophically and medically inappropriate for their elderly patients. *Medical Care of the Elderly: A Practical Approach* attempts to answer this question by describing the important issues in geriatric medical care for primary care practitioners—usually general internists or family practitioners. The chapters are pragmatic; extensive referencing and detailed pathophysiology have to some degree been sacrificed to make the text readable, accessible, and relevant to the needs of the practitioner.

Texts of geriatric medicine all face a common problem: a book that comprehensively covers the skillful care of the elderly must of course include all the knowledge present in a text of internal medicine. Where does an editor make the distinction between general internal medicine and geriatric medicine? I have attempted to draw the line, imperfectly to be sure, throughout this book between the practice of adult medicine and that of geriatric medicine, and have excluded from the text as much of the former as possible—hopefully thereby highlighting what I call the "special" knowledge of geriatric medicine. Some topics, the discussion of diabetes for example, must be generally discussed, with special reference to the elderly patient when appropriate. Others, like skin care, can be directly discussed in terms of the problems encountered by the elderly. Finally, some problems such as syncope or constipation are not different in the elderly, just much more common and often poorly managed.

A great deal of effort was spent on making the style and organization of this book uniform and readable, often at the expense of the patience of my excellent authors. The references in the Suggested Reading lists at the end of each chapter were chosen not for documentation but to serve as resources for further information on the topic covered.

Nearly all family practitioners and internists will care for large numbers of the elderly by the 1990s. This book is designed to prepare us for caring for our elderly citizens expertly and with compassion.

ACKNOWLEDGMENT

This book is primarily a collaborative effort of the full-time, part-time, and clinical faculty of the University of North Carolina at Chapel Hill who practice at The Moses H. Cone Memorial Hospital in Greensboro, North Carolina. Special gratitude is owed the staff of The Moses H. Cone Memorial Hospital and the Area Health Education Center in Greensboro.

1

THE AGING PERSON
AND SOCIETY

Understanding Aging

JACK D. McCUE, M.D.

Editor's note: There is no single aging process. Aging occurs simultaneously among various physiologic and psychological systems at different rates; it interacts with, but is not synonymous with, diseases. Psychosocial malfunction as a result of "unsuccessful" aging may impair the elderly much more than the general decrement in the reserve performance and efficiency of integration of various organ systems from biologic aging. The variation in levels of function in elderly persons is so great that generalizations about aging are usually meaningless.

Aging proceeds simultaneously on many levels. Our external appearance changes and our organs function differently. These macroscopic and gross changes presumably derive from the changes of cellular or microscopic aging. As humans with a complex psychiatric and social existence, we undergo changes in our relationships with others and with society as our bodies age—psychosocial aging. On an even larger scale, our society is now aging demographically, with already evident economic and political effects.

PHYSICAL AGING

Appearance

Height decreases by about 3 inches by the age of 80 years, and body weight, after reaching a peak at middle age, also steadily declines. Fat is redistributed away from the face and limbs onto the trunk; the percentage of body weight that is fat actually increases despite declining weight due to a loss in muscle mass. Bone mass also decreases, and the normal curve of the spine is accentuated by changes in vertebral bodies and vertebral interspaces. Skin loses its elasticity, and

3

hair, both sexual and decorative, changes in color and decreases in quantity. Secondary sex characteristics, in general, diminish in size and firmness. Physiognomy is altered by the changes just described and by sun-related skin damage, loss of teeth, and perhaps even one's outlook on life.

Organ Function

Apart from the cardiorespiratory and gastrointenstinal systems, all organs tend to shrink in size. Except for endocrine organs, all tend to decline in function. Perhaps the most cogent generalization about organic aging is that the functional reserve of all organ systems, which allows adaptation to stress, declines. Cardiac output declines steadily after the age of 20, reaching about 60 percent of baseline levels at the age of 80. Circulation is altered both qualitatively and quantitatively by inelastic blood vessels. The lungs become more rigid, with a consequent decline in maximum breathing capacity. The gastrointestinal tract has diminished motility, greatly reduced enzyme secretion, and probably reduced absorption. The parenchymal mass of the liver and kidneys declines, as does the function they subtend.

Central Nervous System

Mental function in the elderly is spared more than the dramatic microscopic changes in the brain would suggest. Cell loss approaches 50 percent in some cortical areas and 25 percent in the cerebellum. In addition, there are fewer dendritic interconnections among the remaining neurons. All senses decline—visual acuity, hearing, taste, smell, and touch.

Intellectual Function

Intelligence is to a large part determined by personality and character, so it is no surprise that people who exercise their intellect when young tend to retain their mental functioning longer. A small percentage of elderly persons maintain a stable I.Q. even at advanced ages, although the great majority demonstrate a gradual decline. Memory, contrary to myth, is not dramatically affected in the healthy, emotionally stable elderly person; the ability to acquire and integrate new information, however, is more susceptible to aging effects, and changes in eyesight and hearing may adversely affect intellectual performance.

CELLULAR AGING

The complex and interrelated events that accompany physical aging presumably occur through some integrated master plan—a "biologic clock." Distinguishing the various "normal" organic changes of aging from those of a yet poorly understood or unknown disease is one of the central issues of research in geriatrics. Is neuronal dropout, for example, related to an undetected viral infection or to autoimmunity, is it secondary to other aging changes like those in the vascular system, or does the biologic clock by accident or evolutionary design call for successive death of neurons?

The rate of cell division and the time that it takes for the organism to reach reproductive age correlate with an animal's life span. As an animal grows, cells divide rapidly. Coincident with the animal's approaching maximal size, cell division slows and the ability to repair molecular mistakes and cell damage declines. At this point, it seems, the alarm is set on the biologic clock—the ultimate life span is theoretically determined. Some observations that support this conclusion include the following: (1) animals that reach reproductive age quickly have shorter lives; (2) cells from older animals, when cultured, have the capacity for a smaller number of divisions than those from younger animals; (3) large animals take longer to reach maximal size and reproductive age, and tend to live longer; (4) in carefully controlled circumstances, a starved infant animal will delay reproduction until fed properly, and the alarm on its biologic clock is not set until it is ready for reproduction—hence, it lives longer.

Postmitotic cells—for example, heart muscle cells and neurons—have lost the capacity for further division and cannot replace themselves, so they must be able to repair their cellular damage. But just as the capacity for continuing division is gradually lost in other tissues, so does the reparative potential of postmitotic cells decline with age. Cumulative damage without repair may then result in poorer cellular function and eventual death of postmitotic cells.

Interest has recently focused on the aging of the immune system. T-lymphocytes (cells derived from bone marrow lymphocytic stem cells, "instructed" by "thymus-equivalent" tissue to become the modulators of the immune system) lose their capacity for cell division in parallel with aging itself. Their decline in function is closely associated with an increase in neoplasia and infection.

PSYCHOSOCIAL AGING

The diseases of aging and normal biologic aging changes are, to some degree, beyond our control. Of equal importance, however, are the psychosocial changes that occur with aging—and these are very much within our control. The concept of "successful aging" incorporates our acceptance of the inevitability of biologic changes, and a belief in our ability to contain the impact of those changes on our lives.

How a person copes with loss is of central importance to successful aging. The losses incurred with aging are legion—loss of friends and family through deaths and moves, loss of income and the ability to increase income at times of need, loss of social and occupational roles, decreased physical well-being and mobility, loss of the opportunities for gaining self-esteem through work and other activities, and loss of the self-esteem gained from the admiration of other people of one's strength and beauty.

The person who ages successfully adapts to losses by creating new opportunities and exploiting previously unused talents. The person who ages unsuccessfully withdraws from society, becomes depressed and isolated, and must rely on others for care. Maintenance of independence, then, becomes one measure of successful aging. Once independence is sacrificed in the intensely dependent settings of hospitals or nursing homes, essential survival skills are lost, and they may be difficult or impossible to reacquire. Support services from family, friends, the community, or government agencies help the successfully aging person to maintain the independence that retards or prevents psychosocial withdrawal.

SOCIETAL AGING

As we age, so do our nation and our world. Shown in Figure 1 is the startling prediction that the last half of the twentieth century will witness a sixfold increase in the number of people over 85 years old, and the next half-century a further doubling. Figure 2 (p. 8) breaks down by sex and age the population figures of 12 million Americans over age 65 in 1950, 25 million in 1980, and a projection of more than 55 million in 2050.

The needs of this fastest-growing segment of our population must be met. Just as the changes wrought by the post–World War II baby boom affected everyone's life, so will the graying of America affect us all. Tastes, transportation, housing, support services, health care, and many other factors will have to adapt to shifting economic and political power. Perhaps of some consolation to the aging readers of this book is the observation that the elderly will be an increasingly powerful segment of the population in the future, not the weak minority our grandparents were.

FIGURE 1

Percentage of change in the number of elderly in the United States,
1950–2000 and 2000–2050, by age group and race.
SOURCE: U.S. Bureau of the Census

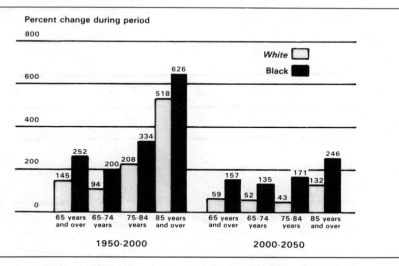

VARIATION IN FUNCTION WITH AGING

The differences in intelligence, independence, appearance, and physical stamina among 70-year-olds are remarkable—much greater than those among members of younger age groups. One 70-year-old college professor may be demented, institutionalized, crippled with chronic illness, or near death from vascular disease, while a colleague of the same age may still be lecturing, writing, administrating, and jogging two miles a day.

Fries, in an examination of the decline of individual performance in marathon records, points out that age alone has less effect on performance than training;[1] an examination of his graph of the increase in record times for marathon runners reveals that at one time an 80-year-old man ran a 26-mile race in under four hours! Generalizations based on age are clearly bound to be inaccurate and unjust when applied to the elderly; variations in function and malfunction are too great to draw certain conclusions from averages, trends, and biases.

---

1. J.F. Fries, Aging, natural death, and the compression of morbidity. *N. Engl. J. Med.* 303:130–135, 1980.

FIGURE 2

Number of elderly in the United States, 1950–2050, by age group and sex. Solid line represents estimate; broken line represents projection.
SOURCE: U.S. Bureau of the Census

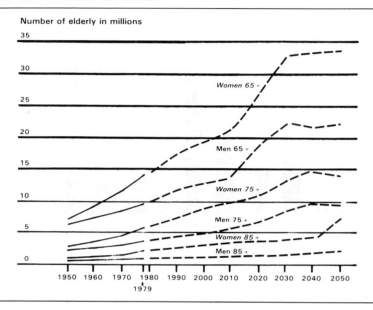

DISEASE AND DEATH

The nearly hundredfold difference in the expected life span of two common mammals, the mouse and man, forces one to conclude that life span and the rate of aging are intrinsic to the organism. One might further postulate that until someone learns how to turn off the alarm and rewind the biologic clock, healthy organisms will have a maximum life span. One can calculate from a variety of data, with remarkably reproducible results, a theoretical maximum life span for man of about 120 years. Under ideal circumstances, ones that omit the accidental deaths of healthy individuals, about two-thirds of persons would die between the ages of 81 and 89, with a mean life span of about 85 years; a practical estimate of the achievable life expectancy of unusual, healthy persons would be about 100 years (4 standard deviations above the mean).

For most of the elderly, the issue underlying medical care is not quantity of life so much as its quality. The hope that treating systolic hypertension will extend the life expectancy of a 70-year-old may be overshadowed for the patient by the inconvenience and embarrassment of having to take a diuretic when bladder control is uncertain. The central nervous system side effects may be too great a price to pay for the theoretical extension of life gained from beta-adrenergic blockers after an acute myocardial infarction.

The quality of death also becomes an issue for the chronically ill elderly person. The loss of independent living skills may outweigh the benefit of an extended life. The pain of surgery and intensive-care-unit hospitalization may need to be considered in the palliative treatment of cancers. The graceful and painless death of an elder may be important to the heirs, who are thus allowed to remember the patient as an independent person.

Psychotherapy and counseling, I believe, are underused for the problems of aging. Successful aging can distinctly improve the quality of life. Most medical and surgical treatment aims to preserve the status quo and only rarely improves the life of the elderly patient.

SUGGESTED READING

1. Fries, J.F. Aging, natural death, and the compression of morbidity. *N. Engl. J. Med.* 303:130–135, 1980.
2. Kohn, R.R. Cause of death in very old people. *J.A.M.A.* 247:2793–2797, 1981.
3. Rossman, I. The anatomy of aging. In Rossman, I. (Ed.), *Clinical Geriatrics.* Philadelphia: J.B. Lippincott, 1979.
4. Stead, E.A., Stead, N.W. Problems and challenges in the treatment of aging patients. *DM* 26:5–41, 1980.

The Special Knowledge of Geriatric Medicine

J. DERMOT FRENGLEY, M.D.

Editor's note: Those who care for the elderly must be more than skillful generalists; they must also be aware of the special issues of geriatric medicine. Perhaps most important among the many ideas highlighted in this chapter is the different "mind set"—the enlightened attitudes and approaches of the geriatrics caregiver toward the illnesses and psychosocial problems of the elderly.

Geriatric medicine encompasses all branches of medicine—perhaps even obstetrics and pediatrics in the sense that events in younger life have an impact on old age. Although geriatric medicine has its origins in internal medicine, ophthalmologists, orthopedists, urologists, psychiatrists, neurologists, dermatologists, and all the subspecialties of internal medicine have much to do with aging patients. Still, my bias is that the attributes of internal medicine are most appropriate for nurturing geriatric medicine as it becomes more securely established.

The diffuse nature of geriatric medicine suggests to some that there is neither a separate discipline of geriatric medicine nor a practical or intellectual need for one. However, the fact that similar arguments were made when pediatrics emerged from internal medicine and that pediatrics achieved a successful separation as a secure discipline argue for the parallel emergence of geriatrics. As with pediatrics, it is likely that geriatrics will evolve further to encompass physicians with highly developed subspecialty skills.

The pressures for the emergence of geriatric medicine as a separate discipline include not only the demographic imperative of an increasing population of aged persons, but also the fact that this is a population in which chronic illness and physical impairment have a high incidence, and one that increases with age. The impact of this old and infirm population on health care services is becoming more

10

noticeable, affecting the nature of the services provided and the overall costs of those services.

CLINICAL CONSEQUENCES OF AGING

The aging process reduces the reserves and resilience of all the physiologic systems and consequently affects pathophysiologic processes. Hence, disease in the elderly has many features that greatly affect clinical practices, and awareness of these special features allows for the appropriate medical management of elderly patients.

Changes in Physiology
The outward physical changes that occur with aging are obvious. The changes that occur within the body are as yet neither fully described anatomically nor understood in terms of changes in function or changes in behavior. Practical decisions of medical management are thus necessarily made with comparatively little understanding of the physiology and metabolism of the elderly patient. The recognition of both normal aging processes and those body functions that are well preserved is necessary for appropriate medical management. For instance, to know that an increased output of antidiuretic hormone is as much a part of the normal stress response in elderly persons as is the increase in cortisol production helps make for more correct fluid management. To know that glucose tolerance decreases with age and that the diagnosis of diabetes requires different criteria is clearly of importance. Similarly, renal function diminishes with age but so does muscle mass, and thus the measurement of creatinine and blood urea levels may well not reflect an elderly patient's renal function. In the elderly the appropriate dose of a drug with renal excretion may not be given if adjustments are made solely on the basis of blood urea and creatinine levels.

Diseases and Disorders Special to Aging
Many diseases occur throughout life, but some have a particular predilection for elderly persons that increases with age. The pathology responsible for these diseases is extremely varied, with no one process common to all of them. Even those diseases largely confined to one system, such as the vasculature, vary enormously in their underlying pathologic processes. Thus, attempting to classify diseases associated with aging sheds little light on the aging process, but it does help to give some order to these diseases and disorders.

Common disorders related to degeneration. These disorders include diverticulitis, abdominal hernias, Parkinson's disease, cataracts, emphysema, macular degeneration, and normal pressure hydrocephalus.

Common disorders related to vascular pathology. These conditions include ischemic heart diseases, myocardial infarction, abdominal aneurysm, angiodysplasia of the bowel mucosa, vertebrobasilar insufficiency, and carotid insufficiency.

Diseases and disorders related to connective tissue changes. These diseases include polymyalgia rheumatica, giant cell arteritis, Paget's disease, rheumatoid arthritis, and degenerative joint disease.

Diseases and disorders related to neoplasia. These disorders include chronic lymphatic leukemia, basal cell and squamous cell carcinomas of the skin, carcinoma of the ovary and body of the uterus, carcinoma of the breast, benign prostatic hypertrophy, and prostatic carcinoma.

Diseases and disorders related to slow organ failure. These conditions include myxedema, renal failure, glaucoma, and achlorhydria.

Diseases and disorders related to metabolic changes. These disorders include osteoporosis, osteomalacia, diabetes, hyperosmolar nonketotic coma, and hypothermia.

Symptom complexes related to aging. Three major symptom complexes occur in elderly patients with such regularity that they can reasonably be considered as disorders related to aging. Dr. Ronald Cape has grouped these together as the "geriatric triad": dementia, falls, and incontinence. Each one encompasses many quite different processes, some of which may be reversible, with improvement of the patient's life. Every physician with elderly patients should be thoroughly knowledgeable about investigating and then managing these three disorders. Granted, much needed information is just not yet available, especially concerning falls and incontinence. Recent emphasis on investigation of dementia has led to improved understanding of this group of disorders, although an explanation for the underlying pathologic changes in the common dementia of the Alzheimer type is still awaited.

Clearly, there is no one pathologic process that accounts for the many facets of the diseases of aging. The likelihood of multipathology must be anticipated: the presence of several chronic conditions simultaneously with an exacerbation of one, a new complication, or the addition of a new diagnosis gives geriatric medicine its singular clinical challenge. The challenge to physicians who have elderly patients is to acquire the good clinical judgment that comes from a knowledge of how the aging processes alter the patient's response to disease and an ability to recognize a multitude of diseases and disorders but to address only those that present important problems for the patient.

Complications of Common Diseases
The alteration of pathophysiologic responses in the elderly results in unusual complications of common diseases. Some may be well known and easily diagnosed, such as postherpetic neuralgia. Others, such as a ruptured empyema of the gallbladder following cholecystitis, are difficult to diagnose. Ischemic bowel lesions, for example, may occur as a complication of congestive heart failure when mesenteric perfusion has already been reduced by atheroma.

Many of the complications of illness in the elderly are banal, yet quite devastating. It is significant that serious complications like fecal impaction, urinary retention, confusion, distraction, and decubitus ulcers can usually be avoided. These conditions occur most frequently in elderly hospitalized and institutionalized patients and require constant attention to detail in order to achieve the meticulous care necessary for their prevention.

Beyond the patient's illnesses and their complications, there is a need for an understanding of the impact of infirm old age on the family and the available social supports, both formal and informal. Even a thoroughly necessary admission to a hospital can have unexpected social consequences, such as a complete change in a patient's normal living arrangements. The anticipation of a prolonged convalescence following any illness can prevent the social and medical complications deriving from readmission to a hospital or an inappropriate placement in a nursing home for reasons of expediency.

Odd Presentations of Common Diseases
Not only do diverse diseases have common complications in the elderly, but the presentation of a disease may be very nonspecific or even thoroughly misleading—thereby challenging all the skills of an experienced physician. For example, depression may masquerade as agitation or dementia. The laboratory or radiography department is quite unable to help the clinician here, and yet to fail to recognize the true clinical situation could be tragic. Myocardial infarction may be painless and present as nonspecifically as unexplained lethargy; early heart failure can present as mere exhaustion; cholecystitis as loss of appetite only; pneumonia as weakness and distraction; thyrotoxicosis as failure to thrive and apathy; pulmonary emboli as loss of energy.

Reduced Responses to Disease

Acute inflammatory conditions may have limited host responses in the elderly. The signs of an acute inflammatory intraabdominal condition may be markedly diminished, thereby masking significant underlying intraabdominal pathology. Similarly, signs of a meningitis may be missing, with acute pneumococcal meningitis presenting only as obtundation. The pain of myocardial infarction may be completely absent, and the diagnosis may be made to some extent accidentally with a routine electrocardiogram.

The fever response may be completely absent in an elderly patient, and infection therefore can go unrecognized. Furthermore, there may be significant impairment of temperature control in general, with some elderly patients capable of becoming hypothermic when in a lowish ambient temperature for some hours. These patients are no longer able to maintain their correct body temperature in a cold atmosphere and have been shown to have a vasodilation response at temperatures much lower than normal. The phenothiazine group of drugs is known to enhance the tendency to hypothermia. The inability of elderly persons to lower body temperature in the presence of a high ambient temperature is also well recognized. For this reason, elderly people are at a higher risk of developing heat stroke than are younger, healthy people.

The white cell response to inflammation may also be absent. Thus, two cardinal indications of an infectious process, fever and leukocytosis, may be lacking in elderly persons. Immune responses are often diminished and may influence the inflammatory response to infection; this may well be an explanation for the muted responses to infection. Tuberculosis may present a diagnostic conundrum in elderly patients in whom a diminished chronic inflammatory response leads to a relatively unchanged chest radiograph even in the presence of extensive pulmonary tuberculosis.

Abnormal But Normal Physical Signs

The anatomic changes of aging alter physical signs. Those that would be interpreted as markedly abnormal in a young adult could well be normal in an elderly patient.

The elongation and tortuosity of aging arteries, especially when coupled with shrinking of the axial skeleton, can result in physical findings that are mistaken as evidence for an aortic aneurysm, particularly in elderly women. While recognition of these aging changes is important, it would also be an obvious error to overlook a true abdominal aneurysm by ignoring abnormal physical signs.

The changes in the skin seen in normal aging are obvious to all, and the absence of wrinkles is thought of as being a sign of youthfulness. The physical characteristics of the skin change in elderly persons, and these changes should be well understood. The normal occurrence of poor turgor and "tenting" of the skin is very often confused with dehydration. Intravenous fluid therapy for a normally hydrated elderly person, mistakenly thought to be dehydrated, is clearly hazardous. Senile purpura on the forearms, a common benign condition, does not require investigation for hematologic disorders.

Changes in the aortic and mitral valves with aging cause physical signs that can easily be confused with significant valvular dysfunction. However, careful and skillful physical examination can usually distinguish these signs from those of hemodynamic importance; an electrocardiogram, chest x-ray, and, if necessary, an echocardiogram can easily confirm the distinction.

These changes are only some of many that occur with aging, but they highlight the need to recognize that the physical examination of elderly persons requires considerable care in separating aging changes from important pathology.

SPECIAL KNOWLEDGE NEEDED FOR THE MANAGEMENT OF ELDERLY PATIENTS

There is little doubt that the management and health care of elderly patients have very special features that are quite separate from the various pathophysiologic changes of aging already mentioned.

Goals
The goals of medical intervention for the elderly are often very different from those of younger patients: the quality of life rather than the quantity usually dominates the elderly patient's own view of how medical care should be managed. Furthermore, the timing and pacing of investigations (as well as their careful selection) are of considerable importance. To proceed by rote schedules and routines rather than to use careful clinical judgment can have dire consequences. A complete gastrointestinal workup of an asymptomatic, frail elderly patient who has been found to have occult blood in the stools, for example, may well incapacitate the patient significantly for a good number of days or weeks.

Most elderly patients are deeply concerned with their ability to maintain independence and their capacity to continue to perform their ordinary daily tasks. Any therapeutic regimen or investigative procedure that mitigates against these very real interests of the patient should be seriously questioned.

Multiple Problems

Most elderly patients have multiple problems. Choosing those that matter most to the patient and distinguishing them from the less important requires recognition that small improvements may make for a great improvement in well-being. The mere clipping of grossly overgrown toenails may have a profound effect on a patient's ability to walk. The simple maintenance of normal bowel and bladder function becomes of considerable importance, for dysfunction in this area may well dominate and even control an elderly person's life. Practical assistance in bowel control, for example, may have much greater value than tight control of exercise angina for a sedentary elderly person with coronary disease.

The multiple medical problems of an elderly patient may well number a dozen or more, with each one causing some impairment of function. Nevertheless, such a patient might still live successfully alone with proper social supports. On the other hand, the same list of problems could force another patient into requiring institutional care. Given the great divergence in capability for independent living by elderly patients with similar diagnoses, it follows that strategies for their management should also be different.

Drugs and Pharmacology

Awareness of altered drug kinetics and tissue sensitivity to drug effects in elderly persons is increasing. Multiple drug regimens designed to deal with the multiple problems of elderly patients are also cause for caution. Drug regimens should be exceedingly simple, and a degree of therapeutic nihilism is justified.

Amelioration versus Cure

Many of the conditions afflicting older patients are chronic and incurable. A therapeutic regimen would often be chosen, therefore, to ameliorate rather than cure. A direct consequence may well be that drug regimens would then continue for the life of the patient, with a steady accumulation of multiple drugs and the sheer inconvenience of a life of taking medicines. When possible, the management of patients through approaches other than drug therapy has much to recommend it.

FOCUS ON FUNCTION

A focus on the patient's capacity to function both physically and mentally is necessary. Few hospital records describe the ability of elderly persons to perform their activities of daily living, their ability to walk or to manage their affairs. An adequate description of their housing and social supports, too, is often lacking. Yet the appropriate decisions for their management require all this knowledge.

Many elderly patients can be considerably helped in their capacity to function. Following any illness, time to convalesce and to regain both the ability and the confidence to perform normal daily tasks, such as eating, bathing, dressing, walking, and managing the toilet, is necessary. This period may well require the skills of physical and occupational therapists as well as nurses in order to achieve these goals. Since patients' ability to manage their house and domestic affairs may be impaired, formal support from agencies and informal support from relatives, friends, or neighbors may be needed after hospital discharge. Thus, planning for the discharge of an elderly patient is often a complex but vital process.

Multidisciplinary Teams
Management of elderly patients requires a multidisciplinary team, whether these patients are in hospital, in outpatient or outreach programs, or in a long-term care setting. Such teams usually consist of physicians, nurses, social workers, and physical and occupational therapists. Physicians need to learn to work within the context of such a multidisciplinary team; thus it behooves the physician to have respect and confidence in the skills of professional colleagues from different disciplines.

Family Involvement
Not only does the aging process affect the patient, it also has an impact on family members who are involved in the care of an elderly patient. It is often necessary to help the family understand the consequences of various aging processes and how best to help the patient. To manage an elderly person without involvement of and discussion with concerned family members may well result in a disservice to the patient.

Naturally the patient must agree to the involvement of his family in medical decisions. The mentally intact elderly person should be in a position to hold a central part in the discussion; never should he be considered to have opinions of no importance. Intrafamily relationships develop over many years, and not necessarily favorably to an elderly patient. Indeed, the opposite may occur, as is seen in situations of physical and mental abuse of an elderly family member. A recent study has shown that family stress may be more marked when three or more generations share living accommodations.

MANAGEMENT OF THE DYING PATIENT

The situation of a patient dying of malignancy appears to be increasingly understood, largely as a result of work of the hospice movement. However, only about 12 percent of elderly patients die of a malignancy. Physicians' concern for the overall well-being of elderly patients should accept the fact that the management of terminal illnesses involves many more conditions than those arising from malignancies. As in the case of terminal malignancies, the inevitability of an impending death needs to be recognized and accepted by all the members of the health care team. When possible, the patient, as well as his family, should be brought into an understanding of the situation. All members of the health care team responsible for the patient should also be involved, and plans should be openly discussed. Thus, unreasonable and futile interventions can be avoided and a dignified death seen as a truly appropriate goal.

THE CHALLENGES OF GERIATRIC MEDICINE

The practice of geriatric medicine presents great clinical challenges to physicians, for the special knowledge needed is extraordinarily wide-based. It is perhaps the best example of the need for facility in both the science and the art of medicine: science provides the knowledge base that informs as to what should be done in any clinical situation; art becomes a debate as to whether that which is indicated by the knowledge base is appropriate for that particular patient. Not only is skilled clinical judgment necessary, but skills in working with a multidisciplinary team and in understanding family interpersonal dynamics are needed.

In this multifaceted challenge, the physician who accepts the obligation to learn the special body of knowledge and clinical skills can find great professional satisfaction. There is little doubt that the special knowledge of geriatric medicine is indeed an important and separate discipline that must be studied, taught, and learned by practicing physicians.

SUGGESTED READING

1. Cape, R.D.T. *Aging: Its Complex Management.* Baltimore: Harper and Row, 1978.
2. Crooks, J., Stevenson, I.H. (Eds.). *Drugs and the Elderly: Perspectives in Geriatric Clinical Pharmacology.* Baltimore: University Park Press, 1979.
3. Fries, J.F., Crapo, L.M. *Vitality and Aging.* San Francisco: W. H. Freeman, 1981.
4. Kohn, R.R. Cause of death in very old people. *J.A.M.A.* 247:2793–2797, 1982.
5. Schneider, E.L., Butler, R.N. Geriatrics. *J.A.M.A.* 245:2190–2191, 1981.
6. Somers, A.R., Fabian, D.R. (Eds.). *The Geriatric Imperative: An Introduction to Gerontology and Clinical Geriatrics.* New York: Appleton-Century-Crofts, 1981.

The Psychology of Aging

WILLIAM R. MARSHALL, PH.D.

Editor's note: *A patient's emotional state and life circumstances affect
all illnesses and diseases; the psychological changes related to aging
can profoundly alter, disguise, and exaggerate symptoms, and can confound
attempts at treatment. The elderly person must adapt to the changes in
his psyche and his circumstances in order to age successfully. The
psychological meaning of these aging changes is "required" knowledge
for all physicians who care for middle-aged or older patients.*

It has been estimated that 86 percent of the elderly in the United
States have chronic health problems, and 15 to 25 percent of people
over 65 have a diagnosable mental illness. If one also considers "adjustment problems" faced by the elderly, this latter figure is certainly
underestimated. But aging and disease, whether physical or psychological, are not synonymous; great difficulties occur in attempts to
differentiate psychological deficits related to age per se from those
attributable to disease processes. This point was clearly elucidated by
Cicero: "So feeble are many old men that they can not execute any
task or any duty or any functions of life whatever, but that truth is
not the peculiar fault of old age but belongs in common to bad
health." The task of understanding the causes of general debility and
disease is made even more complex by the biopsychosocial model,
now gaining acceptance in modern medicine, which asserts that all
health issues, including illness, have an essential psychological component—that is, that environmental and psychological factors maintain, trigger, and even predispose to disease.

Barrett maintains that aging is merely one of the important de-
velopmental periods in the life span.[1] If this is true, then the major

1. J.H. Barrett, *Gerontological Psychology* (Springfield, Ill.: Charles C Thomas,
1972).

20

therapeutic aims of psychological intervention with the elderly become the recognition and acceptance of the biologic shifts and decrements (e.g., sensory and hormonal changes, decreased energy and strength), remediation of reversible dysfunction, and facilitation of coping with these inevitable changes.

To prolong life without concurrently improving its quality is of limited value at best; the plight of the Struldbrugs in Swift's *Gulliver's Travels* would not seem attractive to most humans. Although the Struldbrugs could not die, they had all of the progressive physical and mental disabilities associated with aging.

SOME PHYSIOLOGIC DETERMINANTS OF PSYCHOLOGICAL CHANGE

Declining Physical Ability

Physiologic function generally declines concomitant with aging. This undeniable and irrefutable fact requires recognition of the inevitable deterioration of a mature being. Although no one encounters all of the difficulties related to aging, it is equally unlikely that anyone will be able to elude all the physiologic declines of aging either. The decline in human peak physical ability that starts in the late teens to mid-twenties becomes more rapid as age increases. Good nutrition, exercise, and health care may slow but will not circumvent this process. Examples of physiologic debilitation include loss of physical strength and stamina, retarded reflexes and poor coordination, dulled taste and olfactory senses, and loss of muscle tone. Although it is a difficult task, personal acceptance of the inevitable physical decline and the willingness to make modifications in life-style are probably the first steps in developing a happy, well-adjusted aging process.

Sexual Function

Decreased sexual interest and activity after the age of 60 were thought to be a result of physiologic deterioration. Recent information suggests, however, that even though the female menopause and male climacteric are difficult and sometimes traumatic for the individual, the primary causes of decreased sexual function are psychological rather than physiological. In fact, as a result of the changing attitude toward sexuality in our society, sexual activity is reported to be maintained and enjoyed into the eighties. The range of individual differences concerning interest in sexuality is so great that continuation or reduction of sexual functioning becomes a personal matter. The physician should encourage each patient to make decisions consonant with his chosen life-style, and then "grant permission" to continue sexual functioning if so desired.

Cognitive Function and Performance Changes
It is often difficult to differentiate reduced cognitive function per se from other physical problems. For example, reading comprehension difficulties may be related more to deterioration in visual acuity than to decline in word comprehension. Nonetheless, there are data that suggest a general correlation between age and decrements in intellectual abilities, perception, decision making, problem solving, and attention.

Cognitive decline could influence an individual in at least three ways: skewed perception of events, slowed processing of perceived information and decision making, and limited motor response potential once the decision for action has been made. Presbyopia (decreased accommodation and focus ability) and presbycusis (loss of hearing for high-frequency tones) are examples of perception difficulties occurring with aging. Slowed reaction time, psychomotor integration, and problem-solving skills are examples of deficient information processing. Decreases in strength, coordination, and capacity for continued exertion are examples of performance decrements.

Interestingly, the commonly assumed relationship between old age and diminished memory is not supported by research. Age differences in primary (short-term) memory are minimal, and the observed differences in secondary (long-term) memory are often the result of attentional deficits, changing perceptual abilities and motivation, or organic and psychological problems.

THEORIES OF "SUCCESSFUL" AGING

Either as result of exposure to similar declines in older family members or through personal experience, most people are themselves aware of changes long before reporting them to others. What impact does decline have on an individual? What responses are required for successful adaptation to biologic changes? Disengagement, activity, and compensation are examples of theories that attempt to explain "successful" aging.

Disengagement Model
As people age they tend to limit many of the activities pursued in younger years. According to disengagement theory, if a person is to

be happy during the geriatric period, he must choose to withdraw from the demands, pressures, and responsibilities previously dictated by society, and passively accept reduced function, importance, and status in society. Conversely, a person who attempts to maintain previous goals, activities, and enthusiasm will become unhappy, frustrated, and depressed. Coincident with this retrenchment is a renewed preoccupation with self, the presence of which is often characterized as a person entering a "second childhood." Thus, a new equilibrium characterized by minimal societal contacts yet self-acceptance is needed for successful aging. There is no doubt that disengagement does occur and, in fact, is demanded by declining physical activity. This theory, however, is too negativistic and morose to be universally accepted.

Activity Model
The activity model, which has strong support in both medical and lay communities, suggests that successful aging is equated with maintaining previous attitudes and activity levels as long as possible. When health or society dictates a change in activity level (e.g., retirement), the task is to find adequate and fulfilling substitutes in order to remain psychologically healthy. The person who is unable to find substitutes will become depressed or unhappy.

The activity model, however, also falls short of explaining the many behavioral changes that occur for the majority of the elderly. Satisfaction and happiness are likely to be related to maintenance and substitution of activities for some, and to disengagement for others. For example, people with academic careers tend to remain active and do not disengage to the same extent as manual and skilled laborers.

Compensation Model
According to the compensation model, it is insufficient to assume that an individual's relationship with society during the first 60 years of life is the sole determinant of the diverse adaptations of later life. One's ability to deal with and adapt to the numerous physical and mental changes of the aging process may be the critical component.

Changes (primarily psychological but also some physical changes) concurrent with aging, therefore, are actually compensatory ones as an individual attempts to adapt to the demands of the genetically determined biologic clock. In other words, an individual's method and quality of adaptation are genetically predetermined in such a way that counterphobic activity levels, denial of aging changes, and even the "use" of lifelong psychopathologic defenses could serve as adaptive measures. Avoidance of certain social situations, repetition of familiar behaviors, and the seeking of tighter structuring and scheduling of activities might be a response to genetically determined decrements in sensory activity.

Carried to an extreme, this theory is somewhat akin to a dog chasing its tail. If viewed practically in terms of the specific tasks required of an aging individual, however, this theory has the advantages of acknowledging the unavoidable physiologic changes of aging and providing a foundation for understanding some of the seemingly irrational behavior changes or the persistence of previous behavior patterns.

PSYCHOLOGICAL NEEDS OF THE ELDERLY

The aforementioned theories are only partially useful; they ultimately fail to account for the numerous and varied changes seen in the vast numbers of aging people. Disengagement, for example, proceeds at different rates and in different forms for different people and affects their adjustment in diverse ways. A congruous approach to this issue requires that the needs, status changes, fears, strengths, and weaknesses commonly shown by aging people be studied. The tasks or strategies required for "successful aging" could then be more clearly developed.

Analysis of prior behavior patterns often indicates that those who were happy and well-adjusted throughout most of their lives will have less difficulty accepting inevitable changes and finding later life rewarding—for such individuals adjustment has always been successful. Those who have struggled to find happiness throughout their lives, however, are likely to find old age as another of a long series of hardships. In Plato's *Republic,* Cephalus responds to Socrates' question about old age by noting that "He who is of calm and happy nature will not feel the pressure of age but to him who is of an opposite disposition, youth and age are equally a burden." Individuals whose adjustments and greatest satisfaction in life stem from athletic achievement, physical attractiveness, or occupational achievement and status often approach old age and retirement with great trepidation, and find this stage of life to be one of great unhappiness.

Although the fact is often not recognized, the emotional needs of the elderly are similar to those of younger people. Unfortunately, it is often assumed that since an individual has lived a long life, most emotional needs have been met, have vanished, or are no longer important. Many signs in our society erroneously suggest that if physical comfort is satisfactory, then a person will be satisfied to vegetate and wait for death. A short tour of some nursing homes would illustrate this point.

A primary need for all human beings, but particularly for older people, is security, both economic and emotional. The great strides over the past half-century to ensure some level of economic security during retirement have removed from family members much of the responsibility for the care of their elderly. Unfortunately, this change also may have inadvertently decreased the probability that the emotional needs of the elderly will be met.

Love and affection, self-esteem, and recognition of self-worth are also important. The individual who has had respect, prestige, and authority within the family quickly recognizes the potential for diminution of these rewards. When the utility of an older person to offspring has passed, it is often easy for children to forget the important role once played by the old person. "Nuisance" behavior by an older person may, in fact, be an attempt to regain the support and security afforded by love and affection. Fortunately, many older people are able to find deserved affection through mates and elderly friends.

Older people are sometimes able to continue a rewarding involvement with families as grandparents. In a classic study, Neugarten and Weinstein found five general styles of grandparenting suggestive of different levels of family involvement:[2] (1) formal, clearly demarcated involvement, (2) fun-seeking self-indulgence and child-indulgence, (3) role as surrogate parent, (4) role as respected reservoir of family wisdom, or (5) role as distant figure with minimal and fleeting involvement. Having grandchildren near may alleviate loneliness for elderly people; youngsters can help them to play, relax, and laugh again. In fact, research suggests that older people become less rigid and seclusive and appear happier when in contact with younger people. Care must be taken, however, to ensure that the playfulness of children does not become burdensome or stressful to the older individual.

The physical and intellectual changes accompanying old age constitute in themselves a blow to one's ego. When this affront is intensified by social disapproval, self-esteem quickly declines, and rigidity,

2. B. Neugarten, K. Weinstein. The changing American grandparent. *J. Marriage Fam.* 26:199–204, 1964.

aggressiveness, and withdrawal reactions often result. The common feeling of hopelessness experienced by the elderly is merely a statement that since the individual no longer feels useful to anyone, there is no need for him to make an effort—especially if his only remaining task is to wait to die. Previous feelings of inadequacy and unworthiness become intensified when the objective changes of aging occur.

Many older people cling to memories of what they once were in a search for acceptance, respect, and personal worth. Failure to recognize instead what they are now can result in difficult, demanding, and aggressive behavior. Ruminative stories of bygone days and past achievements, although sometimes irritating to younger people, are an attempt by the elderly to enhance self-importance. Through constant repetition of "old war stories," the older person is reminded of former vitality and potency and consequently is able to live through past achievements.

Perhaps the most significant emotional change facing the aging person is the potential for loneliness. As one gets older, friends and contemporaries die. The death of a friend is the loss of potential emotional support, but, more important, reminds one of the inevitability of one's own death. Feelings of despair, futility, hopelessness, loneliness, and isolation are often intensified. Loss of friends is particularly problematic when an individual has difficulties making new friends, as is frequently true of aging people. People need the companionship of friends of their own age, but fewer contemporaries are available as one ages, and difficulties with locomotion and transportation often make exploration for new friends virtually impossible. Community living settings and recreational and social clubs attempt to restore access to social contacts for the elderly.

From birth to early adulthood, an individual moves from complete dependence to relative independence. Complete dependence in childhood may be deemed appropriate, but if it occurs during adulthood it is viewed as pathological and inappropriate. But as an individual ages further, independence diminishes such that dependent tendencies might once again dominate. Those older people who resist the loss of independence should be encouraged and helped to maintain their dignity and vitality. Unless death intervenes, however, everyone will eventually once again reach the stage of complete dependence.

Increased dependence on family often forces acceptance of a lesser role and status within the family. The worry that inadequate finances might place the individual in a position to accept charity from off-spring may be devastating. The parent who tended to be overprotective, overcontrolling, or dominating may be unable to accept so extreme a parent/child role reversal. The role shift from provider to being provided for, from depended upon to dependent, from caregiver to care receiver, from center of household to outsider is rarely easy. Still, most older people can recognize and accept the inevitable role changes. Difficulties occur, however, when shifts are abrupt, either because of bad health, the death of a spouse, or when they are prematurely imposed by family or society. Aging individuals are often not aware that role changes can cause unhappiness or dissatisfaction; they just recognize restlessness, irritability, or uneasy feelings that may appear as psychosomatic complaints, easy emotional upset, and crankiness.

From the time of early adolescence we are capable of giving at least as much as we recieve, and for many people self-respect depends on the ability to meet their own needs without having to accept assistance from other people. Many older people have difficulty learning to accept help, whether it is in the form of gifts, financial aid, or even assistance with housekeeping. Care givers must be especially sensitive to the need to help an elderly person maintain self-esteem and self-respect when they offer them assistance.

Because of the potential for decreased prestige associated with retirement, occupational disengagement may pose special difficulties. An individual's response to retirement will be determined primarily by previous job satisfaction: people who have been work-oriented or career-oriented and have had a majority of their emotional needs met through an occupation will be likely to consider retirement traumatic, while those who are unhappy with their occupation or who view work just as a way to earn a living are more likely to welcome retirement. Most individuals, but particularly those in the former group, may need encouragement to develop substitute avocations.

Retirement may also have adverse effects on marital relationships. Retirement often means that one spouse must readjust typical routines to accommodate the presence and involvement of the retired individual. Studies have shown that preretirement husbands often look forward to retirement more than their spouses do. Too often couples begin in their thirties and forties to invest and plan financially for retirement, but neglect to plan mutual activities until retirement is imminent.

ADJUSTMENTS TO AGING

The pessimism engendered by viewing aging as characterized by debilitation, decrements, and weakness must be avoided. Many well-known individuals—Winston Churchill, Albert Schweitzer, Senator Sam Ervin, Senator Strom Thurmond—retained their productivity and usefulness into old age. Older people have strengths and talents that younger people do not possess. For example, in early life people often devote so much attention to achievement, productivity, activity, and success that little energy remains to exploit many hidden and undeveloped creative talents. Creativity is particularly relevant because it does not appear to be directly related to measurable intelligence and academic achievements. Clearly, six or more decades provide the resource of tremendous life experience that younger people do not possess. Maturity, wisdom, patience, and freedom from social pressures are all strengths that may be used to the benefit of self and society as a whole. Other cultures tend to take greater advantage of the strengths of their elders than does the American culture, endowing them with higher esteem and prestige.

Making health and dietary adjustments depends, once again, on the individual's adjustment prior to aging. Was the body developed or abused? Has the individual lived a life of moderation or excess? Did he "eat to live" or "live to eat"? Those who have been comfortable with moderation when younger, and who are able to make dietary adjustments such as decreased salt intake, are likely to have the physical abilities to support successful aging.

It seems paradoxical that the largest amount of leisure time is available to those who may be least able, because of financial constraints and physical abilities, to take full advantage of that time. Still, gerontologic adjustment and happiness depend on an individual's ability to use leisure time profitably. Retirement is likely to be less difficult for the person who has developed an avocation in addition to a career than for a person whose entire life revolved around a vocation. Having activities that one looks forward to during retirement does not, however, alleviate the problem. As a person ages, activities that were rewarding earlier in life, such as athletics, may not be available because of declining physical abilities. In most situations a person has to be flexible enough to modify activities and hobbies continually so that at some point, sedentary activities like needlework, coin collecting, or chess might satisfy.

In addition to preventing boredom, the emphasis on activities in the geriatric age group is important for helping the elderly person attain some sense of status and self-worth. Barrett claims that four types of individuals are found among the retired population:[3] Those who acquired status during maturity and have no need for such striving during retirement, those who accept that they have never been able to achieve status, those whose status is achieved through affiliation rather than personal activities and who continue to maintain that affiliation during the geriatric period, and finally, those who in old age still "unhappily seek status." Individuals in the first three categories will age more successfully than those in the fourth group.

The person who believes in himself, is satisfied with his self-worth, and has been happy in his younger years will age happily. Conversely, the person who has struggled to find happiness throughout adulthood is likely to have a difficult adjustment to aging.

THE PHYSICIAN'S ROLE

Regardless of the degree of physiological or psychological success with which one ages, contacts with the medical profession increase with aging. Although only 10 percent of the population is older than 65 years, it is estimated that more than 40 percent of the outpatient and 33 percent of inpatient physician time is devoted to patients older than 65.

As this book attests, the diagnosis and care of geriatric patients are increasingly viewed as a worthy pursuit. Physicians who care for the well-being of geriatric patients must be skilled in attending to the psychological and social as well as the organic aspects of the patient's life. Yet medical training has traditionally emphasized knowledge of the latter to the exclusion of the former.

One issue that physicians must address prior to seeing geriatric patients is their personal "ageism," that is, prejudice against the elderly. Ageism often surfaces in the form of trivializing patient complaints because "nothing can be done." If the physician's expectation is that older patients will be irascible, crabby, unresponsive, or withdrawn, then surely this expectation will be fulfilled, and the patient will receive less than optimal care.

If the physician is able to see beyond the stereotypes and view geriatric patients objectively, the challenging organic, psychological,

---

3. Barrett, *Gerontological Psychology*, pp. 134–135.

and social diversity among geriatric patients is likely to be appreciated. The physician who has known the patient in earlier years has the opportunity to know the patient's typical pattern of dealing with stress. This physician can then have a significant role in anticipatory guidance (e.g., planning for retirement) and in identifying particularly stressful events for the patient. The physician can help the patient put physical and emotional changes into perspective, and above all else, can assist the patient in maintaining independence and self-respect.

SUGGESTED READING

1. Barrett, J.H. *Gerontological Psychology*. Springfield, Ill.: Charles C Thomas, 1972.
2. Birren, J.E., Schaie, K.W. *The Handbook of the Psychology of Aging*. New York: Van Nostrand Rheinhold, 1977.
3. Hussian, R. *Geriatric Psychology: A Behavioral Perspective*. New York: Van Nostrand Rheinhold, 1981.
4. Millan, T., Green, K., Meagher, R. *The Handbook of Clinical Health Psychology*. New York: Plenum Press, 1982.
5. Neugarten, B., Weinstein, K. The changing American grandparent. *J. Marriage Fam.* 26:199–204, 1964.

Elderly Abuse

THOMAS A. CABLE, M.D.

*Editor's note: Physical, psychological, and financial abuse of the
elderly is a growing problem. Prey to harm from a variety of
intentional and unintentional kinds of abusers, the elderly often have
little recourse because of dependence and frailty. Physicians, the formal
caretakers, are often unintentional abusers of the elderly in subtle ways.*

Increased interest in and study of our geriatric population have un-
coverd a newly described problem—abuse of the elderly. As a societal
group, the elderly are generally less visible and more isolated than
children and women, and this fact alone may account for the relative
ignorance of this problem. A University of Maryland researcher stated
in the *Journal of the American Medical Association*'s medical news: "Abuse
of the elderly is at a stage that child abuse was at 20 years ago. People
are horrified at the notion."[1] Physicians and other health care personnel caring for the aged must realize that elderly abuse is now
thought to be as common as child abuse,[2] with an estimated nationwide occurrence of 500,000 to 1,000,000 cases per year. The prevalence of abuse has been estimated to be between 4 and 10 percent
of individuals 60 years of age and older.

Elderly abuse is most often a family problem—indeed, close relatives are known to be the most frequent abusers. Since maltreatment
is a sensitive family issue, it is not surprising that underreporting
may occur and may mask the true magnitude of this form of family
violence. The abused elderly person and his or her family also tend

---

1. The elderly: Newest victims of familial abuse. *J.A.M.A.* 243:1221, 1980.
2. Gerontologists: Innovative living arrangements help offset elderly abuse. *Behavior Today*, July 27, 1981, pp. 4–6.

to deny the existence of the problem. The aged person may fear reprisal from family members (e.g., removal from the home), may be ignorant of avenues of help, and may also be ashamed to admit to such treatment by his own family.

Levine defined abuse of the elderly as follows:

> Abuse is any action on the part of an elderly person's family (family being defined as any relative related by blood, marriage, or adoption and any associated persons who have daily household contact such as a housekeeper or roommate, or any person upon whom the elderly is reliant for his daily needs of food, clothing, or shelter) or a professional caretaker to take advantage of his person, property, or emotional being through threat of violence or use of disciplinary restraint (i.e., physical and chemical strait-jacketing) or negligence on the part of the caretaker to provide basic needs.[3]

With this definition in mind, I propose to review characteristics of the abused and abuser, examine the various types of abuse and possible causes, and offer recommendations to alleviate the problem of elderly abuse.

THE ABUSED

All elderly persons are subject to abuse. The limited data, however, do suggest a common profile of the abused elder as a low- or middle-class Protestant woman with an average age of 84 years who lives with relatives.[4] In fact, the term "granny battering" was coined to emphasize the frequency of ill treatment of elderly women, not only by short-tempered relatives but also by well-meaning hospital staff. One small study found no ethnic predisposition to abuse.[5]

As would be expected, the potential for abuse is directly related to the quality of the relationship and communication between the elderly person and the caretaking family. Those families in which communication systems are already poor are more likely to break under stress, ultimately leading to some form of abuse. This relationship

3. L.R. Kimsey, A.R. Tarbox, D.F. Bragg. Abuse of the elderly—the hidden agenda: I. The caretakers and the categories of abuse. *J. Am. Geriatr. Soc.* 29:466, 1981.
4. The elderly: Newest victims of familial abuse. *J.A.M.A.* 243:1221, 1980.
5. J. Steuer, E. Austin. Family abuse of the elderly. *J. Am. Geriatr. Soc.* 28:372–376, 1980.

can also be affected by the dependent elderly person's health. Many old people suffer multiple illnesses that make them less productive. They may display regressive behavior; become more stubborn, quarrelsome, and untidy; or refuse to eat. They may even become aggressive or combative to the point of provoking the same behavior from their caretakers.

The abused elderly, then, are a segment of our population who suffer both physical and mental disabilities that cause them to be dependent on a care giver for nutrition, medication, cleanliness, ambulation, and, in some cases, even bed care.

THE ABUSER

There are, in general, two groups of caretakers involved with the elderly. Informal caretakers include relatives, friends, and neighbors and account for the greater percentage of the abusers; formal caretakers (e.g., physicians, nurses, social workers) are those who are professionally trained to deliver health care to the elderly, usually in an institutional setting. While either group may be involved in elderly abuse, an antithetical third group I call the "peripheral noncaretakers" commonly is guilty of shameless exploitation of elderly people. From the unscrupulous door-to-door salesperson with products such as insurance or investment scams colored by scare tactics to the grocery boy who charges excessively for carrying an elderly person's weekly groceries, these noncaretakers prey on the vulnerability of the aged. They may even enter the home indirectly through television commercials such as those offering cancer insurance.

TYPES OF ABUSE

The four types of elderly abuse are not necessarily mutually exclusive: physical abuse, verbal/psychological abuse, financial/fiscal abuse, and material abuse.

Physical abuse covers a broad range of behaviors that can be overt and intentional in nature, or may be disguised in a more subtle form as physical neglect. Overt intentional abuse is apparent when the victim is actually deliberately injured in some way. It is not known how frequently overt intentional abuse is inflicted on the elderly, but the Illinois Department of Aging indicated in 1981 that 5 percent of the cases of elderly abuse in their state were serious enough to result in serious injury or death.[6]

Physical neglect, not always readily recognized, is the creation of, or the failure to relieve, physical discomfort, for example, overly hot bath water, decubitus ulcers, inappropriate hanging of a urine bag above the level of a bedridden patient's bladder, improper medication (especially oversedation or polypharmacy), or failure to heed a call for assistance or to change bed sheets and clothing when soiled. Sometimes the neglect becomes even more subtle—for example, leaving an elderly person unattended in a wheelchair for a prolonged period of time.

It is important for the physician to realize that the line between any form of physical abuse and actual accidental injury is often hazy. Elderly people with unstable gait may suffer multiple unexplained falls, fractures, and bruises as a result of slippery ice, darkened stairways, or a gentle shove. The physician as caretaker of the elderly must recognize that to treat an injury without addressing the cause could be to the ultimate detriment of his patient.

Psychological or emotional abuse, both verbal and nonverbal, can be just as damaging as physical abuse. Family threats of institutionalization, abandonment, and even homicide can lead to disintegration of the elderly person's ego. The aged person may become depressed and uncommunicative after repeated verbal abuse, and may even appear to have an organic brain syndrome. Under the stress of repeated verbal abuse, many elderly people with a stable organic brain syndrome become worse and require institutional care or even die prematurely.

Elderly people who are placed in nursing homes against their will can become more dependent in this new and strange environment. Confusion, disorientation, poor vision, and deafness may compound the shock of loss of ties with familiar objects and people, leading to exacerbation of the person's already demoralized and depressed state. Psychological abuse by a caretaker may take the form of infantilization that increases as ego regression becomes more pronounced. This behavior is further exacerbated by a feeling among staff that "these people are going to die anyway." A vicious cycle of regressive and infantilizing behavior can ensue; in nursing homes elderly women have been observed to be playing with dolls which the staff call their "babies."

---

6. Gerontologists, *Behavior Today*, pp. 4–6.

Nonverbal psychological abuse that deprives the elderly of their dignity can be simply an attitude of the caretaker that conveys a feeling of hopelessness. The resulting impersonal and mechanistic care is illustrated by the report of a registered nurse of the care received by her grandmother in a nursing home as follows: "She was treated like a car: lubricated, rotated, aligned, given additives, and no doubt the proper entry was made on the proper checklist initialed by a proper L.P.N. or R.N."[7] A caretaker who leaves medication and other items of daily living just beyond the reach of the bedridden patient is also engaged in nonverbal psychological abuse. Automatically raising one's voice when speaking with the elderly—assuming a hearing impairment that may not exist—can be denigrative to the old person with normal hearing.

Although no age group is immune to poor judgment, the elderly are particularly prone to financial abuse, especially if they have some type of cognitive dysfunction. Family members abuse the elderly financially by spending their personal savings, pension, or Social Security money inappropriately, and formal caretakers within institutions may embezzle patients' funds or improperly charge patients for services that are not even performed. The elderly patient may also be inappropriately reclassified as requiring skilled nursing care, thus ensuring higher Medicaid reimbursement; ironically, this new level of care may actually be necessary because of the inattentive nursing that caused decompensation. Peripheral noncaretakers often find the easily confused elderly person an easy prey on whom they may impose "hard-sell" pressure tactics—for example, for multiple insurance policies or investment scams.

Material abuse, either mismanagement of assets or actual theft of personal possessions, can occur in the home or in an institutional setting. Fearing theft of their belongings, many elderly were reluctant to leave their homes for air-conditioned centers during a recent heat wave in the Southwest; many chose to remain behind locked doors and closed windows, only to die of heat stroke.

In nursing homes, narcotics and sedatives prescribed for the elderly are easily sidetracked into personal use or sale on the street by nursing home personnel. For an elderly person in pain, such a diversion of material (in this case, drugs) becomes simultaneous physical, psychological, and financial abuse. The patient becomes, in effect, a passive participant in illicit drug use.

---

7. Kimsey, et. al., Abuse of the elderly—the hidden agenda, p. 469.

CAUSES OF ABUSE

There are multiple causes of abuse, depending on the situation in which abuse occurs. One prevalent thought is that many abusers may have been battered as children; thus, the abused children of today may become the abusive adults of tomorrow. Abusive adults may become formal caretakers in an institution caring for the elderly, or they may be unwilling members of a family charged with caring for an aging dependent parent.

The introduction of a new disability or the increased severity of a chronic disability often puts stress on stable relationships and creates an atmosphere in which abuse can occur. For example, even in a stable marriage of 50 years, abuse can occur when a change in one spouse's health upsets the equilibrium of the relationship.

The aging process and its associated life changes may also create the potential for an abusive situation. Retirement often brings more idle time to an elderly couple who previously had multiple outlets outside the marriage to stabilize their relationship. A time of rediscovery of the partner may ensue, and unfortunately in some couples this leads to increased marital stress.

Unresolved family conflicts between parents and siblings are a catalyst for abuse. Most families have abuse potential if pushed to the limit. "Role reversal" or "parenting the parent" may be looked upon as a "burden without relief." Unresolved conflict between elderly siblings living together may also result in abuse, especially if one suffers declining health.

The "generational pressure" of middle-aged caretakers—caught between their own retirement, children's demands, and the stress of caring for an elderly disabled relative for whom they feel an obligation—results in emotional, financial, and physical burdens that may create an atmosphere conducive to abuse.

Frustration underlies many abuse situations. Caring for an incontinent person or worrying about an elderly person's nocturnal house roaming can become frustrating even for the most tolerant of caretakers. Within institutions, formal caretakers, frustrated by long hours and excessive bureaucratic paperwork, develop angry or pessimistic attitudes toward their vulnerable wards that make them candidates to become abusers.

Efficient care, on the other hand, may also lead to abuse when elderly patients get lost in the shuffle of activity within a busy hospital, with multiple caretakers following "orders" and "charting" on the appropriate pages of the patient's record. The privacy and dignity of the elderly may be forgotten in the network of a "well-run" hospital.

RECOMMENDATIONS

With no effective method of case identification or long-term management of domestic abuse, and with an obvious lack of consensus of etiology of abuse, no clear solutions to the problems of elderly abuse are apparent. What is known is that the problems are likely to grow. Projected increases in the elderly population, coupled with economic trends that force more generations to live under the same roof, amplify the potential for abuse.

No clear-cut mechanism for detecting abuse of the elderly exists. Perhaps the institutional setting with formal caretakers is most amenable to a reporting mechanism. The loose network of professionals who come into contact with the elderly includes physicians, nurses, social workers, adult protective workers, and mental health professionals, along with police, attorneys, legal counselors, clergy, morticians, and even coroners. Awareness by these professionals of potential abuse would help to bring this problem "out of the closet" and under public scrutiny. Only in this way can we hope to identify the problem of elderly abuse and face its legal and moral implications.

Certainly we need to dispel the notion that the dependent, frail elderly are routinely secure in the care of family or friends in the home. Adult protective services logically should be extended to the home setting. As the elderly population increases and a greater demand is placed on already overburdened long-term care facilities, coupled with family rejection of institutional care, the possibility of domestic abuse increases. Intensive family counseling at the time an aging parent joins an offspring's household and later during times of increased stress on the relationship may relieve some of the burden on the caring family. Likewise, specific training in the skills needed for care of the ailing family member, along with expanded community services such as day-care centers and home helpers, may decrease the potential for abuse.

Respite programs in which the elderly could spend a few days to a week in a particular facility give family members a rest period from the stresses of caring for an elderly person. Adopt-a-Grandparent programs, present in many nursing homes, represent a healthy way to provide advocates or guardians for the elderly. A strong advocate in the community provides a buffer against all kinds of abuse both within and outside of the institution.

Innovative living arrangements, in which three or four older persons buy a four-bedroom house and share common living space, promote elderly independence and help avoid the psychological pressure to surrender independent living. Emergency response systems that provide prompt medical service would enable some elderly persons to continue to live alone, despite serious chronic illness.

Most states have passed extensive legislation dealing with domestic violence. Most of the adult protective service laws mandate reporting by any individual having reasonable cause to suspect abuse and, at the same time, grant immunity from prosecution to anyone who gives a good-faith report to local authorities. Some states authorize social service agencies to investigate reports of abuse and provide needed services. Thirty-five states have passed protection order laws which guarantee any individual in the family setting the right to be free from fear of physical abuse. A protection order is a court order that can remove the abuser from the home and/or require that individual to seek psychological help. The elderly are often ignorant of such laws, and prosecution of flagrant abuse remains difficult. Furthermore, the abused elderly are understandably reluctant to report their family members on whom they are dependent. An effort must be made to encourage the elderly to report abuse and to learn their legal rights and avenues of legal recourse.

SUGGESTED READING

1. Abuse of old people. *Community Outlook,* September 11, 1980, pp. 262–264.
2. Alford, D. The battered older person: Problem identification. *Gerontologist* 17:340, 1977.
3. Baker, A. Granny battering. *Modern Geriatrics* 5:20–24, 1975.
4. The elderly: Newest victims of familial abuse. *J.A.M.A.* 243:1221–1225, 1980.
5. Gerontologists: Innovative living arrangements help offset elderly abuse. *Behavior Today,* July 27, 1981, p. 4–6.
6. Goldfarb, A.I. Prevalence of psychiatric disorders in metropolitan old age and nursing homes. *J. Am. Geriatr. Soc.* 10:77–84, 1962.
7. Hickey, T., Douglas, R.L. Mistreatment of the elderly in the domestic setting: An exploratory study. *Am. J. Public Health* 71:500–507, 1981.
8. Kimsey, L.R., Tarbox, A.R., Bragg, D.F. Abuse of the elderly—the hidden agenda: I. The caretakers and the categories of abuse. *J. Am. Geriatr. Soc.* 29:466, 1981.
9. Kirkland, K. Assessment and treatment of family violence. *J. Fam. Pract.* 14:713–718, 1982.
10. Mancini, M. Adult abuse laws. *Am. J. Nursing,* April 1980, pp. 739–740.
11. McCuan, E.R. *Intergenerational Family Violence and Neglect: The Aged as Victims of Reactivated and Reversed Patterns. Proceedings of the Eleventh International Congress of Gerontology,* Tokyo, Japan, August 1978. Tokyo: Scimed Publications, 1978.

12. Steinman, L.A. Reactivated conflicts with aging parents. In Regan, P.K. (Ed.), *Aging Parent*. Los Angeles: Ethel Percy Andrus Gerontology Center, University of Southern California Press, 1979, pp. 126–143.
13. Steuer, J., Austin, E. Family abuse of the elderly. *J. Am. Geriatr. Soc.* 28:372–376, 1980.

2

DRUGS AND THE
ELDERLY

Pharmacokinetics of Commonly Used Drugs in the Elderly

KAREN S. OLES, PHARM.D.

Editor's note: A knowledge of age-related and disease-related changes in drug response and toxicity is central to the skillful treatment of elderly patients. The data to permit the establishment of such a knowledge base are, unfortunately, incomplete and unavailable. The general recommendations for most categories of drugs included here are preliminary but represent important distillations of the available information and experience.

The choice of an appropriate drug dose regimen for an elderly patient is a challenge to the knowledge and commitment of the busy clinician; it requires an understanding of the relevance of various chronic medical problems and an ability to integrate past responses to drugs into a therapeutic plan. It also requires familiarity with adverse effects and drug interactions, a general appreciation of how the elderly handle drugs—how drugs and their aging organs interact—and awareness of atypical clinical presentations of drug toxicity that at first seem unrelated to drugs. Most important, it demands a commitment to review drug regimens again and again, discontinuing agents that have failed to produce the desirable therapeutic endpoints.

Pharmacokinetic drug profiles, based on mathematical models of rates and patterns of drug movement in the body and their relationship to the pharmacologic effects of drugs, are modified by the aging process. The altered physiology of the healthy elderly person may change the absorptive and distributive characteristics of drugs, and slow the metabolism and renal excretion of drugs. Problems commonly encountered by the elderly, such as confinement to bed and chair, malnutrition, dehydration, congestive heart failure, and thyroid disease, may further modify pharmacokinetics. Unfortunately, few pharmacokinetic studies on either the healthy or the sick

43

elderly person are available to physicians. Further confounding the understanding of pharmacokinetics in the elderly is the unusual heterogeneity of this population. As a result, clinicians must remember to titrate doses to the individual patient's response and not be influenced too much by the usual population norms reported in the medical literature. Monitoring of serum drug concentrations is helpful and often obligatory, particularly for theophylline, salicylates, antiarrhythmics, aminoglycosides, anticonvulsants, digoxin, and lithium. "Cookbook" approaches do not work well in geriatric medicine, and consequently most recommendations for average doses of drugs should be viewed as approximations.

The side effect profile of a drug is often more important than the pharmacokinetic profile in drug selection for the elderly. For example, the neuroleptic or antidepressant with the fewest anticholinergic, sedative, and orthostatic properties, such as haloperidol (Haldol) or desipramine (Norpramin) would be chosen as much for its lack of toxicity as for its pharmacokinetic profile. Still, these are not ideal agents, because haloperidol commonly causes tardive dyskinesia and desipramine is less effective for the insomnia of depression than are some other agents.

SIGNIFICANT ISSUES IN GERIATRIC PHARMACOTHERAPY

Expense
There are large differences in cost between therapeutically similar drugs, such as the many "step-two" antihypertensive agents. The use of generic drug products, with documented bioavailability and made by a reputable manufacturer, can reduce costs without compromising quality for many agents. Switching back and forth between different generic and brand-name products, however, should be minimized because of possible differences in bioavailability as well as patient confusion with different shapes, colors, and names of medication. The physician should also generally avoid generic drugs when prescribing digoxin, quinidine, phenytoin, and sustained-release preparations. Optimal generic prescribing requires communication between the patient, physician, and pharmacist.

Convenience
Geriatric patients typically use four or five prescription drugs daily. Unwieldy regimens should, therefore, be simplified wherever pos-

sible; for example, antihypertensive drugs can usually be prescribed once or twice daily rather than three or four times a day. Cimetidine or sucralfate taken three times a day may be more palatable than a two-hourly antacid regimen. Two tablets of a nonsteroidal antiin-flammatory agent may yield better compliance than sixteen aspirin divided in four daily doses, although the increased cost must also be reckoned with. Combination tablets, generally best avoided, can be helpful when a step-two drug is added to a diuretic in a mildly hypertensive patient.

Compliance

Drug-taking behavior should be integrated with the patient's other routines. Specific times for medication, dosing in relation to food, and how to deal with missed doses should be discussed. The time and interest invested will be repaid with better patient understanding and adherence to the physician's regimen.

Increased Sensitivity to Drug Effects

Elderly patients have more chronic illness and take more medication than do younger patients; commonly they have multiple drug therapies acting on multiple diseased and aging organ systems. Consequent to this often obligatory "polypharmacy," they have more adverse effects and drug interactions and are more often admitted to hospitals with drug-related problems. The altered homeostatic mechanisms in the elderly may cause a loss of the ability to tolerate usually mild untoward effects of drugs. For example, hyponatremia from thiazide diuretics appears to be more frequent in the elderly due to a defect in free water clearance. Postural hypotension and confusion from a variety of antihypertensive drugs, diuretics, levodopa, neuroleptics, and antidepressants are more common and cause more dramatic problems in old people.

The sensitivity of drug receptor sites may change with age. Equivalent concentrations of psychotropic drugs, for example, commonly cause more central nervous system depression in the elderly than in younger patients, and thus must be used in lower doses; paradoxical excitation with these drugs, on the other hand, does not appear to increase with age. Resistance to the effects of beta-blockers and beta-stimulants is seen in the elderly: the unbound concentration of pro-pranolol required to lower the heartbeat by 25 beats per minute increases linearly with age. Similarly, isoproterenol's chronotropic effect is lessened in the elderly. Clinically significant inotropic activity may occur at "subtherapeutic" digoxin serum concentrations in the elderly. In summary, both increased and decreased sensitivity to drugs occur with aging, and often unpredictably so.

Drug-Drug Interactions

Although drug interactions are not well documented in the elderly, one would predict that they are more common in elderly patients due to their high frequency of drug usage and susceptibility to untoward effects. Additive effects are particularly problematic. For example, accumulation of drugs with anticholinergic side effects may cause an "atropine psychosis" or dementia without the usual warning signals of mydriasis, xerostomia, constipation, urinary retention, or tachycardia.

Drug-Disease Interactions

Clinically significant drug-disease interactions and disease-related contraindications may be more important considerations than increased drug sensitivity in the geriatric patient. For example, guanethidine would be a poor choice in a diabetic with autonomic neuropathy and orthostasis. Because of the problem of fluid retention, nonsteroidal antiinflammatory drugs must be used with caution in a patient with a history of heart failure.

Overuse of Medication

The atypical presentation of disease may lead physicians to overmedicate their elderly patients. Nonspecific symptoms such as dizziness and weakness, for example, can be the only manifestations of potentially serious medical problems or can be caused by the stress of loneliness. An unnecessary sedative-hypnotic is often prescribed for the normally diminished duration and depth of sleep seen with aging.

DRUG ABSORPTION

Several age-related physiologic changes occur in the gut. Gastric pH increases with age, possibly affecting dissolution, enzymatic breakdown, and the state of ionization of the drug moiety. Gastric emptying time is slowed, which might be expected to delay the absorption of some drugs, increase degradation in the stomach, and allow more time for the "first-pass" effect. The absorptive surfaces in the stomach and duodenum are reduced in old people. The rates of active transport and passive transport, the latter being the usual pathway for drug absorption, are impaired.

In practice, there are surprisingly few modifications in the pharmacokinetic parameters of absorption to parallel these physiologic changes. The quantity of drug absorbed orally is not usually reduced except in the case of prazosin (reduced by approximately one-third). The bioavailability of levodopa, a mainstay of therapy for Parkinson's disease, is thought to be greater with increasing age, perhaps due to a combination of slowed gastric emptying time and a concomitant reduction in gastrointestinal mucosal dopa-decarboxylase that destroys a portion of the levodopa before absorption.

A slowed rate of absorption could result in a delayed onset of effect for some drugs. The effect of delayed gastric emptying on enteric-coated products designed to bypass the stomach and disintegrate in the intestine has not been studied, but is possibly significant for bisacodyl (Dulcolax), enteric-coated aspirin (such as the usually well-absorbed Ecotrin), and the solid dosage forms of potassium. Oral liquid dosage forms may speed the onset of action and are particularly useful in patients with dysphagia, those requiring feeding tubes, patients with ileostomies or high colostomies, agitated patients, and patients who "cheek" their medications.

While it is often useful to give food with a drug to reduce gastrointestinal discomfort, ingestion of a meal may either decrease or increase bioavailability by stimulating gastric secretion and delaying gastric emptying time. Food decreases the availability of tetracyclines (except doxycycline and minocycline), erythromycin (except the estolate and ethylsuccinate salts and E-Mycin), penicillin, and ampicillin. Food may increase the absorption of diazepam, nitrofurantoin, griseofulvin, and some drugs that undergo the "first-pass" effect, perhaps from increased hepatic blood flow, such as propranolol and hydralazine.

Antacids are the best example of commonly used drugs that interact with other drugs and modify bioavailability by slowing dissolution, destroying enteric coatings, or binding to drugs. It is therefore advisable to administer antacids at least one hour before or two hours after other drugs known to be affected by antacids—for example, digoxin, chlorpromazine, cimetidine, isoniazid, and tetracycline. Other drugs that are known to reduce drug absorption include psyllium, colestipol, cholestyramine, and those with anticholinergic side effects that slow gastric emptying.

Intramuscular and subcutaneous absorption may be delayed in the elderly, especially those who have diminished peripheral circulation such as some diabetics and patients with peripheral atherosclerotic disease. Since muscle mass is reduced in the elderly, intramuscular injections may be technically difficult and painful and should be avoided when possible. A useful practice in hospitals or extended-care facilities is to write the order for medication as "i.m. or p.o.," allowing the nurse to make the best determination.

The intramuscular route of absorption may be less reliable than oral absorption (for example, the delayed and erratic absorption of intramuscular diazepam and chlordiazepoxide) and may result in a highly sedative action days after the effect was intended. Intramuscular phenytoin causes muscle necrosis and is unpredictably absorbed. Digoxin and quinidine are also poorly absorbed by the intramuscular route.

VOLUME OF DISTRIBUTION

As a group, the elderly tend to be smaller than young people. They have more body fat (by approximately 35 percent), less muscle mass, and less body water. By age 65 the average man has 12 kg less of lean body weight, and the average woman's lean body weight has diminished by 5 kg. Drugs that are lipophilic and bind to fat may show increased volumes of distribution in the elderly; those that are hydrophilic or bind to muscle typically show smaller volumes of distribution. As a result, drugs that are dosed by estimated lean body weight may require altered dosages in the elderly.

Serum albumin tends to be reduced in the elderly: the number of patients with normal serum albumin concentrations (4.0 g/100 ml or greater) decreases progressively from about 50 percent of those less than 40 years old to less than 30 percent of those over 80. Thus, in the elderly, drugs that are highly bound to albumin may have a significantly increased unbound (active) fraction which is free to diffuse to the receptor sites. For example, warfarin is 97 percent bound to albumin; if there were 3 percent fewer binding sites, the free fraction of warfarin would double from 3 to 6 percent. A Boston Collaborative study showed a 13.3 percent rate of adverse reactions to phenytoin in patients with serum albumin concentrations lower than 2.5 g/100 ml versus a 1 percent prevalence when serum albumin concentrations were above 4.0 g/100 ml.[1] Other factors affecting vol-

---

1. Boston Collaborative Drug Surveillance Program. Diphenylhydantoin side effects and serum albumin levels. *Clin. Pharmacol. Ther.* 14:529–532, 1973.

umes of distribution are obesity, malnutrition, dehydration, and being bedridden.

DRUG METABOLISM

The overall changes in drug metabolism with aging are poorly quantitated. Metabolism occurs predominantly in the liver but is also known to occur in the plasma, lungs, kidneys, and gastrointestinal mucosa. The rate of hepatic arterial blood flow decreases with age by approximately 2 percent each decade, and liver mass is reduced with age, possibly resulting in a reduced metabolism for some drugs. Liver enzymes can be induced (activated) by drugs like phenobarbital or phenytoin and by environmental stimuli such as smoking. Drugs such as chloramphenicol, cimetidine, and influenza vaccine may act as inhibitors of microsomal enzyme activity. The influence of age on interactions related to microsomal enzyme activity is unknown, but since the elderly receive so many drugs, the potential for untoward interactions is increased.

RENAL ELIMINATION

Unlike metabolism, the effect of aging on renal clearance can be quantified. The creatinine clearance can be easily calculated from formulas using age, weight, sex, and serum creatinine, providing a most clinically useful estimate of renal function:

$$\text{CrCl} = \frac{(140 - \text{age}) \times \text{kg lean body weight}}{S_{Cr} \times 72}$$

multiplied by 0.85 for women, is one such formula. The serum creatinine may remain "within normal limits" because there is a decrease in muscle mass and endogenous creatinine production with age. Both the glomerular filtration rate and tubular secretion usually decrease by approximately 40 percent between the ages of 20 and 90.

Diminished renal clearance is clinically important for drugs primarily excreted unchanged by the kidney (e.g., penicillins, aminoglycosides, cimetidine, and digoxin) and drugs with active metabolites that are predominantly excreted by the kidney (e.g., procainamide and its metabolite, *N*-acetylprocainamide). It is also important for antibiotics that must achieve an inhibitory concentration in the urine; for example, nitrofurantoin is usually ineffective against *Escherichia coli* and other gram-negative organisms growing in the urine when the creatinine clearance is less than 40 ml/min. Drugs that reduce renal blood flow (e.g., some beta-blockers and prostaglandin inhibitors) might require careful observation for drug toxicity in elderly patients with low creatinine clearances.

LIMITATIONS OF PHARMACOKINETIC STUDIES

The heterogeneity of pharmacokinetic data obtained from studies of the elderly reinforces the concept that chronologic age correlates poorly with physiologic age. Two separate groups, at least, must be defined—the young-old (55 to 75 years) and the old-old (85 + years). Longitudinal studies of the elderly are obviously needed, but the cost and difficulty of follow-up are often prohibitive.

Many of the pharmacokinetic parameters are derived from small numbers of ambulatory "well" elderly who may not be representative of the diseased, bedridden patient with multiple problems who often receives the drugs. Although it is appropriate that studies be performed in this "controlled" host environment, data should be collected from "real patients" as well. Conversely, other studies are conducted on patients with so many medical problems that it is difficult to isolate the effect of "normal" aging.

GENERAL OBSERVATIONS ON COMMONLY USED DRUGS

Theophylline. The dose of theophylline should be reduced by an average of 30 percent in the elderly. Congestive heart failure, cirrhosis, influenza vaccine, and viral upper respiratory infections reduce hepatic clearance, and smoking increases clearance. Theophylline serum concentrations are imperative for optimal dosing.

Salicylates. While there are no well-documented changes in salicylate pharmacokinetics with aging, there may be an increased potential for adverse effects.

Nonsteroidal antiinflammatory agents. Few studies have specifically examined changes in the pharmacokinetics of those agents available in the United States, but the data suggest that adjustments may need to be made for age alone. Adverse effects on renal function and fluid retention may be more problematic in the elderly.

Acetaminophen. No major changes in pharmacokinetic parameters with age have been noted, and dosage adjustment is not recommended.

Narcotic Analgesics. Doses should be lowered by one-third to two-thirds, or longer dosage intervals should be used in the elderly.

Cimetidine. Dosage should be based on estimated creatinine clearances. Patients whose serum creatinine concentrations are unknown can be started on a dose of 200 mg four times a day.

Digoxin. Lower doses are frequently necessary. Despite extensive research, digoxin dosing remains largely empirical, with most patients requiring a dose between 0.125 mg every other day and 0.25 mg every day. Atypical presentations of toxicity, including delirium, may be seen in the elderly.

Procainamide and quinidine. Current literature indicates that doses may need to be reduced by approximately 50 percent in the elderly.

Lidocaine. Reduced lidocaine clearance with age has been noted, and the elderly may be more susceptible to toxicity. Lower doses may be warranted.

Anticoagulants. Although the pharmacokinetics of warfarin and heparin are largely unchanged with age, elderly patients, particularly women, are especially prone to bleeding complications. The potential for trauma resulting from unsteadiness or arthritis with secondary bleeding, hematomas, and emergency orthopedic surgery also means that lower dosages are frequently required.

Phenytoin. The average dose may need to be reduced in the elderly by approximately one-fifth. Use of serum concentration measurements are necessary.

Phenobarbital. The use of barbiturates as sedatives has fallen out of favor. Phenobarbital may be used, usually in low doses, as an anticonvulsant in the elderly; measurement of serum levels is advisable.

Antidepressants. The implications of pharmacokinetic data for the therapeutic effects of this class of drugs are as yet unresolved. Side effects, some dose-related, are the greatest concern in the elderly.

Lithium. Elderly patients may be prone to neurologic side effects, often requiring a 50-percent dosage reduction. Measurement of serum concentrations is necessary.

Beta-blockers. Pharmacologic studies show diminished receptor site sensitivity to these agents. Adverse reactions, especially neurologic ones, tend to become more common with age. In general, propranolol should be started at a low dose of 20 mg twice a day, increasing by 20-mg increments as indicated by blood pressure and heart rate.

Benzodiazepines. Most of the long-acting agents show extended half-lives and decreased clearances, but the pharmacokinetics of the short-acting agents are largely unchanged with age. Adverse central nervous system effects of these drugs may be more pronounced in the elderly, and a 50-percent decrease in dosage may be recommended for both long-acting and short-acting agents with elderly patients.

Antibiotics. Aminoglycoside dosing should be based on estimated creatinine clearance and use of serum drug concentrations. Nitrofurantoin should be avoided in patients with creatinine clearances less than 40 ml/min.

SUMMARY

A few global statements can be made with regard to the pharmacokinetic changes that occur with age. Absorption is rarely modified with age. The volume of distribution may increase, decrease, or remain the same depending on the lipid/water solubility and protein-binding characteristics of the drug. Clearance of drugs is frequently diminished, especially when drugs are excreted by the kidney. Liver microsomal enzyme activity is inconsistently affected, and generalizations about the effects of age on drug metabolism are not possible. Half-life, a hybrid parameter influenced by both volume of distribution and clearance, typically rises with age. While pharmacokinetic changes usually act to enhance or prolong drug effects in the elderly, there may be decreased effects (as for beta-stimulants and beta-blockers).

In general, the clinician should anticipate heterogeneity of response in the elderly and an increased incidence of adverse effects, and hence should monitor clinical response and toxicity closely. For drugs in which the concentration–therapeutic response relationship has been defined and levels are available, serum drug monitoring is helpful.

SUGGESTED READING

1. Gibaldi, M., Levy, G. Pharmacokinetics in clinical practice. *J.A.M.A.* 235:1864–1867, 1987–1992, 1976.
2. Greenblatt, D.J., Shader, R.I. Pharmacokinetics in old age: Principles and problems of assessment. In Jarvik, L.F., Greenblatt, D.J., Harman, D. (Eds.), *Clinical Pharmacology and the Aged Patient.* New York: Raven Press, 1981.
3. Lamy, P.P. *Prescribing for the Elderly.* Littleton, Mass.: John Wright-PSG, 1980.
4. Ouslander, J.G. Drug therapy in the elderly. *Ann. Intern. Med.* 95:711–722, 1981.
5. Vestal, R.E., Drug use in the elderly: A review of problems and special considerations. *Drugs* 16:358–382, 1978.

Physician Drug Abuse of the Elderly

PETER P. LAMY, PH.D.

Editor's note: In geriatric medicine, care most often supersedes "cure." Clinical experience is still the most important factor in drug treatment, since guidelines for geriatric drug use are still largely lacking. Drug regimens not only should be designed for their therapeutic advantages but also must be integrated with the patient's physical, nutritional, and psychological needs. Yearly drug "checkups," including a survey of those agents purchased without the physician's knowledge, help keep the drug regimen safe and rational.

Although data to support the statement that there is drug abuse/ misuse in the care of the elderly are still largely lacking, there is ample presumptive evidence that older adults often get poorly conceived drug treatment. Drug abuse is likely to be a shared responsibility between provider and patient. Both the use of drugs, either prescription or nonprescription, for reasons other than clearly justified ones and the overuse of drugs for symptomatic treatment could be classified as drug abuse. An important type of drug abuse in the elderly is "polymedicine," a term I use to refer to the treatment of multiple ailments by multiple providers acting independently of each other. Such multiple providers, for example, were responsible for the following drug regimen of an elderly female patient. The duplications, overlapping of pharmacologic actions, and complexity of the regimen are obvious.

Motrin, 400 mg	Two/day
Digoxin, 0.25 mg	One/day
Lanoxin, 0.125 mg	One/day
Lasix, 20 mg	One/day with juice

53

Hydrochlorothiazide, 50 mg	One/day
Dyazide	Two/day
Quinidine, 200 mg	One q.6h.
Papaverine, 150 mg	Two/day
Pavabid	Two/day

WHAT KIND OF DRUG ABUSE?

The elderly patient often presents with confounding multiple diagnoses, complications, and disabilities. In caring for elderly patients who are often "hoarders of subclinical illness," the physician must be a clinical detective. Physicians may be hampered in the diagnostic process and subsequent therapeutic decisions by an inadequate knowledge of the natural course of a chronic disease and of the similarities of the effects of disease, drugs, and aging.

Many factors can contribute to drug abuse/misuse. The most important ones are listed here.

1. Poor or insufficient drug history
2. Incorrect diagnosis
3. Unclear decisions to treat or not to treat
4. Inappropriate drug/chronic drug use habits
5. Failure to consider alternate treatment modalities
6. Failure to consider potential drug interactions
7. Failure to ensure patient compliance

THE MEDICATION-RELATED HISTORY

Unless questioned in detail, the elderly patient often fails to relate all pertinent facts. Consequently, many conditions may be overlooked that can affect drug compliance and toxicity, such as sight and hearing impairments, incontinence, and confusion. A detailed drug history, for example, should elicit all the agents a patient uses, including those bought in the supermarket or the health food store, which are often not viewed as drugs by either the patient or the physician.

CONFUSION IN THE DIAGNOSTIC PROCESS

The diagnostic process in the elderly is often complex and time-consuming because their disease presentation may change with age and their diseases may inhibit precise information gathering. The range of normal laboratory test values may vary by ±5 percent ordinarily, but this variation is considerably widened in the elderly—as much as 15 percent. The serum creatinine concentration may not rise significantly in the elderly, for example, in spite of significant kidney function impairment. The multitude of drugs the elderly take may interfere with laboratory determinations. For example, ascorbic acid can alter the urine pH, thereby affecting the results of some tests for urine sugar, and a number of drugs can interfere with creatinine secretion, thus incorrectly indicating acute renal failure.

Another important diagnostic confusion is the accumulation of side effects of the numerous drugs used in the elderly. Patients might receive a number of drugs with an anticholinergic side effect, such as a phenothiazine, an anticholinergic antiparkinsonian drug, an antihistamine for sleep (possibly diphenhydramine), and a cold preparation containing a belladonna alkaloid. The cumulative side effects of such a combination could lead to paralytic ileus, urine retention, an atropine-like psychosis, and cognitive impairment from additive sedative effects. The psychosis might then be mistakenly treated by increasing the dose of phenothiazine rather than by withdrawing all drugs with anticholinergic side effects.

Therapeutic and toxic blood levels overlap widely, especially in the elderly, so overreliance on blood level determinations of drugs may lead to an inaccurate diagnosis. Digoxin blood levels, for example, are overused to rule out digoxin toxicity or to document therapeutic doses, and digoxin toxicity correlates poorly with its described signs and symptoms in the elderly. Psychiatric side effects are often the presenting symptoms and, since physicians do not commonly associate them with digoxin toxicity, they may be overlooked.

TO TREAT OR NOT TO TREAT—THE THERAPEUTIC GOAL

An unrealistic therapeutic goal may result in inappropriate drug use. It might be better not to treat all complaints at once, but to address only the most serious ones first. In fact, patients may not always choose to have their complaints treated; they may just want to know the seriousness of a symptom. The treatment of one illness may have a beneficial effect on another (e.g., a psychotropic drug helping angina) or an adverse one (e.g., timolol for glaucoma inducing heart failure).

Because elderly patients are likely to suffer from multiple illnesses, the decision to prescribe must involve an assessment of the whole patient. For example, strict control of diabetes can best be achieved with insulin, and strict control appears to reduce the risk of nephropathy and retinopathy. Yet for an elderly, sight-impaired patient with arthritis, living alone and on a restricted income, a judicious blend of an oral hypoglycemic and diet may prevent dependence and institutionalization while the use of an injection may force institutionalization.

Once a decision to treat has been made, a flexible and reasonable therapeutic goal should be set. Often the goals of antihypertensive treatment are too rigidly pursued; in lowering a patient's systolic hypertension with diuretics, one may also lower the diastolic pressure to unacceptable levels, causing syncope and serious disturbances of electrolyte balance. Similarly, one must recognize that no drug treatment will be able to restore a patient with Parkinson's disease to predisease effectiveness. Certainly, palliation rather than cure or restoration of normal function is also an appropriate therapeutic goal.

The decision to prescribe an indefinite course of medication should be made only when there is reasonable expectation that the overall morbidity/mortality of the disease process will be decreased, and that the beneficial effects of the drug are not outweighed by its toxicity. Commitment to a chronic drug regimen should be undertaken only with the full knowledge and agreement of the patient, whose lifestyle and financial resources may be strongly affected by the proposed regimen. Examples of drugs that are often inappropriately used chronically are the anticholinergic antiparkinsonian drugs, iron therapy, digoxin, phenothiazines, sedatives/hypnotics, antidepressants, and cimetidine. Frequent reevaluation of a specific regimen—a yearly "drug checkup"—can help avoid this problem.

INAPPROPRIATE DRUG USE

Both prescription and nonprescription drugs may be used inappropriately and excessively by physicians for their elderly patients. Many of the elderly are being overmedicated because of physician acquiescence to patient or family demands; nonprescription drugs are often selected by patients and not monitored by the primary provider.

The physiologic changes that accompany aging can present as signs of a disease process and are often incorrectly treated with drugs. For example, insomnia may be a normal change in patterns seen with aging or may result from bad habits such as daytime napping and lack of activity that are amenable to nondrug treatment. Pain, other diseases, and many drugs (the diuretics, for example) can also be responsible for sleeplessness in the elderly. All of these problems should be ruled out or treated before hypnotics are considered. Once hypnotics are prescribed, it is important to avoid long-term use, which can lead to physical and psychological dependence. Withdrawal may cause agitation, autonomic hyperarousal, and rebound insomnia.

Constipation, another frequent complaint of the elderly, is more difficult for the physician to manage because of the wide availability of nonprescribed medications. Many factors can contribute to constipation, including the normal aging process, insufficient fluid and roughage intake, lack of exercise, and many drugs and diseases. Before laxatives are considered, all of these need to be ruled out as causative factors.

Asthenia, lack of energy, fatigue, and similar complaints often prompt the provider or the patient to begin iron therapy. Although iron is widely viewed as an innocuous "pep pill," it can cause considerable trouble. In nursing homes the start of iron therapy commonly leads to the use of laxatives and, very shortly thereafter, to the use of antacids to ameliorate the stomach upset caused by the first two treatments.

Duplication in medication is a serious and dangerous problem in geriatric medicine that often results from patients' consulting more than one physician. A diuretic prescribed by one physician under a trade name and by another under a generic name will look different, and the patient may be unaware of the duplication. Patients must be encouraged to carry a medication record listing all current medications and to use one pharmacy only, preferably one that provides patient medication records and personal attention.

Duplication may be seen in the use of psychotropics, despite the general opinion that there is rarely an indication for the use of more than one phenothiazine or more than one antidepressant at a time. Appropriate prescribing practices would lead to the trial of one tranquilizer or antidepressant at a sufficient dose for a sufficiently long time. If there is no appropriate therapeutic response after the trial, the first drug should be discontinued and another drug tried.

Most adverse drug effects in the elderly occur because of inappropriate dosing or inappropriate duration of treatment. Age-related biologic and physiologic changes in the elderly may lead to altered pharmacodynamic drug properties, and indeed, elderly patients are more sensitive to the action of many drugs, particularly central nervous system drugs. Changes in liver and kidney function slow metabolism and excretion; if the elderly are given the same dose and dosage schedule as younger patients, drugs are likely to accumulate to toxic levels, causing increased adverse drug effects. If the changes in kidney function in the elderly were recognized more often, adverse drug reactions could be reduced by as much as 50 percent. Altered dosage schedules or reduced doses may be necessary especially for drugs with a narrow therapeutic-to-toxic ratio—for example, digoxin, the diuretics, and the psychotropic drugs. An across-the-board dosage reduction, however, may lead to underdosage.

NONUSE OF ALTERNATIVE TREATMENT MODALITIES

Patients, it is believed, expect to receive a prescription. Also, there is an unfortunate belief that new and powerful medicines are always inherently superior to nondrug or to older modalities in disease management.

Humidification, however, may be superior to many over-the-counter cough preparations. The use of moist heat and increased activity may be more helpful than drugs in managing arthritic stiffness. Dietary changes, including increasing fiber and fluid intake, may be helpful in preventing or treating constipation. In the management of exogenous or situational depression, frequently encountered among the elderly and attributed to the effect of cumulative losses, empathic listening, reassurance, and community social services are likely to be more valuable and successful in the long run than antidepressants, which may, in addition, be toxic and sedating.

OTHER DRUG-RELATED PROBLEMS

Institutionalization and Deinstitutionalization
The patient may be at great risk for inappropriate drug use when released from an institution. On admission, all of the patient's "old" drugs may have been stored as "private property." On release, the patient will most likely have a set of new drugs and new dose regimens, and will also be given his private property, including his old drugs. Lacking instructions, he may continue taking his former medications along with his new drugs.

Standing orders, numerous p.r.n. orders, or both can easily lead to drug misuse in nursing homes. For example, standing orders for two or three different laxatives ultimately lead to the continuous use of two or three laxatives. Any drug started as a p.r.n. drug can find its way into regular use, and multiple p.r.n. drugs such as pain medications are often used simultaneously.

Cost Factors

Only about 70 percent of all drugs prescribed for the elderly are actually purchased, probably because of the financial difficulties of elderly persons living on fixed incomes who must contend with increases in costs of prescription drugs. Some of the new nonsteroidal antiinflammatory drugs are very expensive, particularly if they are used for both their antiinflammatory and analgesic actions. Combining these drugs with acetaminophen, for example, may permit a lesser dose and thus a reduction in cost. Although the use of nitro-paste may be messy, it may be much less expensive than the new transdermal units, which can cost up to one dollar daily. Liquid antacids can have as much as a tenfold range of potency and an almost fortyfold range in cost. Dermatologics can be dispensed in the form of expensive perfumed cosmetics or as inexpensive and practical therapeutic preparations.

Self-Medication

Up to 60 percent or more of the elderly use self-medication, most frequently analgesics, laxatives, vitamins, and cough and cold preparations. Recent statistics imply that self-medication is increasing, probably as an attempt to reduce the overall cost of medical care. Nonprescription drugs, although often not regarded as drugs by patients or health care providers, are by no means innocuous, and their use can interfere with prescribed drug regimens and laboratory test values.

Dosage Forms

It is generally recognized that different dosage forms have different bioavailability and thus may exhibit differences in duration and intensity of action. Rarely recognized is the fact that a particular dosage form can alter the clinical outcome of therapeutic regimens in other ways. For example, it matters to the hypertensive patient whether a regular or effervescent bulk laxative is used—the latter contains too much sodium. Certain tablets or capsules can be a bane to elderly patients who have problems swallowing them. In nursing homes, this problem is sometimes overcome by crushing all oral solid dosage forms and administering them in applesauce. Such a procedure would yield an overdose when a slow-release dosage form is prescribed. It is relatively simple to prescribe eye drops, but one must consider whether a patient afflicted with poor vision, Parkinson's disease, or arthritis will be able to self-administer them.

SOME SOLUTIONS

Provider-Patient Interaction

Adverse drug effects and interactions may occur frequently in a complex therapeutic regimen but are difficult to differentiate from the effects of aging or disease. One way to reduce the hazards of drug therapy is to improve the interaction between provider and patient—patients cannot remain passive recipients of health care but must become active participants. Informed of the need for a drug and the expected action of drugs, patients can and should report back any unforeseen effect so that adjustments can be made.

Communication may well be the key to good medical care. The common use of professional jargon is equivalent to poor handwriting. The patient simply cannot understand it, and will not, therefore, be an active participant in the treatment. Written instructions should be used only after assessment of eyesight and the patient's ability to read.

Noncompliance must always be assumed. Even though noncompliance may not be higher in the elderly age group, its consequences may be more severe, and the elderly may recover more slowly from adverse drug effects. Compliance requires agreement between provider and patient. It is mandatory to tailor a drug regimen to the patient's activity, rather than to expect the patient to change substantially to adjust to a regimen.

The Therapeutic Goal and Reevaluation

Once a therapeutic goal has been set, the drug regimen should be reevaluated at specified intervals. This is of particular importance in geriatric medicine, since chronic care must be assumed to be constantly changing care.

Awareness of Special Drug Problems

Not so long ago, physicians dispensed psychological comfort more often than cures. Now a vast arsenal of medicines and technologies is available to cure or manage diseases. It is extremely important that physicians become familiar with the pharmacodynamics and pharmacokinetics of new drugs, with their actions and side effects, and, most important, with their behavior in patients with multiple pathology and on multiple drug regimens.

AND FINALLY—THE BROWN BAG

Geriatric care must become multidisciplinary care. Even when health practitioners work together—physician, nurse, pharmacist, and dietitian—something else is needed. This may be provided by scheduled yearly checkups, by reevaluation of the patient and the patient's drug regimen, by close cooperation with the family and significant others— and finally, by the brown bag. Ask your patient to bring in *all* drugs. To reevaluate, you must know what has been "contributed" by friends and neighbors or bought in the health food store, supermarket, and by mail order. This knowledge alone would substantially reduce polymedicine, the incidence of adverse effects, and the general hazard of medicines in geriatric care.

SUGGESTED READING

1. Lamy, P.P. Drug prescribing for the elderly. *Bull. N.Y. Acad. Med.* 57:718–730, 1981.
2. Lamy, P.P. *Prescribing for the Elderly*. Littleton, Mass.: John Wright-PSG, 1980.
3. Lamy, P.P. Special features of geriatric prescribing. *Geriatrics* 36(12):41–52, 1981.
4. Ouslander, J.G. Drug therapy in the elderly. *Ann. Intern. Med.* 95:711–722, 1981.
5. Reidenberg, M.M. Drugs in the elderly. *Bull. N.Y. Acad. Med.* 56:703–714, 1980.
6. Vestal, R.E. Drug use in the elderly: A review of problems and special considerations. *Drugs* 16:358–382, 1978.

3

COMMON NUISANCES
OF AGING

Constipation

R. BALFOUR SARTOR, M.D., and
C. THOMAS NUZUM, M.D.

*Editor's note: Constipation, often thought to be the bane of aging,
may be more a problem of fear than of colonic dysfunction. Increased intake
of fiber, privacy, exercise, and education can make avoidance of the
evils of laxative abuse possible. Knowledge of the fiber content of
various foods is essential for a primary care practitioner.*

The meaning of constipation differs widely among patients and physicians. Strictly defined, it is the passage of less than 35 grams of fecal matter per day; more practically described, it is the passage of fewer than three stools per week. The sensation of incomplete evacuation or the need to strain are common concomitant symptoms. The high prevalence of constipation in Western civilization appears to be directly related to decreased dietary cereal fiber and improper bowel habits.

Although constipation is commonly attributed to the aging process, there is no known age-related degeneration of gastrointestinal function. Connell's surveys of ambulatory subjects show little change of stool frequency with aging but an increasing prevalence of laxative use from 16 percent of persons 10–59 years of age to 50 percent of those over 60.[1] Increased laxative consumption by elderly people seems to be a result of factors such as the conviction that less than one stool a day is abnormal, dehydration, immobility, neurologic disorders affecting both the "gastrocolic reflex" and the voluntary response to rectal distention, and low fiber intake due to poor dentition or depression. Myths and home remedies may reinforce beliefs

1. A.M. Connell, C. Hilton, G. Irvine, et al. Variation of bowel habit in two population samples. *Br. Med. J.* 2:1095–1099, 1965.

that periodic purging is necessary, leading to laxative abuse and dependence.

Constipating drugs frequently used by the elderly include opiates, anticholinergics, psychotherapeutic agents (particularly antidepressants and phenothiazines), aluminum and calcium antacids, and certain antihypertensive agents. Geriatric conditions associated with constipation are hypothyroidism, diabetes with autonomic neuropathy, uremia, hypokalemia, hypercalcemia, stroke, parkinsonism, spinal cord lesions, and scleroderma. For unknown reasons constipation is more common in women than in men.

Three general issues must be addressed in order to treat the constipated patient effectively. (1) Is constipation harmful? Simple constipation is frequently asymptomatic. Symptoms of cramping abdominal pain, nausea, and fullness are more often produced by laxatives taken for perceived "irregularity" than by accumulating fecal matter within the left colon. However, chronic constipation, usually in conjunction with laxative use, has been associated with colonic diverticulosis, hemorrhoids, and colonic dilatation which predisposes such patients to sigmoid volvulus. Long-standing impactions may present as incontinent "diarrhea" or cause stercoral ulcers. (2) Is regular laxative use harmful? Repetitive use of certain laxatives can produce motility disturbances manifested by decreased propulsive activity of the right colon. Agents incriminated in this syndrome, the "cathartic colon," include cascara, senna, castor and croton oils, and phenolphthalein. In addition, frequent purging can result in electrolyte and renal disturbances, particularly hypocalcemia, hypokalemia, and hyperaldosteronism. Side effects of specific cathartics are cited later in the chapter. (3) What are the relevant cultural and dietary factors? A customary low-fiber diet diminishes stool distention of the rectal ampulla and the resulting afferent impulses for defecation. Suppression of the urge to defecate, due to real or fancied exigencies, diminishes the responsiveness of this reflex arc, leaving more residue in the distal colon with subsequent stool desiccation and rectosigmoid dilation. The large bowel appears to function optimally when supplied with voluminous stool, as occurs on high-fiber diets.

DIAGNOSIS

Evaluation should determine whether constipation is actually present; search for intrinsic gastrointestinal pathology, particularly of colonic origin; diagnose systemic diseases that might present as constipation; and detect easily remediable causes, such as constipating drugs or poor dietary habits.

History

The history, usually more valuable than the physical examination or tests, should focus on when and under what circumstances constipation first became a problem. Constipation beginning in adolescence or early adulthood without abrupt change in bowel function is more compatible with a functional disorder. Constipation may date from the time of immobilization in the patient who has become bedridden or chair-confined due to another disease, or it may correlate with the use of certain drugs. Recent onset dictates a more aggressive search for gastrointestinal disorders, especially carcinoma of the colon, but the patient with habitual constipation cannot be considered safe from other bowel diseases. Fibrosis from ischemia, Crohn's disease, diverticulitis, or prostate cancer may impede stool transit. Colonic diseases causing constipation by partial obstruction may also cause rectal bleeding, abdominal distension, weight loss, anal pain, and vomiting. A history of surgery suggests the possibility of a secondary anal stricture or obstructing intraabdominal adhesions. The metabolic and neuromuscular diseases just listed can often be excluded by a directed review of systems, examination, and selective use of laboratory tests.

Family and social histories reveal attitudes toward constipation and laxative use, genetic risk of colon cancer, and rare cases of familial pseudo-obstruction. A dietary history should include a detailed recall of all food and fluid intake over the past 48 hours. This information is often helpful not only in establishing an etiology for constipation, but also in planning therapy and teaching the patient the importance of dietary factors in the pathogenesis of constipation. A meticulous history of intake of both prescribed and over-the-counter drugs is essential, with emphasis on laxatives as well as on compounds known to induce constipation. Frequently patients are reluctant to admit the extent of laxative use, so the physician must be persistent in his questioning.

Physical Examination

Rectal palpation should include evaluation of perianal sensation, anal sphincter tone, amount and consistency of stool in the ampulla, and rectal dilatation. Painful anal disorders reinforce constipation by spasm of the sphincter. Strictures and masses (extrinsic, mural, or luminal) should be identified. The stool should be tested for occult blood.

Anoscopy and proctosigmoidoscopy are integral to the physical examination of the constipated patient and essential to find anal fissure, carcinoma of the lower colon, rectal distension, and melanosis coli. Melanosis coli is an apparently benign darkening of the colonic mucosa produced by pigment-engorged macrophages in the lamina propria of patients who chronically use anthraquinone laxatives (senna and cascara). Patients with a large amount of stool in the rectum on digital examination can be most thoroughly evaluated after a Fleet's enema.

Diagnosis
Idiopathic or habitual constipation is a diagnosis of exclusion. The extent of laboratory or radiographic evaluation depends on the degree of clinical suspicion that an associated disorder is present. Serum calcium, glucose, potassium, thyroid function, and blood urea nitrogen determinations are not routinely indicated but are useful in patients with indications of possible systemic disease. All patients should have three separate stools tested for occult blood. A barium enema is not always indicated but should be performed in patients with recent onset or abrupt worsening of constipation, stools positive for occult blood, weight loss, or evidence suggesting bowel obstruction. Elderly patients with chronic or recurring constipation, as well as those with more urgent indications, should have a barium enema unless their other diseases make detection of colon cancer unimportant. Radiographic abnormalities of the "cathartic colon" are usually confined to the right side and include lack of normal haustration and bizarre contractions. Rectal manometry is useful only in patients with fecal incontinence not related to impaction or obvious neuropathy. Colonoscopy is rarely indicated in constipation unless a stricture or other focal lesion is suspected.

TREATMENT

Increase in Fiber
Idiopathic constipation in the ambulatory patient is treated by increasing dietary fiber intake, cessation of laxatives, and reeducation. The bulk of colonic contents may be augmented with cereal, vegetable and fruit roughage, bran, and commercial psyllium preparations. Fiber increases stool mass by holding water, and it may have secondary cathartic effects through increasing the colonic bile salt concentration and enhancing bacterial production of short-chain fatty acids.

Bran, the outer coat of grain removed by modern milling, has higher fiber concentration than any other dietary constituent. Bran has been demonstrated to increase stool frequency, bulk, water content, and dry weight and to decrease intestinal transit time in numerous studies of constipated patients, including the immobile geriatric population.

The best sources of fiber in ordinary diets are whole-grain breads, bran cereals, and rye crackers (Table 1). Brown bread contains twice the fiber content of white bread, and whole-grain bread contains

TABLE 1
Dietary Fiber in Some Common Foods

Food	Amount	Dietary Fiber (g)	Kilocalories
Bread			
White	1 slice	0.8	70
Brown	1 slice	2.0	70
Whole wheat	1 slice	2.4	65
Cereals			
All-Bran	1 ounce	9.0	70
Cornflakes	1 ounce	3.0	100
Rice Krispies	1 ounce	1.3	90
Total	1 ounce	2.0	110
Oatmeal (dry)	½ cup	4.5	130
Raw fruits			
Apple	1 small	3.1	70
Banana	1 medium	1.8	100
Grapefruit	One-half	2.6	45
Orange	1 small	1.8	65
Peach	1 medium	1.3	35
Pear	1 medium	2.8	100
Raisins	1½ tablespoons	1.0	40
Vegetables			
Green beans	½ cup	1.2	15
Cabbage, cooked	½ cup	1.5	15
Carrots, raw	1 medium	3.7	40
Celery, raw	1 stalk	1.2	12
Corn	½ cup	3.2	85
Lettuce	1 cup	0.8	8
Peas, cooked	½ cup	3.8	60
Potatoes, cooked	½ cup	2.3	90
Rice, white, cooked	1 cup	0.4	225
Summer squash, cooked	½ cup	2.2	15
Meats and milk products			
Beef steak	6 ounces	0	345
Whole milk	1 cup	0	160
Egg	1 large	0	80

TABLE 2

Representative Methods for Adding Supplemental Fiber to the Diet

Agent	Average Amount per Day	Dietary Fiber (g)	Cost per Day (cents)
Metamucil	2 tablespoons	?	31.0
Miller's bran	3 tablespoons	10	2.2
Fibermed cookies	2 cookies	10	24.0
All-Bran cereal	1 ounce (⅓ cup)	9	8.5

three times as much. Leafy green vegetables contain little fiber, being 90 percent water. On a weight basis, legumes (beans and peas) contain more fiber than root vegetables (carrots and potatoes), which contain more fiber than leafy green vegetables. Fruits and nuts contain moderate amounts of fiber, particularly blackberries, dried dates, prunes, raisins, peaches, apples, and oranges.

Mild constipation of short duration usually responds to a high-fiber diet alone, but patients who have been using laxatives for a long time will require at least 10 grams of supplemental fiber per day. This can be accomplished by the daily intake of 20 grams of miller's bran (3 heaping tablespoons), 2 tablespoons of commercial bulk laxative agents (psyllium plantago ovata powder—Metamucil, Konsyl, and Effersyllium—also available in generic form), or two high-fiber cookies (Fibermed). Of these options (Table 2), miller's bran is the cheapest (50 cents per pound); it can be mixed with hot cereals or sprinkled on food, and it has been found to decrease the colonic transit time more than bulk laxatives. Nearly all patients experience temporary sensations of gaseousness, abdominal distension, and cramping during the first few weeks of fiber supplementation; if the physician fails to explain these side effects, patients may discontinue the regimen before it takes effect. Fiber binds calcium and iron, reducing absorption, but additional mineral intake is rarely necessary. The effects of fiber persist with less supplementation as the colon is gradually "retrained" over a period of months.

Education

Patient education is essential to bring about the life-style changes necessary for lasting benefit. Normal colonic phsyiology should be explained, with emphasis on the wide variation in stool frequency of the normal population and the fact that a daily bowel movement is not essential for health. The patient should learn to respond to the urge to defecate whenever it occurs. The physician should emphasize the benefits of a high-fiber diet, capitalizing on its current vogue. The reasons for avoiding laxatives should be reiterated. Fluid intake must be adequate; if no contraindication exists, 40 to 50 ml/kg/day should be consumed. Exercise seems to enhance colonic motility. Some patients respond best to a daily ritual with prescribed amounts of fiber, fluid, exercise, and time at toilet (perhaps after a morning walk and breakfast).

Use of Laxatives
The majority of patients are able to stop the use of laxative agents upon beginning a high-fiber diet, but those having full colons may require enemas or peroral enteric irrigation with balanced electrolyte/polyethylene glycol (Golytely) solution. For a few weeks, while adapting to the high-fiber diet, patients will probably experience some discomfort and pass stools irregularly. Fleet's or saline enemas or suppositories can be used to induce a bowel movement for asymptomatic patients who have not had a movement in three days. This treatment has the advantage of stimulating the rectal distension reflex and avoiding cathartics. With continued bowel retraining and physiologic adaptation, enemas and suppositories should become unnecessary for most ambulatory patients.

Patients who are institutionalized with neuropsychiatric disorders, confined to bed or chair with neurologic defects, or, rarely, whose colons are intractably atonic from laxative abuse, scleroderma, or other dysautonomic syndromes respond variably to a high-fiber diet and bowel retraining efforts. They may require an osmotic laxative such as milk of magnesia (30 to 60 ml) or lactulose (15 to 45 ml) every second or third day, or suppositories or enemas. They should be checked regularly for fecal impactions.

The following common laxatives should *not* be used chronically because of potentially serious side effects: senna (Senokot—degeneration of colonic myenteric plexus leading to irreversible cathartic colon syndrome, melanosis coli); mineral oil (aspiration produces lipoid pneumonia, malabsorption of fat-soluble vitamins)[2]; dioctyl sulfosuccinate (Colace, Dialose—increased absorption of concurrently administered drugs); and those producing the cathartic colon,

---

2. In selected patients not prone to aspiration and refractory to fiber alone, the colon may be retrained by using mineral oil in addition to fiber. A starting dose of 4 tablespoons twice a day may be increased as needed to produce mushy stools. After a satisfactory pattern is established, the dosage of mineral oil can be tapered and fiber alone usually will suffice.

including cascara, castor oil, and phenolphthalein. Soapsuds enemas should never be used because of the irritant action which occasionally causes hemorrhagic colitis. Rectal trauma from enema administration is common. A recent outbreak of amebiasis with several fatalities was traced to colonic irrigation as practiced in a chiropractic clinic.

Numerous studies have shown bran therapy to diminish the use of laxatives in nursing homes. A 300-bed geriatric facility saved $44,000 in expenses for laxative drugs in a year after instituting fiber supplementation. The recipes used, including a tube feeding formula of bran buds in prune juice, are given in a study by Hull and colleagues.[3] A trial of fiber therapy is safe except in obvious cases of obstruction or pseudo-obstruction.

Enthusiasm on the part of the physician is essential to the success of these treatment programs. One must be supportive during the initial adjustment period, but firmly committed to complete weaning from laxatives in all but a few cases. The risk of constipation should be recognized in patients confined by other illnesses. Dietary bulk (fluid and fiber) and provision for easy defecation (access to the toilet, privacy, and so on) may prevent the vicious cycle of laxative abuse and colonic dysfunction.

SUGGESTED READING

1. Andersson, H., Bosaeus, I., Falkheden, T., Melkersson, M. Transit time in constipated geriatric patients during treatment with a bulk laxative and bran: A comparison. *Scand. J. Gastroenterol.* 14:821–826, 1979.
2. Connell, A.M., Hilton, C., Irvine, G., et al. Variation of bowel habit in two population samples. *Br. Med. J.* 2:1095–1099, 1965.
3. Cummings, J.H., Jenkins, D.J.A., Wiggins, H.S. Measurement of the mean transit time of dietary residue through the human gut. *Gut* 17:210–218, 1976.
4. Fingl, E., Freston, J.W. Antidiarrhoeal agents and laxatives: Changing concepts. In Freston, J.W., (Ed.), *Clinics in Gastroenterology*. Philadelphia: W.B. Saunders, 1979.
5. Hull, C., Greco, R.S., Brooks, D.L. Alleviation of constipation in the elderly by dietary fiber supplementation. *J. Am. Geriatr. Soc.*, 28:410–414, 1980.
6. Oster, J.R., Materson, B.J., Rogers, A.I. Laxative abuse syndrome. *Am. J. Gastroenterol.* 74:451–458, 1980.
7. Sanders, J.F. Lactulose syrup assessed in a double-blind study of elderly constipated patients. *J. Am. Geriatr. Soc.* 24:236–239, 1978.
8. Smith, R.G., Rowe, M.J., Smith, A.N., et al. A study of bulking agents in elderly patients. *Age and Ageing* 9:267–271, 1980.
9. Southgate, D.A.T., Bailey, B., Collinson, E., Walker, A.F. A guide to calculating intakes of dietary fibre. *J. Hum. Nutr.* 30:303–313, 1976.

---

3. C. Hull, R.S. Greco, D.L. Brooks. Alleviation of constipation in the elderly by dietary fiber supplementation. *J. Am. Geriatr. Soc.* 28:410–414, 1980.

10. Thomas, G., Bronzinsky, S., Isenberg, J.I. Patient acceptance and effectiveness of a balanced lavage solution (Golytely) versus the standard preparation for colonoscopy. *Gastroenterology* 82:435–447, 1982.

The Care of Aging Skin

BRYAN R. DAVIS, M.D.

Editor's Note: Aging skin loses turgor, its ability to resist damage, and its capacity to heal quickly. Still, the greatest changes are sun-inflicted. Most benign changes and malignant skin disorders would be largely eliminated by avoidance of solar damage. Many of the common discomforts of the elderly can be ameliorated by simple, commonsense skin care measures.

Both environmental factors, such as sunlight, and the passing of time express themselves on the genetic constitution of the individual. Many of the qualities that we think of as representing aging skin are not, in fact, representative of the aging process at all. Our misconception is the result of the limited portions of the skin of another individual that we are ordinarily permitted to view. It is the privilege of physicians to examine those areas of skin that seldom, if ever, see the light of day. It is, in fact, exposure to sunlight that produces many of the changes that most people think of as typical of aged skin. Wrinkling and the appearance of senile lentigines are sun-related changes, whereas loss of turgor and the development of seborrheic keratosis are examples of changes primarily due to age itself. Other factors, such as nutrition and systemic disease, that may in themselves be related to aging can also have pronounced effects on the skin.

A 1977 report by the U.S. Public Health Service found that two of every three people over the age of 65 surveyed had "significant" cutaneous problems, and one-half of those had more than one problem.[1] Other studies have found that the prevalence of benign tumors

---

1. M.L.T. Johnson, J. Robert. Relevance of dermatologic disease among persons 1 to 74 years of age. Advanced data from *Vital and Health Statistics*. National Center for Health Statistics, Publication no. 4. Bethesda, Md.: U.S. Department of Health, Education and Welfare, 1977.

such as actinic and seborrheic keratosis was one-third, that of tinea pedis four-fifths, while that of asteatosis (dry skin) and lax skin approached 100 percent.[2] Despite the high incidence of cutaneous problems in the elderly, there has been little research on cutaneous aging as compared with the amount of attention given to other organs.

NORMAL CHANGES IN HEALTHY AGING SKIN

Looking first only at those portions of the skin that have not been exposed to the sun, one finds by microscopic examination that the epidermis is thinned and the rete ridges, those finger-like projections of epidermis down into the dermis, are less apparent. The morphologic changes in the dermis include damage to the elastic fibers, both in the superficial and in the deeper portions of the dermis; the collagen fibers of the dermis, its major constituent, change diameter and show subtle changes in their chemical structure. The significance of these changes is uncertain. It may be that the important changes occur in the ground substance, the proteoglycans (mucopolysaccharides). Proteoglycans probably are involved in "structuring" water, or determining the way that it is held in the skin.

The net result of these microscopic and chemical changes is the rather dramatic change in the viscoelastic properties of the skin with increased age. The skin is less resilient, less able to restore itself quickly after either momentary or prolonged force, with an inherent loss of turgor and an increased translucency. The gums, for example, only gradually return to their normal thickness and shape after dentures are removed. The inherent lack of restorative forces may also contribute to the ease with which bedsores develop. In addition, aging causes increased pigmentation of some light-protected parts of the body, such as the breast areola and the anogenital region, that is of negligible significance.

The epidermal atrophy noted earlier leads to the most important practical and clinically important consequence of aging: the relative inability of the skin to keep itself moist. Essentially all elderly people have asteatosis or dry skin. In northern climates during the months of January and February nearly one-fifth of a dermatologist's office visits may be for dry skin, and nearly all elderly patients will complain of it if asked.

---

2. J.P. Tindall, J.G. Smith. Skin lesions of the aged. *J.A.M.A.* 186:1039–1042, 1963.

Aging of the Cutaneous Appendages
Of the appendages, it is the hair that most noticeably shows its age. Graying of the hair is a normal process that is under genetic control. In the Caucasoid races it normally begins at age 34 ± 10 years; by age 50, 50 percent of the population have hair that is 50 percent gray. In the Negroid races the onset of graying is 44 ± 10 years. Japanese men start to gray between 30 and 34 years of age, with Japanese women beginning five years later.

The nails, particularly those of the toes, may become thicker and typically become dull and opaque with longitudinal ridging. Some believe that onychogryphosis, the very thick, curled nails commonly seen in the elderly, is due to age itself, but others claim that it is a result of previous injury. Although these nails can be surgically removed and the nail matrix destroyed in younger people, in the elderly treatment should be more palliative because of poor healing of wounds on the feet. The nail may be filed down, or it may be softened and removed with a paste of 40 percent urea applied under occlusion. The latter method allows the nontraumatic, although temporary, removal of a bulky nail that tears stockings and limits walking.

SUN-DAMAGED SKIN

Solar Elastosis
The name *solar elastosis* derives from the tinctorial qualities of the sun-damaged dermal collagen, which picks up the same basophilic dyes that elastic tissue does; unfortunately it does not also acquire its resilient properties. The most conspicuous changes in elderly skin are those induced by excessive and prolonged sun exposure. The skin of the face and neck, in particular, shows wrinkling from minor to major degrees; the wrinkling is particularly prominent on the back of the neck where deep furrows cut the diamond-shaped patterns of cutis rhomboidalis nuchae or "sailor's neck." The color of this skin ranges from an ivory white through a waxy yellow-brown. Until recently well-tanned skin was considered a mark of the peasantry; the refined lady or gentleman cultivated white skin. With the availablity of increased leisure time, tanned skin was recognized as a sign of a leisure class that had sufficient means to afford a sunny vacation, especially in the winter. In addition to the wrinkling and color changes, one of the most intriguing manifestations of solar elastosis is the development of numerous and prominent open comedones (blackheads) at the temples and below the eyes (Favre-Racouchot syn-

drome). Although the skin puckers into diamond shapes on the back of the neck, on the face and hands it may form nodules and plaques.

Although there is no medical treatment for solar elastosis, prophylactic use of sunscreens with high "skin protective factor" (SPF) of 8 to 15 will probably prevent much of the damage. Once it occurs, however, no quantity of moisturizers, astringents, masks, and vegetable or protein creams will improve it. Chemical face peels, potentially hazardous, or surgical facelifts become the only effective remedies.

Senile Lentigo

Senile lentigo is characterized by usually multiple, hyperpigmented, discrete brown macules scattered primarily over the backs of the hands, the extensor forearms, and the face. The popular name for them is "liver spots." When they appear on the face or neck it is important to differentiate them from lentigo maligna of Hutchinson, one of the in situ forms of malignant melanoma. In any location lentigines may be confused with fairly young, still flat, seborrheic keratoses, but here the difference is immaterial since both are benign. Prophylactic sunscreens will probably prevent them from appearing. The best treatment is only partially successful: twice-daily application of a hydroquinone cream or solution followed by an effective sunscreen. Concentrations of hydroquinone up to 2% are permitted without prescription, while 3% and 4% concentrations are available with it. In either event it must be applied faithfully for at least twelve weeks before the patient gives up; in my experience most do.

DRY, FRAGILE SKIN

Asteatosis

The single most common cutaneous problem that the elderly have is dry skin. Surveys have found that virtually all old people are afflicted with it during the winter, especially in the north. In its mild forms it is characterized by dryness and slight scaling, but as it progresses the surface cracks like a dried mud flat into a tessellated pattern. Once the protective barrier of the stratum corneum has been breached, inflammation with pruritus follows.

Treatment should be easy, but it often is not. Heating the air in one's home lowers its relative humidity, whereas bathing, cooking, and breathing increase it; opening a window lets moist air blow out, to be replaced by cold and eventually drier air. The first step in treatment, then, is to decrease the loss of moist air by closing windows and caulking cracks, as necessary. Plants, hanging laundry, or a humidifier will add water to the air. The patient next should try to prevent his skin from losing its own moisture by applying lotion or oil immediately after a shower or bath, while his skin is still damp. If substances like urea or lactic acid are added to these lotions (oil-in-water emulsions), they will bind more water to the stratum corneum. Although there are several over-the-counter preparations available, white petrolatum or baby oil will often suffice and is far less expensive. Bath oils should be applied directly to the skin and not put into the bath water, where they make the tub slippery and difficult to clean.

If the scaling and fissuring are severe or if they develop suddenly or at the wrong time of the year, they may represent an acquired ichthyosis, an entity that is frequently associated with an internal malignancy.

Senile Purpura

Because of decreased resilience of the skin, it is not surprising that the elderly bruise easily. Dermatologists are commonly asked to evaluate the purpura on the forearms or hands of elderly hospitalized patients caused by innocent and forgotten daily trauma, or the trauma of venous tourniquets and phlebotomy. Patients with no evidence for a bleeding diathesis other than senile purpura need not be further evaluated.

CUTANEOUS NEOPLASMS

The most common cutaneous complaints brought by elderly patients to dermatologists relate to neoplasms and benign tumors.

Benign Tumors

Probably the most common cutaneous tumor found in the elderly is the seborrheic keratosis. Susceptibility to it is under genetic control (the Negroid races seldom develop these tumors, for instance), although other factors may be involved. This tumor most commonly presents in the Caucasian as a gray-brown patch, often described as "smoky candlewax dripped onto the skin." In time the surface usually becomes harder, more pigmented, verrucous, and often crumbly. The hyperpigmentation is usually, but not always, even. When the pigmentation varies, it is imperative to rule out a malignant melanoma, the tumor most often confused with a seborrheic keratosis, as well as a pigmented basal cell carcinoma. Seborrheic keratoses are usually treated by superficial curettage and electrofulguration. The development of a malignancy in a seborrheic keratosis is a decidedly rare event.

"Senile" or "cherry" angiomas actually start in the third decade of life, and by age 50 half of Caucasians will have at least one. They start as a minute red spot which grows to a smooth, globose papule. They do not have prominent spiderlike vessels. Best left alone, they may be treated by electrodesiccation if necessary.

Senile sebaceous hyperplasia occurs on the central part of the face as a flat, waxy-yellow papule several millimeters in diameter. Because of its central depression it is easily confused with an early basal cell carcinoma, but unlike the basal cell, its raised border shows no telangiectasia. It may be curetted off.

Premalignant Neoplasms

Actinic keratoses are scaly patches and papules up to several millimeters in diameter on the exposed skin. The surface may be smooth, slightly atrophied, or raised in an impressive horn; they may be flesh-colored, red, or hyperpigmented. Up to 20 percent are said to become malignant, producing either a basal cell or a squamous cell carcinoma.

There are several effective treatments for actinic keratosis. Since a dermatologist usually has liquid nitrogen available, freezing by a cotton swab or by spray technique is the most common method of treatment. The skin is frozen until there is a halo, or rim of ice, completely surrounding the keratosis and then is kept frozen an additional 10 to 15 seconds. This may produce a hemorrhagic blister or just a crust, which will usually fall off in three weeks leaving little if any scar. If liquid nitrogen is not available the keratosis may also be curetted off, either before or after light electrodesiccation, but there may be more scarring than with freezing. Although a simple shave excision will scar, it is also satisfactory for removal and has the advantage that the tissue can be sent to the pathologist to confirm the diagnosis.

When there are multiple actinic keratoses it is often more efficient to use topical chemotherapy with 5-fluorouracil; this method has the decided advantage of seeking out and treating inapparent, incipient keratoses. It is applied in a 1–5% concentration as a cream or solution, the lower concentrations being used on the face and the highest concentration on the forearms and hands. It is applied with the fingertips twice daily until the keratoses become red, raw, and eroded, which usually takes about two weeks for the face and up to four weeks for the forearms. Once the treatment is stopped the surface reepithelializes in another two weeks, leaving skin that is usually much smoother. The obvious difficulty is the rather marked discomfort and unpleasant appearance during therapy, but patients are delighted with the baby-smooth skin that may result. The improvement may last for several years, particularly if the treatment times are extended, although 6 to 24 months would be more typical. The erythema and discomfort can be reduced by the concomitant use of the highest potency topical steroids.

MALIGNANT TUMORS

In Situ Carcinoma

Bowen's disease, or squamous cell carcinoma in situ, presents as an erythematous, scaly patch on sun-exposed skin. Topical steroids bring about only a slight improvement. Diagnosis is made by punch or shave biopsy. The treatment is essentially the same as for a basal cell carcinoma.

Paget's disease produces a similar erythematous, slightly scaly patch on the nipples that may or may not weep or crust. This probably reflects an underlying intraductal carcinoma. This same process may occur on the genitalia as extramammary Paget's disease. Biopsy is necessary, with either a 4-mm punch or an elliptïcal excision preferred, and if the diagnosis is confirmed the patient should be referred to a surgeon.

Basal Cell Carcinoma

The most common cutaneous malignancy is the basal cell carcinoma, thought to arise from an actinic keratosis. Over a period of months it slowly enlarges and develops its characteristic features: a rolled, pearly border with subtle telangiectasias, or a somewhat translucent, brown to black hue. With time the central, older portion of the tumor ulcerates. Several basal cell carcinomas may arise in the same area, producing a somewhat speckled patch 2 cm or more in diameter—the multicentric, superficial basal cell carcinoma.

There are four methods of treatment that produce essentially equal cure rates in experienced hands: electrodesiccation and curettage, excision, cryotherapy, and radiotherapy. Since radiotherapy often leads to radiation dermatitis in 15 to 20 years, it is usually reserved for patients over 65 years of age or the infirm.

The morphea or sclerosing type of basal cell carcinoma, however, is difficult to treat adequately by any of these methods because of its long, fingerlike projections that penetrate widely and deeply through a sclerotic dermis, making it difficult to determine the actual margins of the tumor. The form of treatment that has a high cure rate with a minimal loss of tissue is the microscopically controlled, histographic surgery developed by Dr. F. Mohs at the University of Wisconsin. This method of treatment should also be used for carcinomas that recur more than once, for recurrent carcinomas near important structures such as the eye, and for recurrences at any of the folds on the face such as the nasolabial crease or the attachment of the ear.

Basal cell carcinomas rarely metastasize to regional nodes or viscera, but they may continue to invade locally, penetrating and destroying underlying structures.

Squamous Cell Carcinoma
Squamous cell carcinomas of the skin occur in two varieties; both, however, appear in their early form as erythematous, scaly patches or plaques progressing to crusted, firm nodules that eventually may have a cauliflower-like surface. The first type, by far the most common, occurs on sun-exposed skin and does not commonly metastasize unless it is long neglected. Like the basal cell, it starts as an actinic keratosis; the methods of treatment discussed for the basal cell are equally appropriate, with the provision that one be especially careful that the margins are free of tumor after resection, since metastasis can occur.

The other type of squamous cell carcinoma is far more aggressive. It occurs on a mucous membrane such as the lip, or in a scar, but the etiology of the scar itself makes little difference: chronic draining sinus tracts from osteomyelitis or a suppurative lymphadenitis, burn or radiation scars, or scars from intrinsic cutaneous disease such as epidermolysis bullosa dystrophica. Thorough investigation for metastasis is in order for this type of squamous cell carcinoma. Whether or not prophylactic node dissection is indicated is controversial, but the carcinoma must be treated as seriously as any other internal carcinoma. Again, Mohs' histographic surgery may be useful in assuring that there is no residual local tumor.

Melanoma
The most malignant of the cutaneous neoplasms is the melanoma. There are several clinical types, but they have a common denomi-

nator: they must be found before they are 1.5 mm thick to ensure the reasonable chance of a cure.

The most common type of melanoma is the superficial spreading melanoma. It has a prolonged, radial growth phase, lasting months to years, in which it spreads along the epidermal basement membrane before it begins its vertical growth phase. It is recognized as a hyperpigmented macule with uneven color, with areas where pigment seems to be diffusing into the surrounding skin; other portions of the border may have lost their pigment, producing a "notch" of decreased pigmentation; there are often red, gray, or black components. When the melanoma begins to invade vertically, a papule or nodule results.

Similar to the superficial spreading melanoma, if not identical with it, is the lentigo maligna. This is a hyperpigmented macule that most commonly occurs on the head or neck of elderly people, often reaching several centimeters in diameter. Like the superficial spreading melanoma, it has a long radial growth phase with a varied color margin. Once the vertical phase begins and the basement membrane is breached, the term *lentigo maligna melanoma* is customarily used.

The second major type of melanoma is the nodular melanoma, a tumor that seems to have vertical growth from the onset. It usually presents as a hyperpigmented papule or nodule, often with a blue or black hue. Amelanotic melanomas are not uncommon and may be flesh-colored or red. It is decidedly uncommon for the patient to present with a nodular melanoma that is less than 1.5 mm deep, and hence the cure rates for this melanoma are disappointing.

Melanomas are more common on the sun-exposed parts of the body. Since in the last few decades children have exposed nearly all of their skin to the sun, melanomas are now being seen with increasing frequency on all parts of the body. Their incidence is also inversely related to the geographic distance from the equator.

The cure rate for melanomas is inversely and dramatically related to their depth of invasion. Melanomas less than 0.75 mm have cure rates with simple excision that exceed 95 percent. There is a gray zone between that size and 1.5 mm. when the success rates fall precipitously. Improvements in melanoma survival rates will occur when physicians and the general public know how to recognize the early, superficial melanomas.

So far all the cutaneous malignancies I have discussed, with the exception of Paget's disease and extramammary Paget's disease, are rarely seen on heavily pigmented individuals. Carcinomas arising in scars or in the depigmented lesions of discoid lupus erythematosus can strike anyone. Occasionally, basal cell carcinomas arise on the genitalia or around the anus.

OTHER SKIN DISORDERS

Dermatophytoses

Ranking just behind skin tumors in incidence are several chronic superficial fungal infections: tinea pedis, tinea cruris, tinea corporis, and tinea manuum. As in all age groups, the hallmark is scaling; in the elderly there may be little or no pruritus and few if any vesicles. The high incidence and lack of symptoms undoubtedly are due to the lowered immunologic resistance of the elderly; eradication and cure are nearly impossible for the same reason. If symptomatic or of concern, tinea pedis should be treated with long-term, daily application of a modern antifungal agent such as clotrimazole or miconazole topical preparations. The solutions spread the farthest and are therefore the most economical, but in unsteady hands they may drip through the fingers and lubricate the floor. In this situation the creams are preferred.

Seborrheic Dermatitis

Especially common in the elderly with neurologic disease, particularly Parkinson's disease, is seborrheic dermatitis. In fact, after tumors and dermatophytosis, it is the third most common cutaneous disease of the elderly. It is recognized in its florid state as the accumulation of greasy (hence its name), pruritic yellow scales on a macular, erythematous background which the patient considers "dry skin." It is located on the scalp, at the eyebrows, temples, and paranasal area, and also on the sternal area of the chest, the center of the back, and the sacral and genital areas. Although seborrheic dermatitis is usually only a localized and annoying problem, it can evolve into a total body exfoliative dermatitis. The simplest form of therapy is 1% hydrocortisone cream. Occasionally this does not suffice, and 3% iodochlorhydroxyquin, 1–3% tar, or 1–3% salicylic acid must be compounded into it. The use of fluorinated corticosteroid preparations should be reserved only for severe flares.

Bullous Pemphigoid

Bullous pemphigoid is an intriguing autoimmune blistering disease seldom seen except in the aged. It usually starts in one or more intertriginous areas as a pruritic, erythematous plaque, and a few days later the bullae begin, perhaps spreading to cover much of the body. Bullous pemphigoid must be distinguished from the less common diseases pemphigus and dermatitis herpetiformis, as well as from erythema multiforme, which is most unusual in the elderly.

The sequelae are those of a second-degree burn of the same extent: if the condition is not treated, fluid and electrolyte abnormalities and sepsis result. Fortunately this disease responds well to high-dose systemic coricosteroids. When the number of new bullae is markedly diminished the steroids can be reduced, often to an alternate-day regimen, over a period of months.

Stasis Dermatitis

One of the most common dermatoses, stasis dermatitis, occurs in the setting of incompetent, varicose veins or chronic edema of the lower extremities. Initially the skin is erythematous and, if the condition is severe, weeping. Eventually the characteristic brown hyperpigmentation of stasis dermatitis results, mainly on the anterior lower leg; it seldom involves the foot. With prolonged involvement, particularly if there is vascular compromise, diabetes, or trauma, an ulcer may develop.

Treatment of stasis dermatitis should first be directed at the etiology. Peripheral edema should be minimized. Well-fitting elastic stockings are essential for those with varicose veins. The acute dermatitis responds well to topical corticosteroids. Initially fluorinated steroids may be necessary, but often hydrocortisone will suffice. When there are vesicles or weeping, compresses should be followed with a cream vehicle. Once the surface is dry and scaly an ointment base may be more effective, but because the petrolatum will quickly degrade the rubber in an elastic stocking, an approach similar to that discussed for asteatosis should be tried.

The treatment of stasis ulcers is often frustrating. I have had most success with the continued application of an Unna paste boot. It seems to be important that the ulcer be thoroughly soaked and debrided at once to twice weekly intervals depending on the amount of drainage. Secondary infection with gram-positive pyogens (e.g., *Staphylococcus aureus*) should probably be treated, but the gram-negative organisms (e.g., *Escherichia coli*) that inhabit the ulcer are inevitable and not eradicable. If granulation tissue does not appear after several weeks, the application of 10% benzoyl peroxide *lotion* compresses, without the Unna-type boot, may hasten its development.

SUGGESTED READING

1. Domonkos, A.N., Arnold, H.L., Odom, R.B. *Andrews' Disease of the Skin,* 7th ed. Philadelphia: W.B. Saunders, 1981.
2. Johnson, M.-L.T., Roberts, J. Skin conditions and related need for medical care among persons 1–74 years. Bethesda: Public Health Service, U.S. Department of Health, Education and Welfare, 1978.
3. Kligman, A.M. Perspectives and problems in cutaneous gerontology. *J. Invest. Dermatol.* 73:39–46, 1979.
4. Korting, G.W. *Geriatric Dermatology.* Philadelphia: W.B. Saunders, 1980.
5. Montagna, W., Kligman, A.M., Wuepper, K.D., Bentley, J.P. (Eds.) Special issue on aging. Proceedings of the 28th Symposium on the Biology of Skin (vol. 20, Advances in biology of skin). *J. Invest. Dermatol.* 73(1):1–134, 1979.
6. Rook. A., Wilkinson, D.S., Ebling, F.J.B. (Eds.) *Textbook of Dermatology,* 3rd ed., vols. 1 and 2. Oxford: Blackwell Scientific Publications. 1979.

The Treatment of Chronic Venous Disorders

C. STEWART ROGERS, M.D.

Editor's note: Chronic venous diseases of the legs are common sources of discomfort, yet they have been largely ignored in the education of primary care practitioners. The two recognized syndromes, varicose veins and chronic venous insufficiency, share the same functional pathology and therefore overlap clinically. Both are more common with aging.

The physiologic anatomy is central to understanding the chronic venous disorders. Leg veins divide into deep and superficial systems connected by venous perforators, all of which are valved to direct cutaneous drainage into the deep system and thence cephalad. There is little axial flow in the saphenous veins (trunk lines of the superficial system); rather, these veins are local collecting channels for the skin.

The deep veins must have a system to overcome gravity; this antigravity system is the calf muscle pump or "peripheral venous heart." Its functional units consist of segments of calf muscle in which contraction expresses blood from venous sinusoids into a deep vein between two valves; it also compresses the deep vein, forcing the blood upward through the valves. Relaxation of the calf muscle creates a vacuum, draining in blood from the foot or through valved perforators from the superficial veins. The system is able to handle a pressure that reaches 120 cm H_2O in the upright adult, and to reduce that pressure dramatically with normal ambulation.

The pathophysiology of both varicose veins (VV) and chronic venous insufficiency (CVI) involves failure of this system, resulting in sustained venous hypertension. Ultimately, both syndromes result from valve failure, but the causes are different. Varicosities are dilated and tortuous superficial veins, usually caused by incompetence

86

of the proximal pelvic and thigh valves, which allows gravitational pressure into the thin-walled, unsupported saphenous veins.

Chronic venous insufficiency, on the other hand, usually begins with an often unrecognized episode of deep venous thrombophlebitis (DVT) that heals with recanalization of the lumen, causing permanent loss of the proximal valves. Again the weight of blood in the vein, unsupported and uninterrupted by normal valves, raises venous pressure. Perhaps more destructive, however, are the pulsatile forces of misdirected muscle pump action; these pressures further damage the remaining deep valves and divert venous flow through incompetent perforators into the superficial veins and the cutaneous capillary beds. This pressure produces secondary varicose veins, chronic edema, dermatitis, and ulceration—the presenting features of CVI.

CLINICAL MANAGEMENT OF VARICOSE VEINS

By convention, the syndrome of VV refers to primary superficial valve failure with a basically normal deep system. This is an important point, because the only purpose of evaluation is to prove that this situation truly obtains in a patient so that treatment aimed at the superficial veins will arrest the problem. Such evaluation is usually quick and noninvasive.

If there is no history of DVT, trauma, or casted fractures, if the patient is under 50 years of age, and if the degree of superficial varicosity greatly exceeds the degree of chronic edema and skin disease, it can be reasonably assumed that the VV are primary. If confirmation is needed, noninvasive studies using Doppler or plethysmographic techniques will clarify the patency of the deep system and its valvular competence. (Further details of these techniques are beyond the scope of a geriatrics book but may be obtained from the Suggested Reading list at the end of the chapter.) One important responsibility of the primary care physician is to be sure that VV surgery is not performed in patients with signs of deep venous insufficiency.

Varicose veins can be treated by surgery or by injection of sclerosing solutions. The latter approach, often favored in Europe, is not even available in many American surgical communities. Most studies show equal short-term results (one year) with both options, while surgical results are better at three years. The advantages of sclerotherapy are that it is much less expensive, it can be repeated *ad libitum*, and the saphenous veins are not lost as potential bypass grafts for future coronary surgery.

CLINICAL MANAGEMENT OF CHRONIC VENOUS INSUFFICIENCY

Chronic venous insufficiency is basically a skin disease of the lower calf and ankle caused by venous hypertension and mediated by edema. Edema interferes with normal delivery of nutrients and removal of metabolic products, producing a tissue that is easily damaged and heals poorly.

The most common complaint is stasis pain, a "bursting" sensation, aggravated by prolonged standing and relieved by elevation or compression. This is an exaggeration of a common complaint in healthy people, and its management simply requires an exaggeration of the common solution of elevation of feet or support hose. Other common and easily managed problems are hemosiderosis, chronic low-grade eczema, and secondary varicosities (which are usually not pronounced).

Treatment of the complaints of CVI requires a permanent regimen of frequent and prolonged elevation or the use of medical-strength support stockings, or both. The elevation must be above chest level and should be used sufficiently to relieve pain and minimize edema. It seems reasonable to avoid constricting garments that might impede venous return, and to correct constipation to avoid venous engorgement from straining (Valsalva's maneuver). Diuretics are probably of little help unless there is a systemic cause for edema.

Support hose must provide 30 to 50 mm Hg of pressure to the ankle and calf. Department store brands do not come close to this; most patients must buy products from a surgical supply house. They have some obvious disadvantages: they are expensive, ugly, hot, and hard to put on. Even though the deep venous pathology may extend to the thigh and pelvis, the purpose of stockings is to reduce edema in the affected skin, so knee length is usually adequate. Special fitting is usually not required, although a tourniquet effect at the knee should be avoided. There is only one medical caveat about the use of compression hose, but it can be a major consideration in older patients. In the presence of severe arterial insufficiency the added pressure of these stockings can lead to ischemia in the feet; in such cases venous edema is best treated with elevation alone.

The typical lesion of CVI is the venous ulcer, usually located 5 to 15 cm above the ankle over the region of the lowermost perforators. Most ulcers are above the medial malleolus, but lateral and circumferential ulcers are found. About 90 percent of lower leg ulcers are caused by venous hypertension, the balance being ischemic or due to a long list of rare conditions. Arterial ulcers are found in a setting of ischemic tissues and are usually painful, especially with elevation. Venous ulcers are usually painless; if there is pain, it is relieved with elevation.

If the patient is bedridden for other reasons, prolonged elevation may heal the ulcer. In other cases ambulation can be preserved with the use of an Unna boot—a light cast, applied like an Ace wrap from toes to knee, to a leg that has been partly drained by overnight elevation. Topical ointments are not needed, and the boot is applied directly onto the ulcer. The boot is changed weekly as long as healing is observed. Large ulcers (more than 4 cm) may require skin grafting, and refractory cases may necessitate ligation of venous perforators, although direct surgical approaches to CVI are not usually employed. Definite infection with suppuration and cellulitis that requires systemic antibiotics is uncommon. After healing of an ulcer, the permanent antiedema measures described earlier are reinstituted and intensified.

A common problem is the exclusion of a superimposed acute DVT when the edema and pain worsen. Chronic venous insufficiency may be asymmetric, and it probably predisposes to DVT because of stasis. Venography is difficult to interpret because of chronic changes from old, healed DVT, but it is often performed anyway, with some risk of overdiagnosis. I^{131} fibrinogen scanning can identify active thrombosis and is more specific for acute DVT, but it is less widely available and is less sensitive for disease confined to the calf. Some authors advise using both venography and fibrinogen scanning for high-risk situations.

SUGGESTED READING

1. Harris, W.H., Waltman, A.C., Athanasoulis, C., et al. The accuracy of the in vivo diagnosis of deep vein thrombosis in patients with prior venous thromboembolic disease or severe varicose veins. *Thrombosis Research* 21:137–145, 1981.
2. Hobbs, J.T. *The Treatment of Venous Disorders.* Philadelphia: J.B. Lippincott, 1977.
3. Hobbs, J.T. The management of varicose veins. *Surg. Ann.* 12:169–186, 1980.
4. Nabatoff, R.A. Ambulatory management of lower extremity venous disease in the aged. *Mount Sinai J. Med* 47:218–223, 1980.

Urinary Incontinence Due to Bladder Instability

SIGMUND I. TANNENBAUM, M.D., and
DANIEL T. VETROSKY, P.A.-C.

Editor's note: Incontinence, due to a variety of potentially treatable etiologies, may cause patients otherwise capable of independent living to be institutionalized. Strokes, prostatic enlargement, and female pelvic relaxation are common in the elderly, for example, and may result in hazardous and embarrassing incontinence. Evaluation of urodynamics and precise diagnosis may make specific pharmacologic and surgical treatment possible.

MALE URINARY INCONTINENCE

Of the causes of urinary incontinence outlined in Table 1, neurogenic disease is the best known, but other conditions may be responsible for the same clinical presentation. Pelvic crush injury from industrial, farm, or automobile accidents frequently tears the most fixed portion of the lower urinary tract, the membranous urethra, or may disrupt the entire bladder neck. Urinary fistulas may result from a diverticular or appendiceal abscess that causes an enterovesical or enterourethral fistula, or from gunshot wounds or infected sutures; the associated inflammation interrupts normal continence. Radical cancer surgery of the lower urinary tract, primarily radical prostatectomy, may necessitate restructuring of the bladder neck and may cause injury to the internal urethral sphincter mechanism; urinary incontinence can be avoided by careful anatomic dissection and postoperative perineal exercises.

THE CONCEPT OF BLADDER INSTABILITY

The urinary bladder (detrusor) and vesical neck musculature are controlled by both the autonomic and the voluntary nervous system. The primary neural control is a simple reflex originating in the spinal

90

cord (autonomic), while secondary control comes from higher mid-brain and cortical centers (voluntary). The bladder functions as both a storage and a voiding organ. During filling, the bladder should remain acontractile until a voluntary voiding contraction is initiated; the smooth muscle sphincter of the bladder neck should open only during a voluntary voiding contraction. Bladder stability is present only if this ideal detrusor–bladder neck synergism is maintained.

Bladder instability results in inappropriate and uncoordinated detrusor contractions and bladder neck opening; continence can then be maintained only by the distal skeletal sphincter mechanism. If this muscle is poorly developed it cannot maintain enough urethral tone to effect continence.

Symptoms Detrusor instability usually causes the nonspecific urinary complaints of frequency, nocturia, enuresis, urgency, and urge incontinence. It is possible that bladder instability can remain asymptomatic or coexist with other anatomic causes of incontinence. In general, patients with stress incontinence who do not complain of frequency, nocturia, or urgency may be assumed to have a stable bladder. When frequency and nocturia accompany stress leakage, however, 50 percent of patients will have an unstable bladder.

Common Causes Neurologic disease and bladder outlet obstruction are two of the major causes of bladder instability (see Table 2). Neurologic diseases cause bladder instability by destroying peripheral nerves (e.g., diabetes), interrupting pathways (e.g., trauma), and by blocking both voluntary and autonomic control (e.g., stroke). Obstructive instability is almost exclusively a problem of males; the instability is responsible for the symptoms of bladder irritation that occur early in outlet obstruction (e.g., dysuria, frequency).

Idiopathic instability occurs in at least 10 percent of the general population, presumably from the inability to achieve voluntary neurologic detrusor control. Enuresis, diurnal continence problems, recurrent urinary tract infections, and reflux are problems that have been associated with this type of dysfunction.

Sequelae Recurrent urinary tract infection is probably the most common complication of bladder instability. Faulty detrusor-sphincter function increases urinary residual and allows contamination by organisms from the perineal or vaginal introitus to cause infection. Patients with neurogenic bladder instability are also subject to the risks of vesicoureteral reflux, recurrent pyelonephritis, and sepsis.

Diagnosis A thorough history and physical examination are required to establish the causes of bladder instability. Peripheral neuropathies, diminished rectal tone, motor weakness, and an absent bulbocavernous reflex are important physical findings. Diabetes, Parkinson's disease, stroke, spinal trauma, transient ischemic attacks, and birth defects are problems that may lead to bladder instability. Many drugs can affect detrusor function, for example propranolol (Inderal) and psychotropics.

Urodynamic evaluation is the most reliable tool in establishing the diagnosis of bladder instability and may direct intervention with specific pharmacotherapy. Provocative cystometry, urethral pressure profilometry, and video urodynamic studies are the most sensitive components of this evaluation. Upper tract evaluation, in the absence of clues from the history or physical examination that suggest disease, is rarely needed.

Treatment About one-third of cases of recent-onset incontinence resolve spontaneously within a few weeks. Seventy percent of men with benign prostatic hypertrophy and bladder instability regain normal detrusor function after prostatectomy. Poorly controlled diabetics are likely to develop instability and ultimately detrusor neuropathy; diabetics who are discovered and treated early with tight control have an impressively decreased incidence of instability. Urinary tract infections must first be treated, of course, before any form of diagnostic or therapeutic plan is instituted.

Pharmacotherapy with alpha-adrenergic and cholinergic stimulators and with anticholinergics is the mainstay in treating neurogenic causes of incontinence (Table 1). Anticholinergic agents block acetylcholine neurotransmitter release and convert an unstable detrusor to predominantly a storage organ. An intermittent self-catheterization program in conjunction with such therapy may be needed.

Flavoxate hydrochloride (Urispas) is beneficial in patients with hypersensitive bladders by urodynamic criteria, and anticholinergics such as oxybutynin chloride (Ditropan), propantheline bromide (Pro-Banthine), and methantheline bromide (Banthine) are of benefit in cases of neurogenic bladder instability.

Biofeedback, psychotherapy, and surgical denervation procedures have all had limited success in the treatment of bladder instability, and their role in patient management is under continued investigation. Other agents are under study and are reputed to benefit some patients.[1]

---

1. M.E. Williams, F.C. Pannill. Urinary incontinence in the elderly. *Ann. Intern. Med.* 97:895–907, 1982.

TABLE 1
Drug Treatment of Incontinence

Specific Condition	Drug Category	Commonly Used Drugs and Dosages
Sphincter weakness	Anticholinergics	Imipramine,[a] 25–75 mg at bedtime
	Alpha-adrenergic stimulators	Phenylpropanolamine, 25 mg twice daily
		Ephedrine, 10 mg twice daily
Bladder instability	Anticholinergics	Imipramine,[a] 25–75 mg at bedtime
		Propantheline, 7.5 mg three times daily
		Flavoxate, 100 mg three times daily
		Oxybutynin, 5 mg three times daily
Overflow incontinence	Cholinergic stimulators	Bethanechol, 10 mg three times a day
		Phenoxybenzamine, 10 mg daily
	Somatic blockers	Dantrolene[b]
		Baclofen[b]

[a]Also improves sphincter tone as an alpha-adrenergic stimulator.
[b]Dosage must be individually titrated. See *Physicians' Desk Reference* for specific recommendations.

Urinary continence in the adult male requires the anatomic integrity and physiologic coordination of the bladder neck, internal urethral sphincter, and voluntary external sphincter. The bladder neck, an involuntary smooth muscle, is the primary source of urinary continence; it is innervated primarily by adrenergic nerves, responsive to the neurotransmitter acetylcholine. Experience with transurethral prostatectomy, however, has shown that the patient can remain dry even in the absence of a competent bladder neck. The second level of urinary continence, the internal urethral sphincter, is also composed of involuntary smooth muscle. Surgical resection of both the bladder neck and internal urethral sphincter will render the patient incontinent of urine. The third level of urinary continence in males, the external urethral sphincter, is made up of voluntary striated musculature. Although it can cause temporary total urinary retention, the muscle lacks the ability to sustain contraction and tires easily. Thus, under the circumstances of normal filling and low pressure in the bladder, continence results from bladder neck elevation in coordination with internal sphincter contraction.

Bladder outlet obstruction in the adult male is a common cause of overflow or paradoxic incontinence; the causes of bladder, bladder neck, prostatic, or urethral obstructions are outlined in Table 2. As the bladder becomes distended, pressure increases enough to overcome the resistance of the partial obstruction and the urinary sphincters, resulting in overflow "dribbling" incontinence.

FEMALE URINARY INCONTINENCE

The urinary bladder in the adult female has mechanisms of continence different from those of the male, being dependent on the interaction of four urethral factors: (1) urethral closing pressure, (2) urethral length, (3) urethrotrigonal anatomy, and (4) influence of intraabdominal pressure on the urethra. The urethral closing pressure is a function of coordinated smooth and striated muscle activity, although little is known of the exact anatomic nature of the sphincter or its innervation. While it was long maintained that urethral length is paramount to female continence, it has been shown that a shortened urethra does not necessarily produce incontinence, and that some women with proven stress incontinence do not have urethral shortening. A normal urethrotrigonal anatomy with a proper relationship between the bladder base descent and the urethral axis is necessary. The major continence mechanism in the female, however, is a passive phenomonon, the transmission of intraabdominal pressure to the urethra. Additionallly, as in the male, proper detrusor function is required.

TABLE 2
Causes of Bladder Instability

I. Neurologic disorders	5. Blood clots
A. Stroke/spinal cord trauma	6. Ureterocele/diverticulum
B. Diabetic neuropathy	B. Bladder neck obstruction
C. Multiple sclerosis	1. Contracture
D. Parkinson's disease	2. Dyssynergy
E. Myelomeningocele/spina bifida	C. Prostatic enlargement
II. Idiopathic/psychogenic instability	1. Benign prostatic hyperplasia
III. Outlet obstruction	2. Carcinoma
A. Bladder obstruction	3. Prostatitis
1. Calculi/foreign body	D. Urethral stricture
2. Tumor	1. Postgonococcal
3. Neurogenic	2. Chronic catheterization
4. Postoperative fibrosis	

Evaluation

Involuntary loss of urine may be classified as stress or urge incontinence, but often combined or mixed types are found. Careful historical documentation of the patient's urinary incontinence may yield significant diagnostic information. Isolated urinary incontinence following a cough, laugh, or sneeze is primarily of the stress type of incontinence. If symptoms of frequency and nocturia are present, there is about a 45 percent incidence of bladder instability; adding the symptoms of urgency and urge incontinence raises the instability rate to 80 percent. In patients with urgency and urge incontinence alone, without stress incontinence symptoms, more than 95 percent are found to have unstable bladders.

Physical examination includes both neurologic and gynecologic evaluation, as well as urinalysis. The finding of significant uterine descent may justify simultaneous hysterectomy. The Marshall test[2] helps confirm the presence of stress incontinence and is an indication of the potential success of an antiincontinence procedure. Cystography and endoscopy give information concerning the posterior vesicourethral angle, bladder neck competence, the urethral axis, bladder mucosa, presence of diverticuli, and urethral abnormalities. More than 75 percent of women who fail to achieve symptomatic relief from surgical correction of incontinence have unstable bladders. Urodynamic evaluation, therefore, is indicated in all these patients as well as patients with urgency or urge incontinence.

Treatment

Urinary incontinence in the female, regardless of type, may be influenced by pharmacotherapy (see Table 1). Because periurethral musculature is innervated by alpha-adrenergic nerves, low-grade stress incontinence may be controlled with ephedrine or phenylpropanolamine. Side effects or patient compliance may limit the long-term use of these drugs, but therapeutic responsiveness seems to predict a good response to surgery.

STROKE AND SPINAL CORD INJURY

Neurologic diseases cause bladder instability by destroying peripheral nerves (diabetes, multiple sclerosis), interrupting nerve pathways (spinal cord trauma, spinal cord anomalies), and blocking both vol-

---

2. Described in Williams and Pannill, p. 900.

untary and autonomic control (stroke). Following the acute interruption of the spinal pathway, bladder instability is immediately evident. The patient may be best treated during this unstable period by intermittent catheterization and prophylactic antibiotics. A baseline urodynamic evaluation and intravenous pyelography, repeated at 6 to 12 months, help determine the need for or allow the discontinuation of pharmacotherapy and intermittent catheterization programs.

It is essential that patients with neurogenic events be evaluated for detrusor stability early in their clinical course and urinary tract infections avoided. During the rehabilitation phase, dryness becomes an important facilitator of neurologic recovery.

CONCLUSION

Adult urinary incontinence, whether caused by obstruction, anatomic variability, or neurologic dysfunction, is treatable. By utilizing basic history and physical examination techniques, the primary care practitioner can have a significant impact on the clinical aspects of incontinence and can also prevent considerable deterioration of upper urinary tracts.

SUGGESTED READING

1. Raz, S., Maggio, A.J., Kaufman, J.J. Why the Marshall-Marchetti operation works or does not. *Urology* 14:154, 1979.
2. Stamey, T.A. Urinary incontinence in the female. In Harrison, J.H., Gittes, R.F., Perlmutter, A.D., et al. (Eds.), *Campbell's Urology*, 4th ed. Philadelphia: W.B. Saunders, 1979.
3. Webster, G.D. Urodynamic studies. In Resnick, M.I., Older, R.A. (Eds.), *Diagnosis of Diseases of the Genitourinary System*. New York: Thieme-Stratton, 1982, pp. 173–204.
4. Webster, G.D. Neurogenic bladder disease. In Resnick, M.I., Older, R.A. (Eds.), *Diagnosis of Diseases of the Genitourinary System*. New York: Thieme-Stratton, 1982, pp. 487–515.
5. Webster, G.D. Female urinary incontinence. In Glenn, J.F. (Ed.), *Urologic Surgery*, 3rd ed. Philadelphia: J.B. Lippincott, 1983, p. 665.
6. Williams, M.E., Pannill, F.C. Urinary incontinence in the elderly. *Ann. Intern. Med.* 97:895–907, 1982.

Sleep Disorders in the Elderly

DAN BLAZER, M.D., PH.D.

Editor's note: Patterns, timing, duration, and quality of sleep change with aging. Most sleep disorders can be diagnosed with a thorough knowledge of a patient's sleeping habits, health, and general circumstances. Treatment varies from commonsense advice to sophisticated manipulation of psychotropic and hypnotic drugs.

A common complaint to the clinician by older people is "How can I get more sleep?" The frequency of this complaint has desensitized clinicians, causing them to attend less to the symptoms of sleep disorder than to other symptoms such as chest pains or hallucinations. Older people are generally dissatisfied with their sleep. Difficulty in sleeping, frequent awakenings during the night, and the use of sedative hypnotic medications increase with advancing years. For example, 15 percent of older people report that they sleep less than 5 hours per night, and 25 to 30 percent report frequent night awakening. In one community survey, close to 50 percent of the elderly reported trouble in getting to sleep or staying asleep during the night.[1]

Sleep problems in late life may not be benign, as demonstrated by recent studies of the association of sleep time and mortality. Even among men and women with no history of heart disease, hypertension, diabetes mellitus, or stroke, there was an increased risk of mortality among those who slept more than or less than 7 to 8 hours per night. Men and women who "often" took sleeping pills died 1.5 times as frequently as did matched subjects who never used sleeping pills.[2]

---

1. A. McGhie, S. Russel. The subjective assessment of normal sleep patterns. *J. Ment. Sci.* 108:642, 1962.
2. I. Karacan, J. Thornby, M. Arch, et al. Prevalence of sleep disturbance in a primary Florida community. *Soc. Sci. Med.* 10:239, 1976.

During the last 25 years there has been a proliferation of research concerning the various processes related to sleep, with more recent studies concentrating on the sleep of the elderly. These investigations are proving to have direct clinical relevance to practicing physicians. The foundation of the diagnosis and management of late-life sleep disorders rests on a thorough understanding of the changing psychobiology of sleep with aging. In this chapter, a description of normal sleep in the elderly will be followed by an outline of an appropriate diagnostic workup. Finally, the treatment of late-life sleep disorders will be reviewed, with special attention directed toward the use of sedative hypnotic agents in the elderly.

NORMAL SLEEP IN THE ELDERLY

The typical night of sleep in late life begins with stage I sleep and is followed successively by stages II, III, and IV. This initial sleep stage cycle is similar throughout life. Following the first episode of stage IV sleep, the older adult gradually ascends through stage III and stage II and then will typically enter the first episode of rapid eye movement (REM) sleep for the night. This episode usually first occurs about an hour and a half following sleep onset and typically lasts 5 minutes.

The second sleep cycle begins with the initiation of stage II sleep, and the pattern is repeated throughout the night. As the night progresses, there is less propensity to enter stages III and IV sleep and a greater likelihood of intense and slightly prolonged REM sleep. In adults over the age of 40, REM sleep constitutes about 20 percent of the total sleep time.

Most studies have found total sleep time to either decrease or remain unchanged in late life, as compared with younger age groups, and to average between 6.5 and 7 hours per night. There is, however, considerable variation around the mean total sleep time. Time in bed must not be confused with total sleep time. Time spent in bed generally increases with age, since older persons may go to bed early at night, lie in bed unsuccessfully trying to sleep, and remain in bed in the morning without attempting to sleep. Resting or napping in bed may occur during the day. Therefore, sleep efficiency (the ratio of total sleep time to time in bed) is reduced in the elderly.

Most sleep researchers have found sleep latency—that is, the time from "lights-out" (the decision to sleep) to sleep onset, to increase in late life from an average of 3 to 5 minutes for 25-year-olds to 10 minutes at the age of 65. Both the young and the old awaken during the night, usually on more than one occasion. Younger adults tend to fall back into sleep very quickly after awakening and do not remember these awakenings the next morning. The elderly are more prone to awakenings, often three to four times a night, and have a greater recall of these awakenings. One factor contributing to greater recall is nocturia, for the older person wakes up and becomes aware of the need to urinate. Once he or she has left the bed and then returns, this awakening is remembered.

The portion of time spent in the different stages of sleep also changes throughout the life cycle. There is an absolute and relative decrease in stage IV, or delta, sleep and an increase in the number of shifts into stage I sleep with increasing age. The reduction in slow-wave sleep is thought to be an indication of increased sleep disturbances with the aging process. Rapid eye movement sleep decreases dramatically during childhood but then remains relatively constant through the adult life cycle. A reduction in REM sleep in older people is usually associated with reduced intellectual functioning, as in the presence of an organic mental disorder or changes in cerebral blood flow. Rapid eye movement sleep has been related to dreaming, and some have noted that the dreams of older people are qualitatively different from those at earlier stages of development. These changes, however, should be expected. As individuals traverse the life cycle, certain biologic drives decrease in intensity, such as the sexual drive, and other concerns are heightened, such as concern about death. The changes in dream content through the life cycle may well reflect the age-related conflicts of the older adult.

In general, elderly men appear to have more "disturbance" in the objective measures of sleep described earlier than do women. One example of an age-related disturbance more common in men is the increased prevalence of snoring. Snoring usually indicates some impairment, often serious, of upper airway functioning. Hemodynamic abnormalities occur in all individuals demonstrating snoring, and snoring almost always precedes development of an upper airway sleep apnea syndrome (and is the most important symptom of the illness). Almost 60 percent of men and 45 percent of women in their sixties are habitual snorers.

Sleep distribution also changes throughout the life cycle. Men tend to increase the number of daytime naps with age, irrespective of employment status, though the tendency to nap among women is confined to those who are not fully employed. Clinicians must consider the propensity to napping when making an assessment of total sleep time in older people. Napping is more common in elderly persons who are suffering from chronic physical illnesses that disrupt normal nighttime sleep.

DIAGNOSTIC WORKUP OF SLEEP DISORDERS

The first step in managing sleep problems in late life is an effective evaluation of the sleep disorder. An outline of a routine evaluation is presented in Table 1. The diagnostic workup will vary with the nature of the sleep problem, but a thorough history is essential.

Many sleep disorders are a result of medical and psychiatric illness, so the clinician should take a general history of medical and psychiatric problems. The medical contribution to a sleep problem is often obvious, such as the interrupted sleep patterns resulting from the severe pain of a carcinoma. In some cases, however, sleep difficulties may be the first evidence of an underlying medical illness, for example, hypothyroidism. Some psychiatric illnesses present initially with sleep disturbances, for example, early morning awakening in the patient suffering from a recurrent unipolar depressive disorder. Disruption of normal sleep patterns can be seen in many neurologic conditions, ranging from brain tumors to carbon monoxide or lead

TABLE 1
Diagnostic Evaluation of Sleep Disorders

General medical and psychiatric history
History from the patient
  Onset and development of the sleep problem
  Sleep latency
  Total sleep time
  Total time in bed
  Sleep pattern (wake time after sleep onset)
  Sleep benefit
  Special problems
History from a family member
Medication history
Physical examination
Laboratory tests
  Polysomnograph (if available)
  Electroencephalogram
  Electrocardiogram
  Thyroxine (T_4)
  Pulmonary function studies

poisoning. Occasionally sleep problems precipitate the recurrence of a medical illness; sleep deprivation can induce a seizure in epileptic patients who were previously well controlled by medications.

Following the general medical and psychiatric history, the clinician should inquire into the specific nature of the complaint. Gathering a detailed sleep history is especially important in the identification of sleep pathology. Questions to be asked include the following: When do you usually turn the lights out and try to go to sleep? When do you get up in the morning? Do you read or listen to the radio in bed? How long does it take you to fall asleep? Do you awaken frequently during the night? Do you nap during the day? Do you dream or have nightmares? What do you do before you go to bed? Is the room warm or cold? What do you do if you cannot go to sleep? Do you feel rested in the morning after a night's sleep? Do you have difficulty staying awake during the day? How much does the sleep problem bother you? Does your sleep pattern vary on weekends or on trips away from home? What helps you to reduce the insomnia? What medications have disturbed your sleeping? Do you have muscle twitching or jerks?

A description of sleep from a family member or "bed partner" is most helpful. Specifically, this person should be asked if the patient snores, has respiratory or gagging problems during the night, experiences leg twitching in sleep, or has noticeable periods of irregular breathing.

Because older patients are often incapable of relating an accurate history of their drug intake, a number of procedures may be of benefit in determining what medications the patient is taking or has taken in the past. First, the patient should bring all medications to the clinician's office. For each medication, the physician should determine when it was prescribed, how often the patient takes it (i.e., whether it is taken continuously, intermittently, or irregularly), and what effects the patient experiences from the use of each drug. Second, a color chart, available in the *Physicians' Desk Reference,* can assist patients in identifying medications not brought to the office. Third, and possibly most valuable in obtaining an accurate drug history, the clinician should question a close family member to determine how well the patient's and family's perceptions of drug intake correspond. Although obtaining a medication history is time-consuming, it is essential in the treatment of sleep disorder in late life. This task may be delegated to well-trained paraprofessionals.

Excellent techniques are now available for all-night electrophysiologic (polysomnographic) monitoring of multiple central nervous system and somatic functions. Polysomnographic monitoring has expanded from the three basic techniques for identifying sleep stages: the sleep electroencephalogram, the electrooculogram, and various instruments for measuring air exchange, respiratory effort, and electrical activity from the heart and leg movements. Tracings are used to verify a history of disturbed nocturnal sleep and to explore its source. They are not necessary for the diagnosis of all sleep disturbances and are, in fact, unavailable in many communities. Nevertheless, referral to a sleep disorder clinic where such tracings are available is indicated when a disabling sleep disturbance cannot be diagnosed. If the primary care physician suspects a sleep disorder, electroencephalographic and electrocardiographic tracings, thyroid function tests, and pulmonary function studies are essential.

The most common sleep disorders in late life are listed in Table 2. Clinicians will immediately be struck by the length and variety of diagnoses that must be considered, as outlined in the first edition of the *Diagnostic Classification of Sleep and Arousal Disorders*.[3] This classification system has been heralded by sleep researchers as a major step toward developing more operational diagnoses of sleep disturbances that reflect the most recent concepts of sleep disorder. As can be seen, the classification system characterizes four major types of disorders: disorders of initiating and maintaining sleep (insomnias), disorders of excessive somnolence (hypersomnia), disorders of the sleep-wake schedule, and dysfunctions associated with sleep, sleep stages, or partial arousals (parasomnias).

INSOMNIA

Of all the sleep disturbances, insomnia is the one most frequently treated by the primary care physician. Symptoms of insomnia include problems in falling asleep, difficulty staying asleep, or final awakenings that occur too early in the morning. Psychophysiologic and psychiatric disorders account for about 50 percent of the insomnias, with drug-related and alcohol-related disorders accounting for 15 to 20 percent and the physiologic-organic-medical-neurologic group for 30 to 35 percent of the total. A major cause of the psychophysiologic

---

3. Sleep Disorders Classification Committee, Association of Sleep Disorders Center. Diagnostic classification of sleep and arousal disorders. *Sleep* 2:1–137, 1979.

TABLE 2
Differential Diagnosis of Sleep Disorders

Disorders of Initiating and Maintaining Sleep (Insomnias)
  Subjective complaints without objective evidence
  Psychophysiologic (transient or persistent)
  Psychiatric disorders
    Affective disorders
    Anxiety disorders
    Dementia
  Drug and alcohol use
    Tolerance to and withdrawal from CNS depressants
    Sustained use of CNS stimulants
  Sleep-induced respiratory impairment
    Sleep apnea syndrome
  Sleep-related myoclonus
  "Restless legs" syndrome
  Medical and toxic conditions
    Chronic obstructive pulmonary disease
    Acute and chronic pain syndromes
    Thyroid disorders
Disorders of Excessive Somnolence (Hypersomnia)
  Sustained use of CNS depressants
  Sleep apnea syndrome
  Narcolepsy
Disorders of the Sleep-Wake Schedule
  Irregular sleep-wake pattern
  Delayed or advanced sleep phase syndrome
Dysfunctions Associated with Sleep, Sleep Stages, or
  Partial Arousals (Parasomnias)

CNS = central nervous system.

insomnias is the transient disruption of sleep that generally occurs in reaction to acute disappointment, loss, or perceived threat. Acute emotional arousal and unfamiliar sleep environments may also induce this condition. Persistent psychophysiologic insomnia not related to an identifiable stress is often associated with psychosomatic disorders. Such older persons experience high levels of anxiety and tension, but without classic psychological conflicts.

Insomnia from Affective Disorders
Affective disorders are a major contributor to sleep disturbances in late life. The depressed older person generally maintains the ability to fall asleep but has a sleep maintenance disturbance with a decreased sleep time or early morning arousal. Stage IV sleep is remarkably diminished. In fact, some researchers consider older subjects free from serious depressive symptoms to be comparable to young

mature subjects in the percentage of stage IV sleep during the night. A reduced REM sleep latency in endogenous depression is so consistent that it has reached the status of a biologic marker. Tricyclic antidepressants increase REM latency as they reverse the depressive symptomatology. In mania, a sleep onset insomnia and abbreviated sleep are common symptoms. The anxious older adult, in contrast, presents with a difficulty in falling asleep or with increased sleep latency, but total sleep time is not diminished.

Insomnia From Dementia
The sleep of patients who suffer from chronic organic mental disorders (i.e., dementia) is characterized by definite pattern changes. A strong correlation exists between a decrease in intellectual performance on a typical I.Q. test, such as the Wechsler Adult Intelligence Scale, and the percentage of REM and stage IV sleep. Patients with dementia also appear to have a decreased total sleep time and a marked increase in time spent awake during the night.

Rebound Insomnia
Pharmacologic tolerance to the central nervous system depressant activities of sleep medications increases when such drugs are used on a sustained basis. Patients therefore frequently decide to increase the dose and thus perpetuate a cycle of progressively higher dosage of sedative hypnotic agents and successive periodic episodes of insomnia. Upon sudden termination of a sedative hypnotic agent, an overt drug withdrawal syndrome, with anxiety-provoking dreams and "rebound insomnia," occurs. Therefore, sedative hypnotic agents should be withdrawn over a 7- to 10-day period. The short half-life of ethyl alcohol renders it an ineffective sedative hypnotic agent, with a mild withdrawal period occurring 3 to 4 hours into the night. A progressive disintegration of the sleep pattern, with persistent sleep interruptions, fragmented REM sleep periods, and reduced REM sleep, occurs during drinking episodes.

Apnea Syndrome
The sleep apnea syndrome may lead to either insomnia or hypersomnia. Upper airway obstruction commonly evokes the complaint of excessive daytime sleepiness. Central sleep apnea syndrome, however, is associated most often with the complaint of insomnia. The diagnosis of sleep apnea syndrome has been found to be dramatically higher in older patients complaining of excessive daytime sleepiness. As noted earlier, snorers are prone to the development of obstructive

sleep apnea. The disorder is worsened by the use of central nervous system depressants and by advancing age, and is potentially fatal. The report of interruptions of breathing by the sleep partner may be the only means of making the diagnosis.

Insomnia Related to Muscle Symptoms
Sleep-related myoclonus, or intense muscle jerks that occur primarily in the legs at sleep onset but that occasionally continue throughout the sleep period, can go unnoticed by the patient but be recognized by the sleep partner. At other times the condition induces a severe insomnia. A similar condition, the "restless legs" syndrome, is manifested as an uncomfortable creeping sensation deep in the legs. It is characterized by deep paresthesias and limb movements during extended muscular rest and with falling asleep. Movement gives some relief but also may produce a severe insomnia. Both of these conditions have been treated with some success with tocopherol vitamin E and 5-hydroxy tryptophan.

Insomnia From Other Diseases
Numerous medical conditions produce sleep problems among the elderly. Dyspnea often induces sleep problems, regardless of whether its cause is chronic obstructive pulmonary disease, congestive heart failure, or some other condition. Older persons with a chronic pain syndrome, such as that caused by osteoarthritis or metastatic carcinoma, frequently report disturbed sleep. Chest pain, such as nocturnal angina associated with REM sleep, may awaken the older person. Even though the pain remits, the individual cannot return to a satisfactory sleep because of the anxiety elicited by the pain syndrome. Older persons frequently suffer from thyroid disorders. Hyperthyroidism can present in an apathetic form but often leads to fragmented, short sleep with excessive amounts of stage IV sleep. Hypothyroidism, which is more commonly found in the elderly, leads to a marked decrease in the percentage of stage III and stage IV sleep. These patterns gradually revert to normal following treatment of the thyroid dysfunction.

HYPERSOMNIA

Hypersomnia, manifested by an increase in total 24-hour sleep and difficulty achieving full arousal or awakening, is a much less common complaint but is potentially more serious as a symptom. The sustained use of central nervous system depressants frequently causes hypersomnia and impaired cognitive functioning. Use of drugs such as antihistamines and antihypertensive agents may also produce excessive somnolence. Sleep apnea syndrome may also present as a hypersomnia. Narcolepsy typically begins in the second decade of life, but no evidence exists that the syndrome improves with aging.

SLEEP RHYTHM DISTURBANCES

Disorders of the sleep-wake cycle are most common in late life. Older people not on a fixed schedule will often stay awake during the night watching television or involved in some other project and then will have difficulty readjusting their sleep-wake cycle. If an older person is forced to move to an institution or into the home of a relative, a rather dramatic change in the sleep-wake cycle can occur. For example, the older person may have become accustomed to retiring very late while at home (2:00 or 3:00 A.M.) but, upon moving, may feel obligated to go to bed at 10:00 P.M.

Clinical evidence at present suggests that biologic rhythms in general are significant variables in geriatric medicine. A breakdown of the biphasic pattern of sleep and wakefulness appears to occur in late life, with a return to a more "polyphasic" alteration of sleep and wakefulness (which is often seen in the infant). The phase of sleep may also change. In one study, individuals tended with increasing age to fall asleep and awaken at earlier times.[4] In addition, some researchers have found that older people are less tolerant to phase shifts of the sleep-wake cycle. For example, the older pilot may experience greater cumulative sleep loss on transcontinental flights. Despite the environmental problems frequently encountered by older persons, many of the changes just described are not due to physical confinement or lack of exercise. Remaining in bed during day and night, which is typical of the debilitated older adult, also disrupts the sleep-wake cycle.

The delayed sleep phase syndrome is marked by stable sleep onset and wake times, though they are intractably later than desired. No difficulty is reported in maintaining sleep once it has begun. One approach to therapy is sleep phase delay: over a number of days, the patient progressively goes to bed at a later time and wakes up at a later time. The sleep period is moved "around the clock" and finally

---

4. G. June. Sleep and wakefulness in normal human adults. *Br. Med. J.* 2:269, 1968.

stops when the patient's sleep onset is at the desired time. A history of early morning arousal and evening drowsiness, common symptoms among the elderly, suggests the possibility of an "advanced sleep phase syndrome."

COMPLICATIONS OF SLEEP DISORDERS

Cardiovascular disease, especially cardiac arrhythmias, are more prevalent with advancing age. The older person may be at a greater risk for developing a cardiac arrhythmia during REM sleep, when the heart rate is generally increased. This in turn may lead to a decrease in cerebral blood flow and temporary or even permanent cerebral damage. These complicated interactions, not yet fully understood, must not be overlooked, for older persons are more likely to die suddenly during sleep.

Nocturnal confusion and wandering are common symptoms among older persons who are suffering from delirium or dementia and who have difficulty distinguishing dream material from actual sensory input. If a patient with a chronic organic mental disorder is awakened from REM sleep during the night, a state of extreme agitation and disorientation can occur. This agitation probably results from REM material (dreams) forcing itself into the waking state.

TREATMENT OF SLEEP DISORDERS IN LATE LIFE

Nonpharmacologic Treatment
The concept of "sleep hygiene" outlined by Hauri is justified given our knowledge of the importance of maintaining regular sleep-wake cycles.[5] Irregular sleep habits may adversely influence the quality and effectiveness of sleep. Because older persons may suffer from a relative disruption of their biologic rhythms, regular arousal and bedtimes are important in establishing a circadian rhythm in such areas as temperature and adrenocorticotropic hormone secretion.

Equally important as the biologic value of a regular sleep-wake cycle are the behavioral cues that precipitate conscious or unconscious reactions relevant to sleep. Although certain noises would typically waken anyone—such as an unexpected explosion—the sleeper often will ignore other noises even though they reach a significant level.

5. P. Hauri. *Sleep Disorders*. Kalamazoo, Mich.: The Upjohn Company, 1977.

For example, an elderly woman can ignore the blaring of an automobile horn or excessive traffic outside her apartment but will respond to a low-intensity moan or groan from her husband in another bedroom if she is concerned about his health. A disheveled bedroom can remind the older person of his or her sleep difficulties. Selective techniques for improving sleep hygiene are listed in Table 3.

The clinician must allow a patient to become adapted to a new environment before implementing any changes in the sleep program. Sleep problems that develop on the first few nights in the hospital or upon moving to new living quarters most often do not require intervention after the process of adaptation has occurred.

Individual differences must be considered when the clinician is determining the sleep hygiene program for any individual. A thorough history should serve as a guideline for developing a hygiene program. For example, some older people sleep well with temperatures that are quite low (even reaching 40°F), whereas others complain when the room temperature falls below a level of 65°F. Implementing regular sleep habits can be complemented by a reasonable program of exercise.

Throughout history, attention has been directed to the physical surroundings of the bedroom. Preferences in accoutrements such as beds, mattresses, and sleep clothes have been recognized by Madison Avenue, and many advertisements are directed to Americans who wish to improve their physical environment of sleep. Although excessively soft and poorly constructed mattresses may contribute to orthopedic problems of the elderly, especially spondylolisthesis, a

TABLE 3

Techniques for Improving Sleep Hygiene in Late Life

1. Acquire an accurate assessment of daily sleep needs
2. Keep the bedroom cool rather than warm
3. Keep the bed clean and neat
4. Avoid the bedroom except at night
5. Avoid heavy meals after 7:00 P.M.
6. Develop regular arousal and bedtimes
7. Eat a light snack, but avoid large meals before bedtime
8. Do not fight wakefulness. Instead, occupy self with some restful activity, such as reading or television
9. Avoid frequent changes in the environment
10. Exercise regularly
11. Do not allow time in bed to become substantially greater than total sleep time

hard surface may lead to more body movements during sleep and therefore to more frequent awakenings.

Although no ideal temperature has been established for effective sleep, most people sleep better at a cooler temperature than is comfortable during their waking hours. Sleeping in warm rooms is common among older persons who live in inner-city apartments where the windows are kept closed during the night for security reasons. Frequently these apartments are without air conditioners, or financial constraints restrict using the air conditioner.

Older people should be cautioned about eating large meals or snacks before bedtime, especially foods that make them uncomfortable or that contain caffeine (e.g., chocolate). Stimulants such as tea, coffee, or caffeine-containing soft drinks definitely should be avoided. Nevertheless, a light snack can facilitate the onset of sleep. Some preliminary studies have even postulated that milk before bedtime leads to increased levels of tryptophan in the blood, which in turn induces sleep.

Sedative Hypnotics

Although sedative hypnotic agents have been the sine qua non of the treatment of sleep disorders by physicians in the past, prescribing of these agents has decreased remarkably over the last ten years. In addition, changes have occurred in the types of drugs prescribed for sleep disturbances, with an increase in the use of benzodiazepine derivatives, such as temazepam (Restoril) or flurazepam (Dalmane), and a decrease in the use of barbiturates. Increased concern about the abuse of barbiturates and the potential for accidental or suicidal deaths resulting from an overdose has contributed to this shift in prescribing practices.

The indications for the use of sedative hypnotic agents are presented in Table 4. Some agents have been shown to be objectively effective as hypnotics, though reported successes from these drugs probably exceed the real value of their use, as indicated by a recent report by the Institute of Medicine.[6] Perhaps of equal value is the fact that sedative hypnotics often promote the subjective feeling of having slept well. The symptomatic relief from insomnia breaks a cycle and enables a person to increase function in his waking hours.

6. Institute of Medicine, *Sleeping Pills, Insomnia, and Medical Practice* (Washington, D.C.: National Academy of Sciences, 1979).

TABLE 4
Indications for Sedative Hypnotic Use in the Elderly

1. Short-term stress reaction manifested mainly by insomnia
2. Fear of poor sleep with a tendency to panic in an insomniac who faces a major event the next day, such as surgery
3. Nightmares in the cognitively clear older adult
4. Patients who have used sedative hypnotic agents safely for years and who gain a significant placebo effect from the medications (i.e., there is little reason to unilaterally withdraw all patients who use long-term sedative hypnotic agents)

Therefore a critical question in evaluating the effectiveness of sedative hypnotic agents is, "Does the patient feel better and function better from their use?" All these agents may produce harmful side effects, so clinicians must ask whether the potential benefits for a medication outweigh the risk in terms of side effects or physical or psychological sequelae.

In general, physicians should attempt a sleep hygiene approach prior to the prescription of sedative hypnotic agents. These drugs are never to be prescribed for an insomniac who continues to use an additional sedative hypnotic agent; the initial drug must be withdrawn before the new drug is prescribed. Paradoxically, sleep may actually improve after an individual has been withdrawn from such an agent. These agents should never be prescribed to demented patients, who can become confused about dosage, or to a potentially suicidal patient outside the hospital setting. For older persons, smaller dosages can be used but repeat dosages should be avoided. For example, both temazepam (Restoril) and flurazepam (Dalmane) are quite effective in most older persons at a dose level of 15 mg.

The potential for tolerance, physical and psychological dependence, and side effects with these agents should be explained to the patient before they are prescribed. No more than two weeks' supply of the medication ought to be dispensed at any given time. There is little evidence that these agents work effectively if prescribed continuously for more than a two-week period. Therefore, after initial prescription, the clinician can choose to withdraw the drug for a period of time and then, if necessary, reinstate it. The doses of hypnotic drugs should be escalated with extreme caution. Sedative hypnotic agents do lead to the development of tolerance and may cause sleep to become even more disturbed. Increasing the dose will temporarily improve sleep but can soon lead to a vicious cycle and the severe problem of addiction. These agents should never be prescribed to heavy snorers because of the danger of sleep apnea syndrome and its complications.

Withdrawal of sedative hypnotic agents from chronic users of such drugs leads to disturbing changes in patterns of sleep. Typically there is a dramatic decrease in the number of hours of sleep each night for the first few nights and an increase in REM sleep (with the possibility of disturbing dreams). Stages III and IV sleep, which are significantly depressed with chronic sedative use, gradually return to their normal state. After one or two weeks, the total sleep time actually increases. Because of the significant sleep problems that follow drug withdrawal, the hospital setting is usually the appropriate place for withdrawal to take place; the readily available relief from "just one pill" is a significant deterrent to outpatient withdrawal from sleep medications.

The potential for grogginess and confusion in the morning, due to the half-life of the longer-acting benzodiazepines in older persons, has led many geriatricians to use shorter-acting benzodiazepines, such as oxazepam. Recently, temazepam has been suggested as a more effective agent in older people because of its specific sedative-hypnotic properties and shorter half-life.

Yet the benzodiazepines are not the only medications that can be prescribed for sleep difficulties in late life. If agitation secondary to a dementia or paranoid reaction contributes to the sleep disturbance, the appropriate use of an antipsychotic agent such as thioridazine, haloperidol, or thiothixene may be indicated. There is little potential for physical or psychological dependence with the use of antipsychotic agents, although they are noted for the increased potential for certain uncomfortable side effects such as secondary anticholinergic effects and tardive dyskinesia. Tricyclic antidepressants are useful as a mild sedative and definitely will correct the sleep disorder secondary to a major depressive episode. As with the antipsychotic agents, there is no potential for physical or psychological dependence, but there are significant possibilities for the development of side effects, primarily anticholinergic effects. In contrast to the antipsychotics, these agents do not lead to the development of tardive dyskinesia.

Diphenhydramine is a widely used medication for its hypnotic effect in both children and older adults. At a dose of 25 or 50 mg it is a relatively safe medication when used alone, but the clinician must be aware of the potential for additive effects when it is used with other anticholinergic agents, such as antipsychotics, tricyclic antidepressants, antihistamines, and antiparkinsonian agents.

112 | *Medical Care of the Elderly*

Tryptophan has been the subject of considerable interest in recent years. The usual dosage is 1 to 5 grams at night. Studies suggest that trytophan may diminish sleep latency in prolonged stage II sleep, and REM sleep may also be suppressed. The hypnotic effect of tryptophan is presumably the result of an increase in levels of 5-hydroxytryptophan in the brain. The relative absence of side effects and the lack of known harmful consequences have increased the popularity of this drug.

Aspirin has also been thought to be of value in inducing sleep. Not only may aspirin decrease the pain of osteoarthritis or other chronic ailments in the elderly and provide a pain-free interval conducive to sleep, but it may also mobilize serotonin. Scopolamine and other over-the-counter preparations serve as hypnotic agents because their anticholinergic effects produce drowsiness. These drugs are not true hypnotics, and in many ways, the potential for adverse side effects is greater than with the benzodiazepines.

Alcohol definitely produces a sedative effect when taken in reasonable quantities before bedtime, but the subsequent sleep is often interrupted. Because the short half-life of alcohol leads to a "rebound" during the middle of the night, it should not be routinely prescribed to older people for sleep induction. Nevertheless, if older adults have used alcohol for years before bedtime without harmful effects, it does not necessarily require withdrawal.

SUGGESTED READING

1. Blazer, D.G. *Sleep Disorders of Late Life*. Omaha: University of Nebraska Medical Center, 1980.
2. Dement, W.C., Miles, L.E., Carskadon, M.A. 'White paper' on sleep and aging. *J. Am. Geriatr. Soc.* 30:25–50, 1982.
3. Harvey, S.C. Hypnotics and sedatives. In Gilman, A.G., Goodman, L.S., Gilman, A. (Eds.), *The Pharmacologic Basis of Therapeutics*, 6th ed. New York: Macmillan, 1980.
4. Hauri, P. *Sleep Disorders*. Kalamazoo, Mich.: The Upjohn Company, 1977.
5. Institute of Medicine. *Sleeping Pills, Insomnia, and Medical Practice*. Washington, D.C.: National Academy of Sciences, 1979.
6. June, G. Sleep and wakefulness in normal human adults. *Br. Med. J.* 2:269, 1968.
7. Kales, A. *Sleep: Physiology and Pathology*. Philadelphia: J.B. Lippincott, 1969.
8. Karacan, I., Thornby, J., Arch, M., et al. Prevalence of sleep disturbance in a primary Florida community. *Soc. Sci. Med.* 10:239, 1976.
9. McGhie, A., Russel, S. The subjective assessment of normal sleep patterns. *J. Ment. Sci.* 108:642, 1962.
10. Roffwarg, H.P., Altshuler, K.Z. The diagnosis of sleep disorders. In Zales, M.R., (Ed.), *Eating, Sleeping and Sexuality: Treatment of Disorders in Basic Life Functions*. New York: Brunner/Mazel, 1982.
11. Sleep Disorders Classification Committee, Association of Sleep Disorders Center. Diagnostic classification of sleep and arousal disorders. *Sleep* 2:1–137, 1979.

Drug Treatment of Musculoskeletal Complaints

PETER M. LEVITIN, M.D., and
VINCENT J. GIULIANO, M.D.

*Editor's note: The variety of drugs, both old and new, available
for the treatment of rheumatic complaints is bewildering. The diagnostic
process is usually straightforward and is well described in standard
texts. The choice of a therapeutic agent, especially in view of the
many adverse effects and drug-drug interactions, is a more difficult
problem that requires an in-depth comprehension of the characteristics
of a few familiar drugs and access to information (not easily available)
on other choices.*

Overall, up to 80 percent of elderly patients will have musculoskeletal
complaints. The causes of arthritis in the elderly include a variety of
common diseases, such as degenerative joint disease, polymyalgia
rheumatica, gout, and rheumatoid arthritis. A specific rheumatic diagnosis is important because there are a number of diseases in which
specific therapy is indicated (e.g., corticosteroids for polymyalgia
rheumatica or giant cell arteritis, colchicine or nonsteroidal antiinflammatory drugs for acute gout). It is best, in general, to avoid
symptomatic treatment of musculoskeletal symptoms without first
diagnosing the cause of the rheumatic complaints.

Choosing a nonsteroidal antiinflammatory drug requires attention
to both the pharmacologic differences among these drugs and their
activity against the specific rheumatic disease to be treated. For example, the drug shown to be most effective for rheumatoid arthritis
is still aspirin. All other nonsteroidal antiinflammatory drugs have
been compared to aspirin as the benchmark of efficacy. Some may
be better tolerated or less toxic than aspirin, but none is any more
effective than maximal therapeutic doses of aspirin. If patients cannot
tolerate aspirin or if their disease cannot be controlled with adequate
therapeutic doses, then other nonsteroidal antiinflammatory drugs,
such as the propionic acids, should be used.

113

FACTORS INFLUENCING DRUG TREATMENT OF RHEUMATIC DISORDERS IN THE ELDERLY

Absorption

There is little evidence that drug absorption is significantly impaired in the elderly, especially in chronic drug administration that aims at easily achieved steady-state blood levels.

Protein Binding

The serum albumin concentration decreases with age, and in patients with chronic inflammatory rheumatic diseases the decrease can be very significant. A secondary decrease in protein binding of drugs can allow more free drug to be available for pharmacologic action or for metabolism and excretion. The effect of hypoalbuminemia on drug availability and toxicity is unpredictable, however, requiring careful clinical observation to determine proper dosage in the elderly patient.

Hepatic Metabolism

Most drug metabolism occurs in the liver. Because hepatic blood flow declines 40 to 45 percent and hepatic microsomal enzyme activity also decreases with aging, reduction in drug dosage may be necessary to compensate for resulting higher blood levels. For example, the nonsteroidal antiinflammatory drugs are metabolized in the liver, and a decrease in liver clearance can increase the potential toxicity for elderly patients taking these drugs.

Renal Excretion

Glomerular filtration decreases by about 35 percent and tubular secretory rates fall with normal aging, which can lead to increased serum drug levels. For the individual elderly patient, the dose of renally excreted drugs is best determined after measuring the creatinine clearance.[1] The serum creatinine concentration alone is insufficient since total muscle mass is decreased in the elderly, and a normal value for serum creatinine may be seen in patients with reduced renal function.

Drug Interactions

Because elderly patients often take several drugs concurrently, the opportunity for drug interactions is increased. For example, one drug

---

1. $\text{CrCl} = \dfrac{(140 - \text{age})}{S_{Cr} \times 72} \times \text{kg} \ (\times \ 0.85 \text{ for women}).$

may interfere with the renal excretion or stimulate the hepatic metabolism of another drug, or may compete for the same protein-binding site, resulting in an increased amount of unbound drug available. An example of a common drug interaction is the increased unbound coumarin in the serum when antiinflammatory drugs such as phenylbutazone are given concurrently.

Adverse Drug Reactions
Elderly patients may be more sensitive to the adverse effects of the antirheumatic drugs, such as the bone marrow toxicity of phenylbutazone (Butazolidin) and the central nervous system side effects of indomethacin (Indocin). In addition, the ability to detect tinnitus as a manifestation of aspirin toxicity is impaired in the elderly, thus making them more susceptible to developing toxic serum levels without warning. There must be an increase vigilance for adverse reactions when prescribing drugs for the elderly.

Compliance
One-third to one-half of patients fail to comply with a medical regimen, and noncompliance may be higher in elderly patients because they often have intellectual, financial, visual or hearing problems that interfere with following instructions. Compliance may improve if medication instructions are written down and discussed with the patient. Drug regimens must be made as simple as possible to follow, and care must be taken to minimize the cost through judicious use of generic preparations and dispensing of large quantities of medication (e.g., 100 tablets at one time).

SALICYLATES

Aspirin (acetylsalicylic acid) and other salicylate preparations have been used for the treatment of rheumatic diseases for over a hundred years. All preparations are derived from salicylic acid.

Absorption and Distribution
Aspirin is an acid with a pKa of 3.5 and therefore is nonionized in the stomach, allowing for rapid absorption. Absorption, however, is also excellent in the neutral pH of the small intestine, possibly because there is an enormous absorptive surface available for absorbing any nonionized drug so that the equilibrium is constantly being pushed toward the nonionized form. The addition of buffering or coating to aspirin may speed up or slow absorption, but once steady state is

reached, the rate of absorption has little effect on salicylate blood levels.

Aspirin and other salicylate preparations are bound to albumin. The proportion of drug bound to albumin decreases as the serum salicylate level increases or the serum albumin concentration decreases. Consequently, elderly patients with hypoalbuminemia will have an enhanced pharmacologic effect from a dosage increase because the albumin binding sites become saturated. Dosage increments should be smaller for these patients than for patients who have a normal albumin concentration. Serum salicylate levels measure both bound and unbound drug and may be low or normal despite an adequate or toxic level of unbound salicylate in the serum.

Metabolism and Excretion

At low doses of aspirin (300 to 600 mg, four times daily) increases result in proportional increases in serum salicylate levels, but at high doses the major metabolic pathway becomes saturated, and a small increase in aspirin dose will result in a relatively large increase in the serum salicylate level and a longer serum half-life. One advantage of the increased serum half-life with large doses of aspirin is that aspirin can be then given on twice daily or three times daily schedules.

Renal excretion of salicylates occurs by passive glomerular filtration of unbound drug and active proximal tubular secretion; this is counterbalanced by passive distal tubular reabsorption. At a high urine pH, most of the salicylate is ionized and not readily reabsorbed through the renal tubule, allowing most of the filtered and secreted salicylate to be excreted. Elderly patients are often taking antacids for peptic ulcer disease or to reduce the gastrointestinal side effects of aspirin; these can alkalinize their urine, resulting in increased renal excretion and a reduced serum salicylate level. Conversely, when antacid treatment is stopped, there can be a significant rise in the salicylate level.

Drug Interactions and Side Effects

When aspirin and other nonsteroidal antiinflammatory agents are given together, there is competition for binding sites, with aspirin usually displacing the other drug. Adding a second drug of this class to already optimal doses of aspirin is, therefore, a questionable practice. Competition for protein-binding sites may cause aspirin to displace coumarin and sulfonylureas from protein-binding sites, thus potentiating their actions.

Because aspirin displaces methotrexate from its binding sites, it must be used only with great caution in patients taking methotrexate for chemotherapy for cancer, psoriasis, or rheumatoid arthritis. Aspirin can block the diuretic effect of spironolactone by inhibiting its binding to the tubular cell receptor, and can inhibit the uricosuric effect of probenecid. Corticosteroids can increase salicylate metabolism and result in a decreased salicylate level, and when withdrawn can significantly raise salicylate levels and thus precipitate acute toxicity. Furosemide can cause salicylate toxicity in patients receiving larger doses of aspirin by competing with the excretion of salicylates at the renal receptor site.

Adverse Side Effects
The potential adverse reactions to therapeutic doses of aspirin (4 to 6 g/day) include allergy, tinnitus, gastrointestinal side effects, decreased platelet count, coagulation defects, and hepatic and renal effects. Tinnitus occurs in patients with normal hearing when the serum salicylate levels are between 20 and 30 mg/dl; elderly patients frequently have high-tone hearing loss and may not experience tinnitus to warn them of the impending toxic salicylate levels. They may also develop a variety of nervous system effects of salicylate toxicity, such as dizziness, confusion, convulsions, stupor, or coma.

Aspirin, but not nonacetylated salicylates, irreversibly inhibits platelet aggregation and increases the bleeding time. Thus aspirin can cause an increase in gastrointestinal bleeding in patients with active peptic ulcer disease, erosive gastritis, or diverticular bleeding. Furthermore, aspirin may cause or aggravate constipation. Aspirin can cause a reduction in renal function in patients with renal diseases (see the section on nonsteroidal antiinflammatory drugs and the kidney).

INDOMETHACIN AND RELATED DRUGS

The indole drugs indomethacin (Indocin) and tolmetin (Tolectin) and the indene sulindac (Clinoril) all have a chemical resemblance to one another. They are all potent antiinflammtory drugs and can be used in a wide variety of rheumatic diseases including rheumatoid arthritis, osteoarthritis, gout, and ankylosing spondylitis.

Indomethacin
Indications for Use in the Elderly Patient Indomethacin (Indocin) has been used with beneficial results in the treatment of rheumatoid arthritis, osteoarthritis, gout, ankylosing spondylitis, and nonarticular

rheumatism. It is especially useful in osteoarthritis of the hip, where it is superior to most other agents in relieving pain. Many clinicians consider indomethacin the treatment of choice in acute gout and pseudogout because of the rapid and usually complete response to 50 mg every 6 hours.

Absorption and Distribution   Indomethacin is rapidly absorbed from the upper gastrointestinal tract. It is highly bound to albumin and has a relatively short half-life of less than 2 hours. Because it is excreted in the bile and recirculates, it is useful as a single bedtime dose for relieving nighttime pain and morning stiffness.

Metabolism and Excretion   Indomethacin is metabolized in the liver to inactive metabolites, the majority of which are then excreted in the urine. About 15 percent of unchanged drug is excreted in the urine. Probenecid may inhibit the renal excretion of unchanged indomethacin, giving increased serum concentrations and clinical efficiency; this interaction has practical implications since both drugs may be used together in the treatment of gouty patients.

Drug Interactions and Adverse Side Effects   It is best not to give indomethacin to anticoagulated patients because of its effects on platelet function and the significant risk of gastrointestinal ulceration with subsequent bleeding. Elderly patients have an increased susceptibility to the central nervous system side effects of indomethacin of headache, dizziness, drowsiness, and confusion. It can produce fluid retention and may precipitate congestive heart failure or striking edema in the elderly; it should, therefore, be used with care if there is underlying heart disease. Acute renal insufficiency can also occur (see the section on nonsteroidal antiinflammatory drugs and the kidney).

Tolmetin

Indications for Use in the Elderly Patient   Tolmetin (Tolectin) is useful in the treatment of rheumatoid arthritis, osteoarthritis, gout, pseudogout, ankylosing spondylitis, and nonarticular rheumatism. Like indomethacin, it is particularly useful in the treatment of osteoarthritis of the hip. Because of the lower incidence of central nervous system side effects, it has become a popular choice for treating acute gout and pseudogout.

Absorption and Distribution   Tolmetin is completely absorbed from the gastrointestinal tract and becomes highly bound to serum albumin. Despite this binding, it does not seem to displace other protein-bound drugs.

Metabolism and Excretion Tolmetin is partially metabolized in the liver. The plasma half-life is 4.5 to 6 hours. It is completely excreted in the urine either as a dicarboxylic acid metabolite or as an unchanged drug.

Drug Interactions and Adverse Side Effects Since tolmetin does not displace other protein-bound drugs from their binding sites, it can be safely used concomitantly with coumarin or sulfonylureas. It has a mild antiplatelet effect. The most frequent adverse reactions are gastrointestinal, predominantly dyspepsia, nausea and vomiting, and peptic ulceration. The central nervous system side effects observed with indomethacin (headache, dizziness, confusion, and so on) are much less frequent with tolmetin; this is one of the advantages of this drug over indomethacin. Fluid retention can occur secondary to sodium retention with the development of edema and potential aggravation of congestive heart failure. Acute renal insufficiency has been described (see the section on nonsteroidal antiinflammatory drugs and the kidney).

Sulindac

Indications for Use in the Elderly Patient Sulindac (Clinoril) is useful in the treatment of rheumatoid arthritis, osteoarthritis, gout, pseudogout, and nonarticular rheumatism. Sulindac has a long half-life, which allows for a twice-daily dosage and perhaps leads to better compliance.

Absorption and Distribution Sulindac is rapidly absorbed from the gastrointestinal tract and reaches peak plasma levels in 2 to 3 hours. However, sulindac itself is inactive until metabolized to a sulfide metabolite that has a half-life of about 18 hours. Steady-state plasma levels are achieved in five to seven days of daily administration. This drug does not displace either coumarin or sulfonylureas from binding sites.

Metabolism and Excretion Sulindac is metabolized in the liver to an active sulfide and an inactive sulfone. These drugs are excreted into the bile and have an extensive enterohepatic circulation. The active sulfide metabolite is excreted in the feces, while sulindac and the inactive sulfone are eliminated by the kidney.

Drug Interactions and Adverse Side Effects Sulindac has no significant effect on platelet function and can be used safely with anticoagulants. Gastrointestinal effects with dyspepsia, nausea, and constipation are the most common adverse side effects; gastrointestinal bleeding occurs rarely. Hepatitis has been reported. Central nervous system effects are very infrequent. Sodium and water retention may occur and can lead to congestive heart failure. Acute renal failure may occur (see the section on nonsteroidal antiinflammatory drugs and the kidney).

PROPIONIC ACIDS

The currently available propionic acid group of drugs includes ibuprofen (Motrin, Rufen), naproxen (Naprosyn), and fenoprofen (Nalfon).

Ibuprofen

Indications for Use in the Elderly Patient Ibuprofen (Motrin, Rufen) has been shown to be of benefit in the treatment of rheumatoid arthritis, osteoarthritis, nonarticular rheumatism, and as an analgesic in disorders such as low back pain, radiculopathies, and postoperative pain. Full therapeutic doses are well tolerated by elderly patients. Antiinflammatory effects require doses of 2,800 to 3,600 mg daily, while analgesia can be achieved with less.

Absorption and Distribution Ibuprofen is rapidly absorbed following oral administration. The drug binds to albumin but has a very low potential for displacing other protein-bound drugs and can be used with coumarin. The plasma half-life is about 2 hours.

Metabolism and Excretion Ibuprofen is metabolized in the liver to inactive metabolites that are excreted through the kidneys.

Drug Interactions and Adverse Side Effects Ibuprofen does not have any clinically significant drug interactions. Its adverse side effects are generally mild and include dyspepsia, nausea, and rarely gastrointestinal bleeding. Rare instances of drug rashes and drug-associated alopecia have been reported. Ibuprofen, like other nonsteroidal drugs, can cause fluid retention that can result in congestive heart failure in cardiac patients and a reversible rise in blood urea nitrogen and creatinine secondary to interference with prostaglandin biosynthesis. Dizziness and cognitive dysfunctions may occur and can be confused with dementia or cerebrovascular disease in elderly patients. Acute renal insufficiency can occur (see the section on nonsteroidal antiinflammatory drugs and the kidney).

Naproxen

Indications for Use in the Elderly Patient Naproxen (Naprosyn) has been shown to be beneficial in the treatment of rheumatoid arthritis, osteoarthritis, ankylosing spondylitis, and gout. Antiinflammatory effects are seen at doses of 500 to 1,000 mg daily. Because of its long half-life it can be given in twice-daily doses, thus aiding compliance. Like ibuprofen, it can be used as an analgesic.

Absorption and Distribution   Naproxen is well absorbed from the gastrointestinal tract. The sodium salt (Anaprox) is absorbed more rapidly than naproxen and thus is marketed as an analgesic for use where quick onset of action is desirable. Naproxen is tightly bound to albumin and has a plasma half-life of about 13 hours.

Metabolism and Excretion   Naproxen is metabolized in the liver and efficiently excreted primarily by the kidney.

Drug Interactions and Adverse Side Effects   Because naproxen is tightly bound to albumin, it may displace other protein-bound drugs such as coumarin and sulfonylureas, but clinical studies have not shown these to be significant interactions. Probenecid can increase the half-life of naproxen because of competition for the glucuronyl transferase metabolic pathway in the liver.

Gastrointestinal symptoms of dyspepsia, nausea, and peptic ulceration are the most common side effect of naproxen. Lightheadedness and cognitive impairment can occur and can be confused with central nervous system disease in the elderly. Naproxen, like ibuprofen, can cause fluid retention and precipitate congestive heart failure in the elderly. Acute renal insufficiency can occur (see the section on nonsteroidal antiinflammatory drugs and the kidney).

Fenoprofen

Indications for Use in the Elderly Patient   Fenoprofen (Nalfon) has been shown to be effective in the treatment of rheumatoid arthritis, osteoarthritis, and acute gout. Antiinflammatory effects are seen with doses of 1,800 to 3,200 mg daily. It should be used with caution in the elderly because of its ability to displace other protein-bound drugs and because of decreased excretion in patients with renal insufficiency.

Absorption and Distribution   Fenoprofen is well absorbed from the gastrointestinal tract, and peak plasma levels are reached in 60 minutes. The plasma half-life is about 3 hours, and steady-state plasma levels are reached in 24 hours. Fenoprofen is strongly bound to the plasma proteins and may displace other protein-bound drugs.

Metabolism and Excretion   Fenoprofen is primarily metabolized in the liver to a glucuronide, and the metabolites are excreted by the kidneys.

Drug Interactions and Adverse Side Effects   Fenoprofen can displace less strongly bound drugs from the protein-binding sites and therefore can potentiate the effects of coumarin, phenobarbital, and the sulfonylureas. Gastrointestinal side effects are the most frequent adverse reaction. Dizziness can occur in 3 to 9 percent of the patients, and fluid retention with precipitation of congestive heart failure can occur in the susceptible patient. Fenoprofen can adversely affect platelet aggregation and thrombus formation. Acute renal insufficiency has been described (see the section on nonsteroidal antiinflammatory drugs and the kidney).

FENAMATES

Mefenamic acid (Ponstel), meclofenamate sodium (Meclomen), and flufenamic acid are anthranilic acid derivatives that have antiinflammatory properties. They are not as effective as aspirin, indomethacin, or propionic acids, and adverse side effects limit their use. They will be considered as a group.

Indications for Use in the Elderly Patient   Mefenamic acid and meclofenamic acid are effective analgesics in the treatment of rheumatic disease but are weak antiinflammatory drugs. The potential drug interactions, high incidence of diarrhea, and caution required in the presence of liver or renal impairment greatly limit their use in the elderly. They are mainly used for pain relief in osteoarthritis and noninflammatory rheumatic disorders.

Absorption and Distribution   Mefenamic acid and meclofenamate sodium reach peak plasma levels in about 1 hour and have a plasma half-life of 2 to 3 hours. The drugs are tightly bound to albumin and will displace other drugs from their protein-binding sites.

Metabolism and Excretion   Mefenamic acid and meclofenamate sodium are primarily metabolized in the liver and are excreted by the kidney, although there is also enterohepatic circulation and biliary excretion.

Drug Interactions and Adverse Side Effects   Mefenamic acid and meclofenamate sodium displace coumarin and sulfonylureas from protein binding sites and potentiate their actions. The most troubling adverse effect of meclofenamate sodium is diarrhea in up to one-third of patients and abdominal pain in 7 percent of patients, disappearing on discontinuation of the drug. The concurrent use of psyllium hydrophilic mucilloid (Metamucil) often controls the diarrhea by aiding in the fecal excretion of meclofenamic acid. Skin rashes, Coombs-positive hemolytic anemias, and bone marrow suppression can also occur. Acute reversible renal insufficiency can occur (see the section on nonsteroidal antiinflammatory drugs and the kidney).

OXICAMS

Piroxicam (Feldene) is a member of a new class of nonsteroidal antiinflammatory drugs that has as its major advantage once-a-day dosage.

Indications for Use in the Elderly Patient Piroxicam has been found to be useful in the treatment of rheumatoid arthritis, osteoarthritis, and gout. It is given only once daily, which may improve compliance. However, its long plasma half-life can also lead to drug accumulation if renal function is decreased.

Absorption and Distribution Piroxicam is well absorbed from the gastrointestinal tract following oral administration and has a plasma mean half-life of 50 hours. The drug is highly bound to protein and may displace other protein-bound drugs. Steady-state plasma levels are reached in 7 to 12 days.

Metabolism and Excretion Piroxicam is primarily metabolized in the liver and excreted predominantly in the urine, although about a third of the metabolites are excreted in the feces. Less than 5 percent of the dose is excreted unchanged.

Drug Interactions and Adverse Side Effects Concurrent administration of aspirin and piroxicam results in a reduction of plasma piroxicam levels to 80 percent of normal values. Although piroxicam is highly protein bound, it has not been shown to interact with coumarin drugs.

The major adverse side effect is gastrointestinal irritation, with a possibly higher incidence of peptic ulcers in patients over 65 years of age. The concurrent use of aspirin with piroxicam may significantly increase the incidence of ulceration. Fluid retention can occur, and congestive heart failure may be worsened. Dizziness that may be confused with primary central nervous system disease can occur in 3 to 6 percent of the patients. Other side effects are reversible elevations of blood urea nitrogen, reversible platelet dysfunction (with elevated bleeding time), and a decrease in hemoglobin and hematocrit without blood loss. Henoch-Schönlein purpura and fatal aplastic anemia have occurred in patients taking piroxicam.

PHENYLBUTAZONE

Phenylbutazone (Butazolidin, Azolid) has been used as an antiinflammatory drug since the 1950s, but its potential for causing adverse reactions limits its use. With the development of safer and equally effective antiinflammatory drugs, there remain only a few indications for prescribing phenylbutazone.

Indications for Use in the Elderly Patient   Phenylbutazone is a potent antiinflammatory drug, effective in the treatment of rheumatoid arthritis, gout and pseudogout, ankylosing spondylitis, and a variety of inflammatory nonarticular rheumatic disorders such as bursitis and tendonitis. Because this drug has a potential for serious adverse effects and drug interactions, especially in the elderly, one of the few indications for its use is ankylosing spondylitis that has been refractory to all other nonsteroidal antiinflammatory drugs.

Absorption and Distribution   Phenylbutazone is less rapidly absorbed from the gastrointestinal tract after oral administration than most of the other nonsteroidal antiinflammatory drugs. Peak plasma levels are achieved in 2 to 4 hours, and the half-life is 20 hours or more; steady-state levels are not reached for 7 to 10 days. Up to two weeks may be required to completely clear it from the plasma after discontinuation. Phenylbutazone is strongly bound to albumin and has a high potential for displacing other protein-bound drugs.

Metabolism and Excretion   Phenylbutazone is metabolized in the liver to two inactive metabolites and one active metabolite, oxyphenbutazone, and is primarily excreted in the kidney.

Drug Interactions and Adverse Side Effects   Many of the adverse side effects of phenylbutazone appear more commonly in the elderly. Bone marrow toxicity, especially aplastic anemia, tends to occur more frequently in the elderly after prolonged treatment with phenylbutazone. Acute hypersensitivity with rash and agranulocytosis is seen more often in younger individuals. Thrombocytopenia occurs as either an acute hypersensitivity reaction or part of an aplastic anemia. Sodium retention may occur and result in cardiac failure in susceptible elderly patients. Gastrointestinal toxicity can occur in 10 to 20 percent of patients on phenylbutazone. Central nervous system symptoms such as vertigo may also occur and mimic primary central nervous system disease. Oxyphenbutazone (Tandearil) is no less toxic than phenylbutazone.

Drug interactions occur as a result of the displacement by phenylbutazone of coumarin and sulfonylureas from their binding sites and the induction of hepatic microsomal enzymes, making other drugs possibly less effective; phenobarbital, prednisone, and phenytoin are examples of drugs in which increased metabolism is induced by phenylbutazone.

DIFLUNISAL

Diflunisal (Dolobid) is a difluorophenyl derivative of salicylic acid. Although it has an antiinflammatory effect, the drug is marketed as an analgesic in the treatment of osteoarthritis.

Indications for Use in the Elderly Patient Diflunisal is an effective analgesic that can be given on a twice-daily dosage regimen. Its main role in the treatment of rheumatic disease is as a substitute for aspirin in the treatment of osteoarthritis pain syndromes.

Absorption and Distribution Diflunisal is rapidly absorbed from the gastrointestinal tract, and peak plasma levels are reached in 2 hours. It is strongly bound to albumin and has a half-life of about 11 hours. Concurrent administration of aluminum hydroxide antacids may reduce bioavailability.

Metabolism and Excretion Diflunisal is metabolized by the liver and primarily excreted by the kidney. Renal insufficiency can seriously decrease excretion, allowing for accumulation in the serum of this nondialyzable drug.

Drug Interactions and Adverse Side Effects Diflunisal displaces coumarin from its binding sites, prolonging the prothrombin time, but it does not affect platelet function. It has fewer gastrointestinal side effects than aspirin. A Stevens-Johnson skin reaction has been reported.

NONSTEROIDAL ANTIINFLAMMATORY DRUGS AND THE KIDNEY

Nonsteroidal antiinflammatory drugs can produce acute renal insufficiency as a result of one of several mechanisms.

1. Allergic interstitial nephritis. Acute renal failure from allergic interstitial nephritis has been reported in patients taking a variety of nonsteroidal antiinflammatory drugs, including indomethacin, tolmetin, fenoprofen, naproxen, meclofenamate sodium, and ibuprofen. The acute renal failure is often associated with proteinuria and nephrotic syndrome; evidence of acute allergic reaction (e.g., fever, skin rash, arthralgias) may be absent. The occurrence of this syn-

drome is not correlated with either the dose or duration of the drug used. The pathogenesis appears to involve delayed hypersensitivity.

2. Acute renal insufficiency secondary to inhibition of prostaglandin synthesis. The nonsteroidal antiinflammatory drugs modify inflammation through inhibition of prostaglandin synthesis (prostaglandins are compounds involved in mediating the inflammatory response that ordinarily do not play a major role in maintaining renal circulation). However: (a) If renal arterial perfusion is decreased, as in dehydration or cardiac failure, renin release is stimulated and subsequent elevated circulating angiotensin II levels cause a vasoconstrictive effect on renal vessels and reduce renal perfusion. The concomitant increase in angiotensin also stimulates synthesis of renal vasodilator prostaglandins, thereby blunting the increase in renal vascular resistance and helping to maintain renal perfusion. (b) In clinical situations of decreased renal arterial perfusion where there is inhibition of renal vasodilator prostaglandin synthesis by nonsteroidal antiinflammatory drugs, the unopposed vasoconstrictor action of angiotensin II predominates, causes increased renal vascular resistance, and results in reduced renal blood flow. If this situation is prolonged, it can lead to acute ischemic renal failure.

Elderly patients will often have reduced renal blood flow and, when given nonsteroidal antiinflammatory drugs, they become susceptible to the development of prerenal azotemia or acute ischemic renal failure. Therefore, when the clinical setting suggests the possibility of decreased renal blood flow, the nonsteroidal antiinflammatory drugs should be used cautiously with careful monitoring of renal function. If possible, the underlying disorders leading to intravascular hypovolemia or decreased renal perfusion should be corrected before these drugs are administered.

Another group of patients at risk for declining renal function resulting from prostaglandin inhibitors are those with preexistent renal disease (especially with lupus nephritis). In mild renal insufficiency there is increased vasodilator prostaglandin synthesis in the kidney; this mechanism compensates for the loss of renal function. Again, if there is inhibition of renal prostaglandin synthesis by nonsteroidal antiinflammatory drugs, further reduction in renal blood flow to the kidney may occur. Again, too, if this situation is prolonged, acute ischemic renal failure can result.

3. Renal papillary necrosis. Acute renal failure can develop from renal papillary necrosis, which also has been associated with use of

nonsteroidal antiinflammatory drugs. This condition occurs mostly in patients who have developed chronic interstitial nephritis.

The inhibition of prostaglandin synthesis by nonsteroidal antiinflammatory drugs affects renal function in other ways as well.

1. Hyporeninemic hypoaldosteronism with hyperkalemia. Prostaglandins stimulate renin release. If renin release is blocked, hyporeninemia occurs, resulting in hypoaldosteronemia with a secondary hyperkalemic metabolic acidosis.

2. Fluid retention. Renal prostaglandins are natriuretic in the kidney either by inhibiting the tubular reabsorption of sodium in the loop of Henle and the distal tubule or by causing renal arterial vasodilatation, leading to natriuresis by a poorly understood mechanism. Inhibition of prostaglandin synthesis, therefore, may lead to sodium and water retention.

3. Diuretic resistance. When nonsteroidal antiinflammatory drugs are given, there is less sodium in the ascending loop (with furosemide) or the distal tubule (with thiazide), where these diuretics work to block sodium retention, thus causing refractoriness to usual diuretic doses. Hypertension may also be aggravated by the resultant salt and water retention.

CORTICOSTEROIDS

The synthetic corticosteroids prednisolone and prednisone are most commonly prescribed; oral preparations, each containing 5 mg of prednisone or prednisolone, are equivalent to 25 mg of cortisone or 20 mg of hydrocortisone. Prednisone and prednisolone have minimal mineralocorticoid activity. The subsequent discussion will refer to prednisone unless otherwise stated. Indications for the use of corticosteroids in the elderly patient with rheumatic disease are discussed in standard texts and in an article by Garber and colleagues.[2]

Absorption and Distribution Prednisone is rapidly absorbed from the upper jejunum and reversibly bound to plasma alpha-globulin (transcortin) if plasma concentrations are low. With increasing plasma levels of prednisone, the globulin-bound fraction becomes saturated and 10 to 15 percent of the drug binding occurs with albumin. Hypoalbuminemic patients (e.g., elderly patients with inflammatory

---

2. E.K. Garber, P.T. Fan, R. Bluestone. Realistic guidelines of corticosteroid therapy in rheumatic disease. *Semin. Arthritis Rheum.* 11:231–256, 1981.

rheumatic diseases) will have a disproportionate increase in side effects with high doses of prednisone.

Metabolism and Excretion   The plasma half-life of prednisone is 60 minutes, but the biologic half-life (biologic potency in tissues) is 12 to 36 hours. Corticosteroids are metabolized in the liver by irreversible reduction and conjugation and are primarily excreted by the kidneys. An increased rate of metabolism has been noted with concomitant administration of barbiturates, phenytoin, and rifampin, probably due to the induction of hepatic microsomal enzymes.

Prednisone must be converted by hepatic enzymes to prednisolone before it is biologically active. In hepatitis, however, there is decreased metabolism of prednisolone in the liver, so a slightly lower dose should be considered in liver disease to avoid increased steroid toxicity.

Drug Interactions and Adverse Side Effects   The concomitant use of aspirin and corticosteroids may decrease the plasma salicylate level due to increased metabolism and/or renal clearance of salicylate. Therefore, a reduction in steroid dose may increase the salicylate level and result in salicylate toxicity.

Corticosteroids cause sodium and fluid retention, and elderly patients may develop congestive heart failure or worsening hypertension. Potassium loss associated with prednisone may result in digitalis toxicity or may increase hypokalemia in patients on diuretics. Prednisone may also increase the requirement for insulin or oral hypoglycemic agents by increasing blood sugar levels. Corticosteroids can cause alterations in mood and even psychosis in elderly patients.

One of the most devastating side effects of corticosteroid therapy in the elderly is the accentuation of osteoporosis, especially in women, leading to painful vertebral compression fractures and considerable disability. We recommend the prophylactic addition of vitamin D, 50,000 units twice a week, and oral calcium and fluoride supplements daily for long-term steroid treatment. Although it has not been proved that this regimen prevents vertebral compression fractures, recent studies support the rationale of this treatment.

SUGGESTED READING*

1. Dromgoole, S.H., Furst, D.E., Paulua, H.E. Rational approaches to the use of salicylates in the treatment of rheumatoid arthritis. *Sem. Arthritis Rheum.* 11:257–283, 1981.

*Complete bibliography available from the author on request: Peter M. Levitin, M.D., The Moses H. Cone Memorial Hospital, Greensboro, North Carolina 27401.

2. Garber, E.K., Fan, P.T., Bluestone, R. Realistic guidelines of corticosteroid therapy in rheumatic disease. *Semin. Arthritis Rheum.* 11:231–256, 1981.
3. Johnson, W.J. Nephrotoxicity of non-steroidal anti-inflammatory drugs. *Mayo Clin. Proc.* 55:120, 1980.
4. Kelley, W.N., Harris, E.D., Ruddy, S., Sledge, C.B. (Eds.). *Textbook of Rheumatology.* Philadelphia: W.B. Saunders, 1981.
5. Ouslander, J.G. Drug therapy in the elderly. *Ann. Intern. Med.* 97:711–722, 1981.
6. Simon, L.S., Mills, J.A. Nonsteroidal anti-inflammatory drugs (first of two parts). *N. Engl. J. Med.* 302:1179–1185, 1980.
7. Simon, L.S., Mills, J.A. Nonsteroidal anti-inflammatory drugs (second of two parts). *N. Engl. J. Med.* 302:1237–1243, 1980.
8. Wagoner, R.D. Renal effects of the newer non-steroidal anti-inflammatory agents. *Mayo Clin. Proc.* 56:525, 1981.

4

CARDIORESPIRATORY DISEASE

The Aging Heart and Vascular System

SEYMOUR EISENBERG, M.D.

Editor's note: Cardiovascular disease, most common in the elderly, presents the dual problem of uncommon presentations of common disorders and the mimicry of serious disorders like angina by benign problems of the gastrointestinal tract or musculoskeletal system. While treatment is similar to that required by younger patients, drug doses must generally be smaller, and the opportunity for therapeutic misadventure is greater.

Cardiovascular disease is the leading cause of death in elderly patients and is responsible for a major portion of their extensive health care needs. Patients over 65 constitute 11 percent of the population but require 30 percent of the health care administered. Geriatric practice is greatly concerned with cardiovascular disease, and it is imperative that those who are involved in care of the elderly understand the particular features of these disorders encountered in an aging population. Geriatricians are often asked, perhaps appropriately, whether or not there is any substantive difference between middle-aged and elderly persons with the same cardiovascular disorder—are the diseases similar in presentation and is management significantly different? In a certain sense the pathology is the same, yet there are differences in clinical presentation, management, and complications of these diseases between middle-aged and elderly patients. Familiarity with this body of knowledge is essential to enlightened care of the elderly.

In this chapter disease change will be examined against the background of true aging change. To be discussed are the particular problems of the elderly, the frequency with which common disorders present with uncommon manifestations, and the likelihood of therapeutic and diagnostic misadventures if the basic vulnerability of the aged is not kept firmly in mind.

CHANGES WITH AGE

The changes in the aorta with age likely initiate hemodynamic adjustments that ultimately compromise cardiac function. There are both quantitative and qualitative changes in collagen and elastin. The ratio of collagen to elastin increases, and in addition elastin undergoes fragmentation with loss of resilience. The aorta, to preserve the pressure/volume characteristics that protect against severe change in pressure with the volume increments of systolic emptying, increases its capacitance. The net effect is a dilated, stiffer aorta and the flow characteristics of a rigid system rather than the pliable vascular system of the younger patient.

Recent noninvasive studies confirm earlier autopsy studies postulating that cardiac muscle hypertrophy is a true consequence of aging. The increase in left ventricular mass may enhance, or paradoxically, by contributing to myocardial stiffness, may compromise cardiovascular function.

Table 1 lists some cardiovascular performance changes that occur with aging and the consequences of these changes. The clinical significance of the aging changes is largely confined to impairment of the response to exercise. At rest, the aged heart functions well in spite of its performance changes. This apparent cardiac competency at rest conceals a lack of reserve until an illness like pneumonia precipitates congestive heart failure or an acute myocardial infarction.

In summary, the well elderly patient may have mild cardiac enlargement and a stiff myocardium that is limited in stroke volume and maximum rate when stressed. The heart is intolerant of tachycardia—either ectopic rhythm or induced sinus tachycardia. Systole is somewhat protracted, but this poses no problem unless exercise is too violent or tachycardia supervenes. Systolic blood pressure tends to be slightly elevated and will rise even more than anticipated with exercise. The cardiovascular system is, in general, slow to accommodate to change in intravascular volume or pressure and responds poorly when confronted with the need suddenly to augment output.

TABLE 1

Performance Changes in the Aging Left Ventricle and Vascular Tree

Performance Changes	Measurable Consequences
1. Protracted ventricular systole—particularly the relaxation phase	1. Gradual increase in peripheral vascular resistance
2. Decreased sympathetic responsiveness—inotropic, chronotropic, and vasodilator	2. Progressive decrease in maximum oxygen uptake (MVO_2)
3. Decreased left ventricular compliance	3. Progressive decrease in maximum attainable heart rate
4. Increased impedance to left ventricular emptying	4. Prolonged systolic time intervals
	5. Normal resting ejection fraction (EF), but a decline in EF with exercise
	6. Decreased myocardial compliance, or increased stiffness
	7. Inordinate rise in pulmonary capillary wedge pressure with exercise

Source: Adapted from Weisfeldt, M.L., *The Aging Heart.* New York: Raven Press, 1980.

HEART DISEASE IN THE ELDERLY

Coronary Artery Disease

Statistically, the major risk factor for coronary atherosclerosis in persons over 65 is age itself. Diabetes, poorly controlled hypertension, and cigarette smoking are important risk factors and must be addressed. Moderate elevations in serum cholesterol, however, may not require aggressive treatment.

Angina Pectoris

Often elderly patients fail to relate a typical history of pain in the chest with exertion, relieved by rest, as occurs in younger patients. The elderly tend to be sedentary and, unfortunately, some may be incapable of giving a completely orderly and reliable history. Also they may have altered pain patterns, and their chest discomfort may be hopelessly intertwined with the pain of musculoskeletal or gastrointestinal origin. The fact that many myocardial infarctions in the aged are "silent"—or at least undetected—supports the existence of altered sensory pathways.

In managing angina, particular attention should be paid to aggravating factors such as anemia, hypertension, congestive heart failure—correctable disorders that tend to induce an unfavorable oxygen delivery/myocardial oxygen requirement ratio. Nitrites and beta-adrenergic blocking agents are the linchpin of treatment, as they are with angina in younger patients. Beta-blockers must be used with caution in patients with spontaneous, drug-unrelated bradycardia; patients who are diabetic or who have had episodes of congestive heart failure should receive these agents in low doses, if at all.

The use of slow-channel calcium-blocking agents, originally promulgated for coronary spasm, has now been widened to include almost any pain caused by myocardial ischemia. There is no apparent reason why these agents should not be similarly employed in elderly patients; however, untoward effects may surface with time and widespread use.

Older persons may be good candidates for coronary artery bypass surgery; age alone is not a contraindication if the procedure is clearly indicated for pain relief and the patient's general state of health does not impose too great a risk. Symptomatic relief and improvement of the quality of existence are the usual goals of surgery in elderly patients, although considerations of life extension, such as with left main coronary artery disease, may apply as well.

Myocardial Infarction
Myocardial infarction is often a subtle event in the elderly. An uncertain but probably high percentage of myocardial infarctions are "silent" or, at least, pain-free. It may present as sudden left ventricular failure, shock, mental confusion, somnolence, or change in state of awareness. The diagnosis is thus frequently missed, perhaps accounting for the high incidence of myocardial rupture that results from failure to control the patient's activity.

Elderly patients are sensitive to the toxic effects of opiates like morphine and barbiturates. They are somewhat more prone to thromboembolic phenomena, and the utilization of low-dose heparin should be routinely considered. The elderly should be treated in coronary care units, but with the realization that they frequently become disoriented in totally unfamiliar surroundings. One should not, however, ascribe changes in mentation to the "CCU syndrome" or "sundowning syndrome" (i.e., disorientation due to the sensory deprivation and strange surroundings of a coronary care unit) without carefully considering adverse drug reactions and other causes of delirium common in the elderly.

Congestive Heart Failure

Congestive heart failure, an extremely common problem in elderly people, prompted the introduction of the concept of "presbycardia" or "senile heart disease" several decades ago. Actually, the commonest cause of congestive failure in elderly patients is not aging but is the same as that of heart disease in younger patients—largely hypertension or coronary artery disease, or both.

The symptoms of heart failure are often atypical. Many of the more elderly patients may complain only of nocturnal cough, insomnia, nocturia, irritability, and mental confusion. The true nature of the problem will become apparent when they are noted to be tachypneic with tachycardia, S_3, cardiomegaly, moist rales, and edema.

Among the causes of congestive heart failure are several "curable" ones. Thyrotoxicosis may present as an "apathetic syndrome" with little evidence of hypermetabolism; rapid atrial fibrillation that is difficult to control and slight enlargement of the thyroid may be the only clues. Myxedema likewise is usually quite subtle in its presentation; all elderly patients with heart failure should have a profile of thyroid activity.

The most common cause of congestive heart failure in the elderly is undetected or poorly managed hypertension and is, therefore, preventable. Treatment of hypertension in the patient who has developed congestive failure may prevent progression, but by and large, the damage is done and the myocardium will not recover fully. Coronary artery disease, most often following myocardial infarction, is the other common cause of congestive heart failure. Although prevention of progression with control of risk factors—such as hypercholesterolemia, hypertension, smoking, diabetes, and exercise—is important, once heart failure has supervened, survival is largely determined by the degree of deterioration in myocardial function.

Aortic Valvular Disease

Aortic stenosis is more frequent in the elderly than is usually thought, and it is a surgically correctable cause of heart disease. Older patients with a systolic murmur at the base of the heart are likely to have some degree of aortic stenosis. It may lack the typical features of radiation into the neck and a crescendo/decrescendo ejection murmur. The louder murmurs (grades 4 to 6) and those with an associated palpable thrill are more likely to be hemodynamically significant.

Valves that ultimately prove to obstruct outflow significantly almost always exhibit calcification by radiography or fluoroscopy, and most patients will have ventricular hypertrophy by electrocardiography.

Patients with far-advanced disease may have seemingly trivial murmurs, and the usually reliable alterations in the peripheral pulse may be absent in the elderly because of changes in vascular elasticity. Age does not contraindicate surgery. Even patients with depressed ejection fractions must be thoughtfully considered for surgery if relief of a hemodynamically significant outflow obstruction could improve cardiac output and ejection fraction.

COMPLICATIONS AND MANAGEMENT OF HEART FAILURE

Infection
In elderly patients with congestive heart failure, even trivial infections may have serious consequences. Influenza and pneumonia should be considered life-threatening infections. Appropriate immunization, amantidine if influenza supervenes, and aggressive treatment of all respiratory infections are essential for proper management of the elderly cardiac patient.

Vascular Occlusion
Congestive heart failure itself is a risk factor for thrombophlebitis, pulmonary embolism, and thrombotic and embolic strokes. During the diuretic phase of treatment for heart failure, edematous patients are even more vulnerable to these thromboembolic complications; this may be related to the increase in blood viscosity and hematocrit associated with the rapid decrease in plasma volume that occurs. Some have advocated the use of low-dose heparin during this period of rapid diuresis, and perhaps restraint in the vigor of the diuresis is advisable if permitted by clinical circumstances.

The low-flow state associated with congestive failure coupled with atheroocclusive disease of the mesenteric vessels can result in bowel ischemia or infarction. The combination of abdominal pain and quiet abdomen in the elderly patient with cardiac disease should arouse suspicion. The stool is apt to be positive for blood, and radiographic examination of the abdomen may reveal dilated loops of bowel with "thumb-printing" of the bowel wall. Metabolic acidosis with an increased anion gap due to elevated blood lactic acid levels commonly accompanies this complication. The diagnosis must be confirmed angiographically. The only treatment is surgery if infarction has occurred; intraarterial vasodilators can be used if the bowel is thought to be viable.

Renal Failure

The kidneys in elderly cardiac patients are particularly vulnerable to nephrotoxic agents and decrements in renal blood flow. The vasoconstrictive state associated with congestive heart failure compounds this danger, and thus the addition of agents that ordinarily have an acceptable risk/benefit ratio now poses a considerable threat. For example, aminoglycoside therapy and agents affecting prostaglandin synthesis, such as nonsteroidal antiinflammatory agents, must be given with great care because of adverse effects on renal blood flow.

INFECTIVE ENDOCARDITIS

Subacute bacterial endocarditis (SBE) is most common in elderly patients. Because the symptoms, such as fatigability, asthenia, and change in mentation, are usually vague, the diagnosis may not be readily apparent. Fever and anemia might be the only manifestations, and the murmur is often ascribed to increased flow rather than valvular disease. Calcific aortic valvular deformity, usually not of hemodynamic significance, may be the site of origin for the thromboinfective vegetations, although they may develop on previously healthy valves. Preexisting rheumatic valvular disease as the substrate for SBE is becoming less common.

The declining number of postmortem examinations obtained by physicians may account for the seeming decrease in incidence of infective endocarditis, since, unfortunately, this is when the diagnosis is frequently made in the elderly.

SYSTOLIC MURMURS IN THE ELDERLY

The incidence of a systolic murmur in any group of elderly persons is probably no greater than 20 percent among well elderly living at home but is more than 60 percent in those who are institutionalized. There are no truly "normal" aging changes in the heart valves. Most murmurs at the base of the heart and many of those at the apex are due to aortic stenosis. Mild mitral insufficiency is well tolerated, permitting long survival, and thus is relatively common in elderly patients.

Although prolapse of the mitral valve is considered to be a disorder of young and middle-aged persons, it is encountered with some frequency among the elderly. It is not always clear whether this reflects survival with a benign condition or whether prolapse actually appears in later years in association with undetected heart disease, probably ischemic. The frequency of atrial fibrillation, cardiac enlargement, and infective endocarditis would suggest that it represents more than simple valvular prolapse without underlying myocardial disease. Asymmetric ventricular hypertrophy or idiopathic hypertrophic subaortic stenosis is seen in the elderly as often as in the young, with similar symptoms and physical findings. It is increasingly important that this diagnosis be made in elderly subjects who may be given drugs for other illnesses that increase the outflow obstruction by increasing cardiac contractility.

HEART BLOCK AND ARRHYTHMIAS

Heart block and symptomatic bradycardia, usually related to degenerative disease of the so-called cardiac skeleton, calcific aortic stenosis, calcification of the mitral annulus, strategically deposited amyloid, or coronary artery disease, occur frequently enough that pacemaker implantation in elderly patients has become relatively commonplace. When indicated, simple pacemakers should be satisfactory inasmuch as activity is more limited in elderly persons. However, if advanced congestive heart failure is also present, the use of simultaneous or sequential atrioventricular pacing may be salutary.

Patients with atrial fibrillation can be a management problem. If the ventricular response is slow without treatment, the fibrillation may be an escape phenomenon in a person with "sick sinus syndrome," and the slow response is indicative of associated disease in the atrioventricular node. If the ventricular response is difficult to control, thyrotoxicosis should be suspected. Cardioversion in young elderly patients should receive the same consideration as in those who are younger, but in persons who are truly of an advanced age the risk of anesthesia and subsequent long-term administration of quinidine may exceed the benefits. Chronic anticoagulation in patients who remain in atrial fibrillation poses a similar risk/benefit issue because of the great hazard of bleeding in persons subject to falls.

Ventricular premature beats should be managed as conservatively as possible. Complicated antiarrhythmic regimens are difficult for many noninstitutionalized elderly patients, and poor compliance may be riskier than no treatment.

ADVERSE CARDIAC DRUG REACTIONS

Cardioactive drugs comprise a major portion of elderly patients' multiple drug needs. Digitalis intoxication, it should be recalled, is the most common most important adverse drug reaction in the elderly. This is primarily due to their decreased lean body mass, altered body composition, and, most important, diminished renal function. There is suggestive evidence that the use of digitalis in elderly patients could exercise a negative effect on outcome, but this entire issue is blurred by factors such as variations in severity of illness, the presence or absence of atrial fibrillation, and the etiology of the heart disease. In the majority of elderly cardiac patients in normal sinus rhythm, digitalis probably can and should be withdrawn under observation or with careful follow-up, once compensation has been achieved. If digitalis is continued, lower doses and extreme care to avoid toxicity are mandatory. Diuretics should be administered carefully to avoid rapid intravascular volume depletion—which, in turn, may be associated with an increased incidence of strokes and pulmonary emboli. Potassium should not be routinely administered because of the danger of undetected hyporeninemic hypoaldosteronism and general intolerance to oral potassium, but serum concentration in the blood should be routinely monitored in order to avoid significant hypokalemia.

Some other major interactions and adverse effects include the following:

1. Quinidine-induced digoxin intoxication. This has recently received considerable attention and probably occurs with significant frequency.

2. Cimetidine-induced excessive beta-adrenergic blockade with propranolol. This is related to interference with hepatic drug metabolism.

3. Salt retention. This may be induced by vasodilator drugs and by nonsteroidal antiinflammatory agents (prostaglandin inhibitors).

4. Renal failure induced by nonsteroidal antiinflammatory agents in patients with marginal renal perfusion.

5. Digitalis-reduced mesenteric blood flow.

6. Potassium or potassium-conserving diuretics administered to elderly diabetics with undetected—or unperceived—hyporeninemic hypoaldosteronism. This can cause lethal hyperkalemia.

In addition, changes in mentation or new and unexpected symptoms, such as "digitalis delirium," should be regarded seriously as potential adverse drug effects.

SUMMARY

In this chapter I have attempted to present those features of cardio-vascular disease in elderly patients that distinguish them from similiar disorders in younger individuals. The most characteristic feature of the aging process is lack of reserve and vulnerability to stress; on the other hand, the elderly are probably biologically advantaged and possessed of an inner toughness and ability to overcome adversity.

Common disorders may present in an uncommon fashion in the elderly, and uncommon disorders may be difficult to perceive among the more common problems. Age alone is a rare contraindication to a treatment modality; the pitfalls may be more frequent but are still by and large avoidable. Convalescence is often more protracted for the elderly, and great patience is required on the part of both patient and physician.

One must guard against therapeutic nihilism or token care. Grave circumspection is essential before writing a "do not resuscitate" order or before discontinuing needed treatment. The patient may have a misperception of what can be gained and may demand cessation of treatment when cure is feasible. The wishes of the family must be carefully weighed, because there may be complicated relationships and motives that are counter to the patient's well-being.

SUGGESTED READING

1. Finegan, R.E., Granelli, R.E., Harrison, D.C. Aortic stenosis in the elderly. *N. Engl. J. Med.* 81:1261–1264, 1969.
2. Howell, T.H. Cardiac murmurs in old age: A clinico-pathological study. *J. Am. Geriatr. Soc.* 15:509–516, 1967.
3. Landowne, M., Branfonbrenner, M., Shock, N.W. The relation of age to certain measures of performance of the heart and circulation. *Circulation* 12:567–576, 1955.
4. Weisfeldt, M.L. *The Aging Heart.* New York: Raven Press, 1980.

Treatment of Angina and Arrhythmias in the Elderly

PETER GAL, PHARM.D., and
JACK D. McCUE, M.D.

Editor's note: Cardiovascular agents effective in the treatment of angina and arrhythmias must be used with care in elderly patients, who have a decreased cardiac reserve and a stiff vascular system that makes them prone to orthostatic hypotension. The goals of treatment must also take into account the decreased physical activity of the elderly (hence the lessened need for treatment) and the often prohibitive expense of the drugs.

The diagnosis of angina in elderly people is confounded by atypical presentations (e.g., dyspnea, weakness, or dizziness) and by the frequent occurrence of noncardiac chest pain due to diseases of the chest wall and gastrointestinal tract. Exercise testing to verify the diagnosis is difficult to perform because of musculoskeletal problems and lack of stamina. Once the diagnosis of angina has been made, cautious consideration of the various therapeutic agents that might be used is necessary since the benefits of treatment, especially since the diagnosis is often uncertain, are not as clear as for younger, more active patients.

The goals of antianginal therapy are to increase coronary blood flow or decrease myocardial work and oxygen demand by reducing left ventricular wall tension, heart rate, and peripheral resistance. The selection of an agent involves consideration of several factors: (1) the type of angina (i.e., stable vs. unstable vs. Prinzmetal's angina); (2) the presence of intercurrent vascular insufficiency elsewhere (e.g., intermittent claudication or Raynaud's phenomenon); (3) the convenience of the dosing schedule; (4) the pharmacologic and adverse effects of the individual medication; (5) concurrent diseases (e.g., chronic lung disease); and (6) cost.

The widespread effects of these various agents on illnesses and

143

TABLE 1

Interaction of Antianginal Agents with Other Disease States

Disease State	NTG	Beta-Blockers[a]			CCBs	
		Propranolol	Metoprolol	Pindolol	Verapamil	Nifedipine
Angina	+2	+2	+2	+2	+2	+2
Congestive heart failure	+1	−2	−2	0	+1	+1
Peripheral vascular disease	+1	−2	−1	0	+2	+2
Hypertension	+1	+2	+2	+2	+2	+2
Diabetes	0	−2	−1	−1	0	−1
Asthma	0	−2	−1	0	+1	+1
Migraine	0	+2	+2	+2	+1	+/−
Tremor	0	+2	+2	+1	−1	−1
Anxiety	−1	+1	+1	0	−1	−1
Hyperthyroidism	0	+2	+2	?	0	0

+2 = good therapeutic effect; +1 = moderate therapeutic effect; 0 = no effect; −1 = moderate aderse effect; −2 = significant adverse effect. NTG = nitroglycerin; CCBs = calcium channel blockers.

[a]Representative beta-blocking agents are listed: propranolol is a nonspecific blocker, metoprolol is a beta₁ specific blocker (but loses specificity above 100 mg/day), and pindolol is a beta-agonist antagonist. See Table 4 (p. 148) for a description of other beta-blockers.

diseases common in the elderly are displayed in Table 1. Drugs available for the treatment of angina include nitrates, beta-blockers, and calcium antagonists. Nitrates and beta-blockers reduce myocardial oxygen demand, while calcium antagonists both diminish demand and increase the supply of myocardial oxygen.

NITRATES

Nitrates are available in rapid-onset, short-acting sublingual preparations used for acute relief of anginal pain, and in longer-acting tablets and topical preparations used to prevent attacks of angina. The available preparations are listed in Tables 2 and 3. Familiarity with only one of each type of preparation is generally necessary for the primary care practitioner; differences in the efficacy of the available preparations are, as yet, lacking.

The short-acting sublingual nitrate of choice is still clearly nitroglycerin (NTG). It acts more rapidly than other sublingual forms and is less expensive. Its shorter duration of action makes it preferable to longer-acting agents for the acute treatment of angina.

TABLE 2

Available Oral and Sublingual Nitrate Preparations

Type of Tablet	Trade Name	Strengths	Average Dose (range)	Wholesale Cost[a]
Sublingual Tablets				
Nitroglycerin	—	1/100, 1/150, 1/200	1/150 p.r.n.	$2.17/100
Isosorbide dinitrate	Isordil, Sorbitrate	2.5, 5 mg	2.5 mg p.r.n.	$6.67/100
Erythrityl tetranitrate	Cardilate	5, 10, 15 mg	10 mg p.r.n.	$4.13/100
Oral Tablets				
Isosorbide dinitrate	Isordil, Sorbitrate	5, 10, 20, 30 mg	20 mg q.i.d. (5–30 mg)	$0.52/day
Erythrityl tetranitrate	Cardilate	5, 10, 15 mg	10 mg q.4h. (5–15 mg)	$0.37/day
Pentaerythritol tetranitrate	Peritrate	10, 20, 40 mg	20 mg q.i.d.	$0.31/day
Long-Acting Tablets				
Nitroglycerin	Nitro-Bid (Caps)	2.5, 6.5, 9 mg	6.5 mg b.i.d.	$0.36/day
Isosorbide dinitrate	Isordil, Tembids	40 mg	40 mg q.i.d.	$0.61/day
Pentaerythritol tetranitrate	Peritrate SA	80 mg	80 mg b.i.d.	$0.37/day

[a]From 1983 Bluebook, AWP prices. Patient cost is usually about wholesale cost plus 60 to 100 percent.

The preventive treatment of angina requires longer-acting tablets or transdermal preparations. Generally the cheapest and simplest regimen is the use of a transdermal NTG preparation, shown to maintain constant serum NTG concentrations for at least 24 hours. With these preparations the skin's outermost surface, the stratum corneum, controls the rate of drug absorption, so they should not be used on damaged or irritated skin.

Three transdermal nitroglycerin preparations are currently available: Nitro-Dur, Transderm-Nitro, and Nitrodisc. Transderm-Nitro and Nitro-Dur actually contain excess NTG beyond that required for 24 hours, and could clearly provide good serum NTG levels for two to four days. If the patient can tolerate having the patch in the same place for several days, the cost of transdermal NTG could be reduced to below 50 cents per day. For patients with skin sensitivity to tape, Nitro-Dur uses tape that is less likely to irritate the skin. The transdermal units should be applied to a hairless area of skin, avoiding scars, skin folds, or wounds.

TABLE 3
Transdermal Nitroglycerin Systems

Product (Mfr.)	Product Surface Area (cm²)	NTG Content (mg)	NTG Delivered Over 24 Hours (mg)	Cost per Day[a]
Transderm-Nitro 5 (CIBA)	10	25	5.0	$0.96
Transderm-Nitro 10 (CIBA)	20	50	10.0	$1.06
Nitro-Dur 5 (Key)	5	26	2.5	$0.84
Nitro-Dur 10 (Key)	10	51	5.0	$0.87
Nitro-Dur 15 (Key)	15	77	7.5	$0.90
Nitro-Dur 20 (Key)	20	104	10.0	$0.94
Nitrodisc 16 (Searle)	5	16	5.0	$0.90
Nitrodisc 32 (Searle)	10	32	10.0	$0.96

[a]Wholesale cost from 1983 Bluebook, AWP prices. Patient cost usually equals AWP cost plus 60 to 100 percent.

Side effects from nitrate therapy are the same as for younger patients and are generally transient. Particularly important is orthostatic hypotension, which is often already a problem in the elderly. The use of NTG patches should not be abruptly discontinued to avoid the possible precipitation of angina symptoms or even a myocardial infarction. For unstable patients, it is best to put the new NTG patch in place before removing the used patch. Used patches, incidentally, must be removed each time a new patch is placed, because they continue to release NTG for five to seven days. Note that Nitro-Dur 10 has the same amount of NTG as Transderm-Nitro 5 (see Table 2), so switching preparations must be done with caution.

Adhesion of the Transderm-Nitro system may be poor in the elderly, and the patches have been observed to fall off the skin of nursing home patients. Nitro-Dur, on the other hand, may adhere too strongly, thus damaging or tearing the fragile skin of some elderly patients. This problem may be avoided if lotion is rubbed over the adhesive part of the patch and allowed to stand for 30 minutes before the patch is removed. When these problems arise, NTG ointment may be the preferred topical nitrate.

BETA-ADRENERGIC BLOCKERS

Three types of beta-blockers are available: nonspecific blockers that affect both beta$_1$ and beta$_2$ adrenergic receptor sites; cardioselective blockers that block only beta$_1$ receptors; and those with intrinsic sympathomimetic activity (agonist-antagonists) that both block and stimulate the beta receptors. These agents are summarized in Table 4.

One might expect problems with beta-blockers in elderly patients, since they have been observed to have a diminished beta-receptor response. More important, elderly patients have diminished cardiac contractile reserve and must rely more on beta-adrenergic drive during stress. Hence beta blockade can result in cardiac failure, especially during stressful illnesses such as pneumonia.

Reduced peripheral blood flow in patients with peripheral vascular disease is particularly a problem with nonspecific beta-blockers because unchallenged alpha-adrenergic activity results in vasoconstriction, with subsequent worsening of intermittent claudication or Raynaud's disease. Prinzmetal's angina may also be adversely affected by beta-blockers by a similar mechanism. Long-term use of beta-blockers results in impaired glucose tolerance and may cause some elderly persons to receive treatment for diabetes when they might otherwise be controlled by diet.

Important adverse central nervous system (CNS) reactions include drowsiness, fatigue, hallucinations, vivid dreams, and depression. They occur most frequently with the preparations that readily cross the blood-brain barrier (e.g., propranolol) and least commonly with preparations that have lower CNS penetration (e.g., atenolol). Other adverse effects are similar to those in younger patients, for example, worsening of chronic lung disease or asthma. Finally, as with younger patients, when beta-blockers are being discontinued they should be tapered to avoid rebound angina or an acute myocardial infarction.

None of the three categories of beta-blockers appears superior to the others in preventing anginal episodes. The maximally effective dose of beta-blockers can be gauged by exercise heart rate, the usual goal being to maintain the heart rate below 100 beats per minute after exercise. The resting heart rate is a poor indicator of beta blockade because the major determinant of resting heart rate is para-

TABLE 4
Summary of Beta-Blocking Agents

Generic Name	Trade Name[a]	Nonselective Blocker	Selective Beta₁-Blocker	Beta Stimulant	CNS Penetration	Daily Dose (mg)	Dose for Cost Calculation (mg)	Daily Cost
			Activity					
Propranolol	Inderal	+	−	−	High	40–960	160	$0.47
Alprenolol	NA	+	−	+	High	400–800	—	—
Nadolol	Corgard	+	−	−	Low	40–560	160	$1.21
Oxprenolol	NA	+	−	+	High	40	1200	—
Pindolol	Visken	+	−	++	Low	2.5–60	20	$0.43
Timolol	Blocadren	+	−	−	Low	15–60	30	$0.67
Sotalol	NA	+	−	−	Low	80–480	—	—
Metoprolol	Lopressor	−	+	−	Low	50–450	100	$0.28
Acebutolol	NA	−	+	+	Moderate	200–1200	—	—
Atenolol	Tenormin	−	+	−	Lowest	50–200	100	$0.67

− = no effect; + = moderate activity; ++ = strong activity.
[a]NA = not currently available.

TABLE 5
Calcium Channel Blockers

Generic Name	Trade Name	Vasodilator	Cardiac Depression	Daily Dose (mg)	Dose for Cost Calculation (mg)	Daily Cost
		Activity				
Nifedipine	Procardia	+++	+/−	40–160	80	$1.66
Verapamil	Isoptin	++	++	160–480	320	$0.82
Diltiazem	Cardizem	+	+	90–240	180	$1.20

+ = mild activity; ++ = moderate activity; +++ = strong activity; − = no effect.

sympathetic activity, not the sympathetic activity that is affected by beta-blockers.

In general, beta-blockers are best avoided in the elderly. When they are used, special attention must be given to toxicity and effects on concurrent diseases.

CALCIUM CHANNEL BLOCKERS

Calcium channel blockers (CCBs) are a relatively new pharmacologic class of drugs (Table 5). The three agents currently available, verapamil, nifedipine, and diltiazem, are chemically unrelated. Some of the numerous excellent reviews on these drugs state that these agents are now the drugs of choice for treating angina, especially vasospastic angina. While all three agents appear to be equally effective for the treatment of angina, they have pharmacologic differences that affect their indications.

Verapamil inhibits the sodium-dependent fast inward current (diltiazem also does this, but only at higher doses), accounting for its efficacy in treating supraventricular tachyarrhythmias. Its negative inotropic effect, on the other hand, may cause heart failure. The risk of heart failure is further increased when verapamil is combined with a beta-blocker, and this combination is best avoided in the elderly, who have a diminished cardiac reserve. Constipation occurs more frequently as a side effect than with other CCBs. Nifedipine is the most potent vasodilator of the CCBs and consequently causes orthostatic hypotension, which may be intolerable for elderly patients. Ankle or leg edema due to peripheral vasodilation, rather than heart failure, may also occur.

The problem of impaired glucose tolerance noted with beta-blockers also occurs with CCBs, although it is usually of a lesser degree. Nifedipine reduces insulin secretion in response to an oral glucose load in both nondiabetics and patients with non-insulin-dependent diabetes mellitus. One study of verapamil found no decreased insulin secretion,[1] so verapamil may be preferable for elderly patients with diet-controlled diabetes; the role of diltiazem for these patients is unknown. Both verapamil and nifedipine have been reported to raise

---

1. D.E.H. Andersson, S. Röjdmark. Improvement of glucose tolerance by verapamil in patients with non-insulin-dependent diabetes mellitus. *Acta Med. Scand.* 210:27–33, 1981.

serum digoxin concentrations as much as 50 to 80 percent and may predispose to digitalis toxicity.

TREATMENT OF ARRHYTHMIAS

Arrhythmias (affecting up to one-third of nursing-home patients) are caused by a variety of diseases and stresses and are often best managed by treating the underlying etiology (e.g., angina, pneumonia, hypokalemia, anxiety). Other asymptomatic rhythm disturbances, such as unifocal atrial, nodal, or ventricular premature beats, or those due to chronic obstructive lung disease which are not causing symptoms may not require treatment at all. The selection of antiarrhythmics is limited; the choice depends not only on the type of arrhythmia but also on the toxicity and cost of the different agents.

Atrial tachycardia and atrial fibrillation are still best managed with digitalis. The addition of a beta-blocker, quinidine, or verapamil may be useful in refractory cases. The least expensive choice is a beta-blocker; unlike quinidine and verapamil, beta-blockers do not elevate the digoxin level.

Procainamide and quinidine are generally considered the agents of choice for ventricular arrhythmias. Both can cause significant toxicity, and neither appears safer in elderly patients. Careful monitoring of blood levels is necessary with both agents to assure adequate antiarrhythmic effect and avoid toxicity. For quinidine the optimum plasma concentration range appears to be about 3 to 8 μg/ml. Active metabolites are not measured with current assays for quinidine; in patients with renal failure these may accumulate and cause toxicity at apparently safe quinidine levels. Procainamide has a reported therapeutic range of 4 to 12 μg/ml, although in some cases higher levels may be used. The active metabolite, *N*-acetylprocainamide (NAPA), should also be assayed since it may accumulate in elderly patients with compromised renal function.

The long-acting quinidine and procainamide preparations are easier to dose because they give effective serum levels for 8 to 12 hours. Possible poor bioavailability with sustained-release forms of both preparations in older patients with heart disease, however, requires careful monitoring of serum levels. An important consideration with these antiarrhythmic drugs is cost, which often exceeds $1,000 annually for either drug.

Disopyramide (Norpace) is an effective antiarrhythmic, but its adverse effects may make its use in elderly patients too risky. It causes congestive heart failure in a large percentage of patients with heart disease, and its potent anticholinergic properties may cause urinary retention, CNS symptoms, and orthostatic hypotension.

Phenytoin (Dilantin) is usually considered a weak antiarrhythmic, primarily useful in the treatment of digitalis toxicity or as an adjunct to other antiarrhythmics. Nevertheless, some patients will have a therapeutic response to phenytoin alone when blood levels between 10 and 20 µg/ml are achieved. The major advantages of phenytoin are that it can be given as a single bedtime dose to most patients and that treatment will cost less than $200 per year for most patients.

Beta-blockers may also be useful for treatment of arrhythmias, but most elderly patients experience intolerable or troublesome adverse effects. Their primary role is as adjunctive therapy for other antiarrhythmics and as arrhythmia prophylaxis after an acute myocardial infarction.

SUGGESTED READING

1. Andersson, D.E.H., Röjdmark, S. Improvement of glucose tolerance by verapamil in patients with non-insulin-dependent diabetes mellitus. *Acta Med. Scand.* 210:27–33, 1981.
2. Black. C.D. Transdermal drug delivery systems. *U.S. Pharmacist* 49–75, 1982.
3. Brown, J.E., Shand, D.B. Therapeutic drug monitoring of antiarrhythmic drugs. *Clin. Pharmacokinet.* 7:125–148, 1982.
4. Charlap, S., Frishman, W.H. Comparative effects of verapamil and beta-blockers in the therapy for patients with stable angina pectoris. *Cardiovasc. Rev. Reports* 4:66–80, 1983.
5. Federman, J., Vlietstra, R.E. Antiarrhythmic drug therapy. *Mayo Clin. Proc.* 54:531–542, 1979.
6. Leonard, R.G., Talbert, R.L. Calcium-channel blocking drugs. *Clin. Pharmacokinet.* 1:17–33, 1982.
7. Mautner, R.K., Phillips, J.H., Katz, G.E. Managing coronary spasm in the elderly—a new way to prevent MI? *Geriatrics* 36(10):40–48, 1981.
8. Moses, O.W., Borer, J.S. Beta adrenergic antagonists in the treatment of patients with heart disease. *DM* 27:7–61, 1981.
9. Scheidt, S.S. Angina pectoris: Pathophysiology, precipitating factors, prognosis, and therapy. *Cardiovasc. Rev. Reports* 4:83–99, 1983.
10. Schwartz, J.B., et al. Adverse effects of antiarrhythmics. *Drugs* 21:23–45, 1981.

Evaluating Syncope

WISHWA N. KAPOOR, M.D.,
DAVID MARTIN, M.D., and
MICHAEL KARPF, M.D.

Editor's note: The high mortality associated with cardiac syncope contrasts sharply with the low mortality of idiopathic syncope. The morbidity of both, however, through falls and the development of a fear of independent living, is potentially great. The expense of an extensive evaluation can often be avoided with the use of a commonsense protocol that optimizes the findings of a careful history and physical examination.

Syncope, a temporary loss of consciousness associated with loss of postural tone, is a common problem in the geriatric population. Appropriate therapy, based on a diagnosis of the underlying cause of syncope, not only can prevent recurrences but also could reduce mortality and prevent serious complications such as trauma from falls, household accidents, and loss of independence because of fear of fainting.

The spectrum of the diseases that cause syncope ranges from common benign problems to severe life-threatening disorders (Table 1). Vasodepressor or situational syncope (e.g., syncope resulting from fear or anxiety, heat, or related to venipuncture) may require only limited assessment. More serious causes of syncope (e.g., cardiovascular or cerebrovascular disease) may require extensive in-hospital evaluation to establish a definitive cause. Physicians are frequently confronted with elderly patients whose usual initial evaluation screen after a syncopal episode (history, physical examination, electrocardiogram, routine blood chemistries) is not helpful in resolving the complex differential diagnosis. Preexisting cardiac, arterial, central nervous system, or metabolic diseases and medications that could be responsible for the syncopal symptoms often compound the diagnostic difficulties. Because geriatric patients do not tolerate the prolonged hospitalizations often needed to sort out a complex differential

152

TABLE 1
Causes of Syncope

1. Vasodepressor (vasovagal)
2. Situational syncope
   Micturition syncope
   Defecation syncope
   Cough and Valsalva syncope
   Swallow syncope
3. Syncope due to orthostatic hypotension
   Idiopathic postural hypotension and Shy-Drager syndrome
   Secondary causes of orthostatic hypotension
4. Reduced cardiac output
   Obstruction to left ventricular outflow: aortic stenosis and hypertrophic
     subaortic stenosis
   Obstruction to pulmonary flow: pulmonic stenosis, pulmonary hypertension,
     pulmonary embolism
   Pump failure: massive myocardial infarct
   Cardiac tamponade
   Atrial myxoma, ball valve thrombus
5. Arrhythmias
   a. Bradyarrhythmias
      Second- and third-degree AV block
      Ventricular asystole
      Sick sinus syndrome
      Carotid sinus syncope
      Glossopharyngeal neuralgia
   b. Tachyarrhythmias
      Ventricular tachycardia
      Supraventricular tachycardia
6. Cerebrovascular disease (syncope is an uncommon presenting feature)
   Subclavian steal syndrome
   Takayasu's disease
   Diffuse extracranial vascular insufficiency
   Cerebral vasculitis

AV = atrioventricular.

diagnosis and because they are at substantial risk when subjected to invasive diagnostic procedures, we systematically investigated the utility of the various diagnostic studies used in the workup of syncope (Table 2) to develop a goal-directed diagnostic strategy (Fig. 1) that avoids unnecessary hospitalizations and procedures.

DIAGNOSTIC METHODS

History and Physical Examination
An invaluable first step in investigating the cause of syncope is to obtain a meticulous history and physical examination. Vasovagal syn-

TABLE 2
Commonly Employed Diagnostic Procedures

1. History and physical examination
2. Carotid sinus massage
3. Electrocardiogram (ECG)
4. Prolonged cardiac monitoring (Holter) or telemetry
5. Electrophysiologic studies (EPS)
6. Echocardiogram (ECG)
7. Cardiac catheterization
8. Electroencephalogram (EEG)
9. Head computed tomography (CT) scan
10. Brain scan
11. Cerebral angiography
12. Glucose tolerance test (GTT)

cope, more common in younger patients but also occurring in the elderly, is frequently diagnosed on historical grounds alone. It usually occurs in the standing position and has up to several minutes of prodromal features, including weakness, pallor, sweating, nausea, increased gastrointestinal peristalsis, yawning, belching, and dimming of vision. Loss of consciousness is associated with hypotension and bradycardia. If the patient is kept recumbent, the blood pressure, pulse, and mental status return to normal within minutes. Unless an obvious precipitating factor is present, however, syncope should not be attributed to a vasovagal attack; alternate causes for the symptom should be investigated. Some types of situational syncope can only be diagnosed by a careful history and physical examination—for example, syncope ascribed to swallowing or deglutition, heat, tight girdles, television viewing, coughing, and micturition or defecation. These are important diagnoses, since an appropriate history may eliminate the need for extensive diagnostic testing. The incidence, etiology, and significance of these forms of syncope are not well known.

Some bits of historical information are useful in limiting or enlarging the differential diagnosis. For example, syncope with exertion is classically described in severe aortic stenosis but may also occur with hypertrophic cardiomyopathy, pulmonary hypertension, and cyanotic congenital heart disease. Syncope associated with lateral movement of the head may indicate carotid sinus hypersensitivity or a mechanical obstruction such as a cervical rib. Arm exercise that induces syncope may indicate the presence of a subclavian steal syndrome.

FIGURE 1

A schematic diagnostic approach to the evaluation of syncope. EEG = *electroencephalogram;* EPS = *electrophysiologic study;* + = *positive;* − = *negative.*

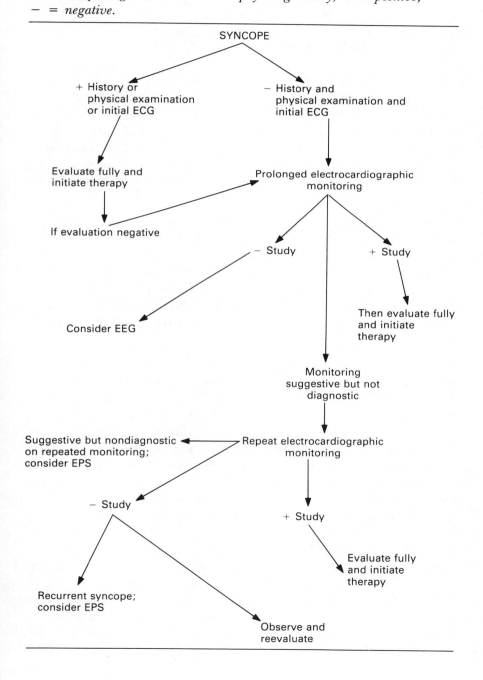

A complete medication history is essential, since diuretics and antihypertensive drugs are well-recognized causes of orthostatic hypotension. Antiarrhythmic drugs such as quinidine, procainamide, and disopyramide are known to produce a prolonged QT interval thus predisposing to ventricular tachycardia (known as torsades de pointes) and resulting in recurrent syncopal episodes.

The physical examination may narrow the search for a cause of syncope. Finding symptomatic postural hypotension suggests drug toxicity, volume depletion, or neuropathy. A significant difference in the pulse and blood pressure in both arms is suggestive of a subclavian steal syndrome. Auscultatory cardiovascular findings may be suggestive of aortic stenosis, asymmetric septal hypertrophy, pulmonary hypertension, or congenital heart disease, and neurologic findings may help focus the evaluation on the central nervous system.

Electrocardiogram

An electrocardiogram (ECG) is essential in the diagnostic evaluation of syncope, especially if the initial history and physical examination do not disclose a definite etiology. The incidence of diagnostic abnormalities on an initial ECG is low, but when found, they can eliminate the need for extensive further evaluation. Significant findings derived from both the initial ECG and prolonged electrocardiographic monitoring are similar; these findings are discussed in the following section.

Prolonged Electrocardiographic Monitoring

Electrocardiographic monitoring is indicated when the initial evaluation including an ECG is suggestive, but not diagnostic, of an arrhythmia or a conduction disturbance as the cause of syncope, or if no etiology can be determined from the initial evaluation. However, because cardiac electrical abnormalities may be episodic, they may not be detected on a single 24-hour monitor recording, and brief episodes of bradyarrhythmias and tachyarrhythmias may or may not cause symptoms (dizziness, syncope, palpitations, chest pain) during monitoring. Despite these shortcomings, we found that prolonged electrocardiographic monitoring is the single most useful diagnostic test in the evaluation of syncope of unknown origin. The information derived from monitoring can be classified in the following manner.

1. *Syncope with transient asymptomatic serious arrhythmias.* Because the majority of patients with syncope have no complaints during the monitoring period, extrapolations often need to be made from monitor findings during asymptomatic periods. Tran-

sient sinus arrests of greater than 2 seconds are rarely seen in normal asymptomatic individuals; consequently, pauses of greater than 2 seconds in a patient with syncope should be considered indicative of sinus node dysfunction. Brief runs of supraventricular tachycardia, on the other hand, have been reported in up to 50 percent of the normal population and thus cannot be considered as the cause of syncope unless they are sustained or accompanied by alterations of consciousness. Similarly, severe sinus bradycardia (<40 beats per minute) has been noted in approximately 25 percent of normal adults undergoing 24-hour Holter monitoring. Thus, discovery of asymptomatic bradycardia may not reflect the cause of syncope.

Supraventricular extrasystoles and premature ventricular extrasystoles (reported in 50 to 75 percent of males) are not helpful in the diagnosis of syncope. Even frequent (>60 per hour) bigeminal, trigeminal, or multiform ventricular extrasystoles, while uncommon in the normal population, should not be considered the cause of syncope unless they are associated with symptoms. An episode of sustained ventricular tachycardia should be considered as the cause of syncope, but when such episodes are isolated and brief (three to five beats), further monitoring is needed to determine whether more prolonged episodes are present.

First-degree atrioventricular (AV) block and Mobitz I AV block also cannot be implicated in the cause of syncope. Mobitz II block, however, is so rarely seen in normal individuals that, when present, it should be considered as the probable cause of syncope. Obviously, third-degree AV block in a patient with syncope should be assumed to be the cause. While the findings of a unifascicular block on Holter monitoring also do not help to define the cause of syncope, patients with chronic or intermittent bifascicular block may require further evaluation, perhaps including electrophysiologic studies.

2. *Exclusion of cardiac arrhythmias.* Rarely, monitoring may exclude arrhythmias when the patient has syncope with a normal cardiac rhythm. The mere absence of arrhythmias in an asymptomatic period of monitoring does not, of course, exclude intermittent arrhythmias.

Electrophysiologic Studies
Electrophysiologic studies (EPS), including His bundle ECGs, measurement of sinus node recovery time, and attempted induction of ventricular tachycardia, are now commonly done in patients who have ECG or Holter monitor findings that suggest a conduction distur-

bance or arrhythmia as the cause of syncope. In some centers all patients with syncope of unknown origin, even those without suggestive monitoring results, undergo EPS. These procedures require a specialized facility, as well as an experienced cardiologist, and their indications and the utility of results obtained are still controversial. They may be indicated for patients with the following conditions:

1. Recurrent syncope with severe sinus bradycardia (rate <40) to document prolonged sinus node recovery time as evidence for sick sinus syndrome. For this purpose, the test seems to have low sensitivity (40 to 60 percent).

2. Syncope of unknown origin (after thorough evaluation) when bifascicular block is documented on an ECG.

3. Recurrent syncope of unknown origin.

Echocardiography and Cardiac Catheterization
Echocardiography and cardiac catheterization should be reserved for patients with suggestive physical findings and should *not* be a routine part of the evaluation of syncope. They do not in themselves establish the cause of syncope but can be helpful in defining the significance of abnormalities already detected on initial clinical evaluation. As an example, a patient with syncope and the murmur of aortic stenosis may require an echocardiogram to define better the evidence for aortic stenosis and then a cardiac catheterization to assess the hemodynamic significance of the aortic stenosis.

Carotid Sinus Massage
Carotid massage should be performed in elderly patients only if other diagnostic studies have not been helpful, because transient and permanent neurologic deficits have rarely been precipitated by this maneuver. The test is initially performed with the patient in the supine position and then repeated, if necessary, in the sitting and standing position, with electrocardiographic monitoring and frequent blood pressure checks. A sinus pause of 3 seconds or more or a decrease in systolic pressure of more than 50 mm Hg with no significant pulse decrease is a positive test, diagnostic of a hypersensitive carotid sinus. Cardiac asystole lasting 2 seconds or a decrease of 30 mm Hg in systolic pressure is a borderline response.

Although elderly patients frequently have hyperactive carotid sinus reflexes, the carotid sinus syncope is a rare condition that occurs in only 5 to 20 percent of persons with a hyperactive reflex; it occurs more often in men than women and is most frequent in the seventh and eighth decades. In most patients a trigger mechanism cannot be demonstrated, but in some patients hyperextension of the neck, head turning, tight collars, carrying shoulder loads, or other postural changes lead to syncope. Occasionally thyroid tumors, carotid body tumors, inflammatory and malignant lymph nodes, and drugs such as digoxin, propranolol, and methyldopa may precipitate carotid sinus syncope. The unequivocal diagnosis of carotid sinus syncope is difficult to establish, but attempts are probably justified in those individuals with a hyperactive carotid sinus reflex whose syncope is clearly related to activities that might press on or stretch the sinus.

Electroencephalography, Brain Scans, Computed Tomography
Scans, and Angiography
The differential diagnosis between syncope and a seizure disorder can occasionally be very difficult, especially if the episode was not witnessed. Electroencephalography is indicated when a seizure disorder is suspected, if there is a neurologic deficit on physical examination, or if the patient has recurrent syncope of unknown origin. If a focal abnormality is detected, further testing with computed tomography (CT) scan and angiography may then be needed.

To our knowledge there are no data available addressing the utility of brain scans and CT scans in the evaluation of syncope. The finding of cerebrovascular atherosclerotic disease on cerebral angiography or dilated ventricles by CT scan does not help to establish the cause of syncope, since such findings may be common in elderly asymptomatic patients. The diagnosis of subclavian steal syndrome requires angiography.

Glucose Tolerance Test
Hypoglycemia can lead to gradual mental changes but does not usually lead to true syncope. A 5-hour glucose tolerance test has no utility in the evaluation of the etiology of syncope.

EVALUATING THE INDIVIDUAL PATIENT

Our approach to the evaluation of patients with syncope is pragmatic and goal-directed (see Figure 1). We rely on a meticulous history and physical examination either to establish a diagnosis or to suggest potential etiologies that need further evaluation. For example, if a patient has situational syncope by history, we try to reproduce the symptoms. If this is successful, then further diagnostic workup is usually not necessary, and appropriate therapeutic measures can be taken. If a patient's history suggests a seizure disorder, we will obtain an electroencephalogram (EEG) first and then undertake further appropriate neurologic workup. In those patients with exertional syncope, our initial evaluation will center on resolving the differential diagnosis of that symptom.

If on physical examination the patient is found to have symptomatic orthostatic hypotension, our efforts will be directed at defining the cause and improving the orthostasis, and thereby hopefully alleviating the symptoms and explaining the syncopal episode. Certainly, patients with auscultatory findings of cardiovascular disease should undergo further evaluation with appropriate studies such as echocardiography, stress testing, or cardiac catheterization. Neurologic findings require an initial investigation of the central nervous system with CT scans, electroencephalography, and other appropriate studies.

At our institution, approximately 15 to 20 percent of patients who present with syncope will have a well-documented cause defined by history, physical examination, or initial ECG. Of the remainder of the patients who then have prolonged electrocardiographic monitoring either by telemetry or ambulatory (Holter) monitoring, approximately 20 percent have findings that suggest a cardiac cause of syncope. We consider doing an EPS only for patients with recurrent syncope and Holter monitoring that suggests sick sinus syndrome or a conduction system disease.

Patients in whom a diagnosis has still not been established are then periodically reevaluated for new clues as to the etiology of their recurrent episodes of syncope, and, if warranted, repetitive ambulatory monitoring is performed. Electrophysiologic studies and electroencephalography are probably justified in patients with multiple recurrences of syncope in whom a diagnosis cannot be established after a period of observation.

Utilizing this approach, we can diagnose a cause for syncope in approximately 50 percent of the patients. Less goal-directed protocols do not increase the diagnostic yield and can potentially increase the cost and duration of hospitalization.

PROGNOSIS OF SYNCOPE

Very little is known about the prognosis and the significance of syncope of unknown origin. We have now followed more than 200 patients prospectively over a one-year period in an attempt to define the natural history of this cohort. Overall, one-year mortality for our entire group of patients was approximately 15 percent. The mortality rate in the patients who were defined as having syncope of unknown origin was only about 3 percent; there are no data regarding the morbidity of syncope, however.

Syncope in patients with cardiovascular disease is associated with a very poor prognosis; 30 percent of our patients died in one year. These findings suggest that patients with cardiovascular disorders and syncope should be investigated aggressively, followed closely, and reevaluated frequently.

SUGGESTED READING

1. Friedberg, D.K. Syncope: Pathologic physiology, differential diagnosis and treatment. *Mod. Concepts Cardiovasc. Dis.* 40:55–63, 1971.
2. Kapoor, W., Karpf, M., Maher, Y., et al. Syncope of unknown origin: The need for a more cost-effective approach to its diagnostic evaluation. *J.A.M.A.* 247:2687–2691, 1982.
3. Kennedy, H.L., Caralis, D.G. Ambulatory electrocardiography: A clinical perspective. *Ann. Intern. Med.* 87:729–739, 1977.
4. Thomas, J.E. Hyperactive carotid sinus reflex and carotid sinus syncope. *Mayo Clin. Proc.* 44:127–139, 1969.
5. Vera, Z., Mason, D.T. Detection of sinus node dysfunction: Consideration of clinical application of testing methods. *Am. Heart J.* 102:308–312, 1981.
6. Wright, K.E., Jr., McIntosh, H.D. Syncope: A review of pathophysiological mechanisms. *Prog. Cardiovasc. Dis.* 13:580–594, 1971.

Hypertension

C. STEWART ROGERS, M.D.

Editor's note: We must reexamine the goals of treatment when hypertension is treated in the elderly. Long-term complications of the disease become less important than short-term ones, and the often worsened quality of life engendered by the use of drugs with disabling side effects may not justify tight control. Familiarity with our limited understanding of the proper treatment of systolic hypertension and its consequences is important for the generalist.

This chapter will address the features of the multisystem disease of clinical hypertension that are most relevant to geriatrics and will suggest an approach to management that combines a basic belief in the benefits of blood pressure control with a respect for the fragility of elderly patients. No attempt will be made to record yet again the enormous volumes of diagnostic and therapeutic information that are widely available.

SIGNIFICANCE OF ELEVATED BLOOD PRESSURE

It is well known that blood pressure rises with age (in Western cultures), but it is not so well appreciated that the prevalence of diastolic hypertension peaks in the sixth decade and actually declines slightly thereafter. Beyond this age the pulse pressure tends to widen, and the major pattern becomes that of systolic hypertension, pure or predominant. Diastolic hypertension (>95 mm Hg) affects 15 percent of older white and almost 30 percent of older black Americans, while an additional 30 percent and 40 percent, respectively, develop pure systolic hypertension.[1]

---

1. Defined conventionally as systolic pressure >160 mm Hg and diastolic pressure <95 mm Hg.

The Framingham Study, comparing risk factor levels (irrespective of treatment) with clinical outcomes over a follow-up period that now exceeds three decades, has clearly demonstrated the morbid effects of systolic and diastolic hypertension. In contrast to the exclusive focus on diastolic blood pressure in later intervention trials, the Framingham group has always highlighted systolic hypertension. As their initial cohort has aged, this study has had more and more to say about the isolated systolic pattern. Here, as with all hypertension, morbidity is striking.

Hypertension exacts four costs: (1) accelerated atherosclerosis leading to coronary and cerebrovascular disease; (2) arteriolar sclerosis affecting the retina and kidneys; (3) vascular mechanical events such as left ventricular failure, aortic dissection, and hemorrhagic stroke; and (4) the expense and morbidity of treatment. The first two generally result from decades of poor blood pressure control and may be less of a consideration for the elderly. Treatment goals in the elderly generally should be more immediate: preventing vascular morbidity at an acceptable cost.

There are special hemodynamic features of essential hypertension in the elderly that have important implications for therapy. Older hypertensive patients usually have compromised left ventricular function as a result of ischemia and increased afterload. Their central arteries are rigid from atherosclerosis and thus manifest poor compliance or a steep pressure rise during left ventricular emptying. These factors, together with a commonly contracted extracellular fluid (ECF) volume, lead to a hemodynamic profile of poor cardiac output, high peripheral resistance, and wide pulse pressure.

This profile forms the basis of the major argument against vigorous treatment of systolic hypertension in the elderly. Reversing the usual concept that high blood pressure accelerates atherosclerosis, this argument holds that established vascular disease is the basis for the high systolic pressure, which cannot be effectively treated without eliminating the underlying mural plaques. Widely believed by practitioners, this conclusion is only partially true and is certainly an oversimplification.

There are many determinants of blood pressure besides aortic impedance: extracellular and intravascular volumes, left ventricular filling and inotropic function, arteriolar and venous tone, and a regulatory system including neural, humoral, and renal components. While atherosclerotic effects on central compliance may determine the form of the pressure wave, they do not negate the contribution of these other components to the blood pressure.

Thus the actual importance of this hemodynamic profile is not that blood pressure cannot be lowered but that unusual problems may be encountered, especially in maintaining perfusion of cerebral, coronary, and renal vascular beds. The dehydrating effects of diuretics can provoke symptomatic hypoperfusion with orthostatic dizziness or even stroke. Since most coronary flow occurs in diastole, patients with coronary disease and isolated systolic hypertension may not tolerate the compromise of diastolic perfusion that follows attempts to trim systolic pressure. Diuretics and drugs that decrease cardiac output can further impair the decline in renal function that occurs with aging and nephrosclerosis.

Social resources are often lost with aging, making obstacles to caring for chronic diseases often insurmountable. The presence of other diseases with their requisite drugs and special costs, lack of transportation to frequent appointments, lack of insurance coverage (including Medicare) for drugs, depression, and loss of sight or hearing may further decrease adherence to management regimens.

Not only do cost and effort increase appreciably in treating older hypertensives, there is a corresponding decrease in the expected benefit, although this point remains poorly defined. There are, to date, no published data of a trial of reducing blood pressure in subjects selected for systolic hypertension. Most of the subjects in the Veterans Administration (V.A.) treatment study of the 1960s and the Hypertension Detection and Follow-up Program of the 1970s had, in addition to a diastolic pressure over 90 mm Hg, systolic pressure over 140 mm Hg. Furthermore, therapy that lowers diastolic pressure will usually also lower the systolic pressure. In younger patients, where the two components of blood pressure usually move together, where any adverse vascular risk factor has many more years to exert its deleterious effect, and where the safety of treatment is usually acknowledged, most authors advise treating systolic pressures above 140. But in elderly patients, especially those with pure systolic hypertension, the benefits remain unknown while the costs are often all too apparent.

Who should be treated? There is a general intuition that everyone with more than borderline or mild hypertension (140–160/90–100) should receive a gentle attempt at partial reduction, even if systolic pressure elevation predominates. It is not easy to predict treatment difficulty from the blood pressure readings, and many patients are surprisingly easy to control at low cost. The V.A. trial suggests, more-over, that partial reduction confers much of the expected benefit from complete blood pressure control. Beyond this, the aggressive-ness of therapy should take into account age, presence of other vas-cular risk factors (smoking, diabetes, high cholesterol), and evidence of developing target organ damage.

EVALUATION

When a person of any age is found to have high blood pressure, five questions must be addressed:
1. Does the patient have sustained hypertension of sufficient severity to require treatment?
2. Is there evidence of target organ damage from hypertension?
3. Are there other risk factors for cardiovascular disease?
4. Is there a surgically correctable underlying cause or one that re-quires special medical handling?
5. Are there coexisting conditions that affect the choice of drugs (e.g., asthma, renal impairment, congestive heart failure)?

There are several adverse effects of the direct and intended action of antihypertensive drugs that are usually more serious in the elderly. These effects are the consequences of decreasing ECF volume with diuretics, of blunting sympathetic tone with adrenergic blockers, of reducing cardiac output with beta-blockers, and, more generally, of lowering blood pressure and thus compromising perfusion. With these effects in mind, the patient must be evaluated (and serially reevaluated on therapy) for orthostatic hypotension, dehydration, and coronary and cerebral hypoperfusion. Several therapeutic op-tions that address these concerns will be described later, but first the patients at greatest risk must be identified.

What about secondary hypertension? The most common cause and the easiest to detect is chronic renal failure. Because old people pro-duce much less creatinine than younger ones (often one-third to one-half as much), a similar serum creatinine concentration represents a one-half to two-thirds reduction in creatinine clearance (or glomer-ular filtration rate) in the elderly. Thus, a serum creatinine concen-tration of 1.0 mg/dl is not "normal," and one of 1.5 to 2.0 may indicate sufficient renal failure to require the substitution of furosemide for thiazide in an antihypertensive regimen.

Other causes of secondary hypertension are uncommon and are not evident on routine examinations. Renal artery stenosis occurs in only about 1 percent of unselected hypertensives, and the other entities such as pheochromocytoma, Cushing's disease, aldosteronoma, or reninoma are even rarer. In the elderly, these lesions should be sought only if strong clues emerge from the history, physical examination, and basic laboratory work, or if the hypertension is abrupt, clearly paroxysmal, very severe, or resistant to therapy. Otherwise, Dr. Edward Freis's statement should serve as advice: "Unfortunately, medical tradition has grossly exaggerated the importance of detecting curable hypertension . . . The physician's responsibility only begins with the ruling out of curable hypertension, and he must not strain unduly his own or the patient's resources in doing so."[2]

By far the major emphasis in hypertension care should lie in cultivation of the patient's adherence to an effective regimen. This process begins with analysis of the traits and resources that have an impact on the necessary behaviors of compliance. These elements, called by L. W. Green and others an "educational diagnosis," consist of predisposing, enabling, and reinforcing factors. The first set consists of knowledge, beliefs, attitudes, and other faculties of mind that predispose the patient to accept the regimen. Enabling factors include financial and social access to care, while reinforcing factors comprise the human support system, usually based on family and physician. It is an absolute obligation of the treating physician to explore these issues and resources and to address any deficits.

There is good evidence that elderly patients respond at least as well as younger ones to educational efforts aimed at improving adherence to chronic disease management. Older patients are far more likely to bond securely with a medical provider because of the high prevalence of symptomatic or serious diseases in this group, or because of a growing sense of infirmity or vulnerability. Factors leading to lack of compliance by the elderly are the high rate of adverse drug effects, complicated drug regimens, and the lack of Medicare coverage for drugs.

MANAGEMENT

The therapy of hypertension has been better standardized in the United States than that of any other chronic disease. A "stepped-care" approach has been heavily promoted to encourage widespread

---

2. E. Freis. *The Modern Management of Hypertension* (Washington, D.C.: Veterans Administration, 1973).

use of effective regimens and to minimize adverse effects. Stepped care is most effectively viewed not as a recipe or rank-ordering scheme, but as a schedule of reevaluation in therapy. Step 1 actually begins with certainty of diagnosis, appropriately targeted evaluation, attempt to achieve weight loss and to decrease sodium when relevant, and finally the decision to use a drug (most often a diuretic). Most important, step 1 includes the establishment of a firm, lasting relationship to promote long-term adherence to the regimen of care.

Advancement to each subsequent step represents a point of treatment failure and requires several considerations, the last of which is the need for an additional drug. Before that final choice is accepted, the diagnosis should be rechecked and the control of excessive salt intake, correct prescribing and dispensing, and patient compliance in drug taking must be carefully evaluated. There is no doubt that large minorities of hypertensive patients will require two or more drugs, but it is impossible to identify them without excluding other causes for failure at each step.

Step 1

There are methods of treating hypertension without drugs, and a surprisingly large body of literature attests to the effectiveness of these methods in small, uncontrolled studies. Most extensively studied are dietary approaches to obesity and high salt intake. Weight reduction lowers blood pressure in obese patients even when salt intake in unchanged. But the most positive and consistent data are on sodium reduction: even rather modest dietary changes can cut sodium intake from 200+ mEq/day to 100 mEq/day, and several studies of this approach have yielded reductions in mean blood pressure of 7 to 10 mm Hg. The American Heart Association provides pamphlets and cookbooks with information, recipes, and menu planning to achieve this goal.

For the occasional patient who wishes to minimize drug use and who is highly motivated to share responsibility for health maintenance, much greater reductions of sodium (to <40 mEq/day) can be achieved with quite ordinary-appearing menus. The contrasts between the left-hand and right-hand columns in Table 1 give a feeling for the range of sodium content in different foods.

Exercise, biofeedback, meditation, and relaxation techniques all have enthusiastic proponents and probably are effective for selected patients. The almost total exclusion of these methods from contemporary medical practice is more a result of professional and societal

TABLE 1
Comparison of the Sodium Content of Common Foods

Food	Sodium Content (mg)[a]	Food	Sodium Content (mg)[a]
Fresh pork (4 oz)	93	Ham (4 oz)	1,400
Fresh or frozen green vegetables	1–3	Canned vegetables	220–320
Orange juice (6 oz)	4	Tomato juice (6 oz)	650
Oatmeal	1	Boxed cereals	250–350
Apples, oranges, pears	2–3	Pickle (1)	1,000–2,000
Ground beef (4 oz)	76	Canned soup (1 cup)	850–1,100
Swiss cheese (1 oz)	74	American cheese (1 oz)	406

[a]1 mEq of sodium = 23 mg.

preference for drugs rather than any clear proof that these non-pharmacologic approaches are ineffective.

Step 1 Drug Therapy
Most physicians begin drug therapy with a diuretic, usually hydro-chlorothiazide. Coexisting heart failure or creatinine clearance below 30 ml/min (serum creatinine >2.0 to 2.5 in older patients) necessitates using furosemide instead. The dosage should start at 25 to 50 mg of hydrochlorothiazide and increase at monthly intervals to 100 mg/day (for furosemide 20 mg at the outset, and titrated over a much wider range). These are short-acting diuretics, but there is excellent evidence that no rebound of hypertension occurs between once-a-day doses.

There are certain aspects of diuretic use that should be emphasized in treating older patients.

1. Dehydrating therapy may succeed all too well. Appetite, thirst, renin secretion, and tubular function, systems to maintain ECF volume within an optimal range, are diminished. Hence, dosing should start low and be increased slowly, and surveillance should be maintained for orthostatic hypotension and prerenal azotemia.

2. Hypokalemia is an overrated problem in treating younger patients with simple hypertension. In the elderly, however, especially those with concomitant heart disease and digitalis therapy, potassium balance requires attention in every case. Studies of serum digoxin levels have repeatedly shown that even mild hypokalemia can lead to toxic arrhythmias in patients with "therapeutic" digoxin levels. Conversely, certain circumstances raise a special danger of hyper-

kalemia. Patients with diminished renal function have a lesser ability to excrete pharmacologic doses of potassium and may not even be able to handle dietary potassium if they are treated with spironolactone, triamterene, or amiloride; it is a maxim that outpatients should not receive concomitantly supplemental potassium and a distal tubule diuretic. Finally, there is a substantial number of older people, usually diabetics with mild chronic renal failure, who have deficient renin and aldosterone secretion in the presence of hyperkalemia. It should be evident that potassium therapy is highly individualized and requires serial observation.

3. All hypotensive diuretics raise glucose levels in diabetics and may occasionally unmask diabetes, but they do not cause the disease or its complications. Antidiabetic regimens may require adjustment when diuretics are added or changed. Hyperuricemia is likewise provoked by all of these drugs but is not usually a clinical problem; if recurrent gout occurs, allopurinol is the treatment of choice. Thiazides alone cause a rise in calcium that is mild, transient, and unimportant except as an occasional source of confusion.

Step 2

If the goal blood pressure is not reached after several months of adjusted diuretic therapy, a step 2 decision is required. Regimens begin to become costly and to be accompanied by uncomfortable side effects at this point. The cost-efficient physician may wish to reconsider investment in compliance testing, salt restriction, and non-pharmacologic methods such as stress reduction, weight loss, or relaxation. A 24-hour urine collection for measurement of sodium and creatinine may be helpful at this point (greater than 100 mEq of sodium per gram of creatinine suggests a need to emphasize diet). Noncompliance is suggested by poor appointment keeping, vague recollection of regimen, erratic refills, and no drop in blood pressure or serum potassium.

When a second drug is indicated, there is a special option in geriatrics that is not usually considered in younger patients. The standard stepped-care approach always selects a sympathoplegic drug like propranolol at step 2 and reserves hydralazine (a direct vasodilator) for step 3. The rationale is this: if blood pressure is lowered with a direct vasodilator, the barosensitive elements of the autonomic nervous system will discharge adrenergic stimulation to the heart, causing so-called reflex tachycardia, which might induce palpitations or angina. If adrenergic inhibitors are used before direct vasodilators, this reflex is blocked.

Two characteristics of older hypertensives recommend reversal of this scheme. First, the baroreceptors become less sensitive in these patients, so reflex tachycardia is less often observed. The second issue concerns the effect of sympathoplegic medication on left ventricular function in the elderly. Most of these drugs decrease cardiac output, and although it falls well within the protective reserve in younger patients, the reduction often leads to symptoms of congestive failure in older persons. Thus, use of hydralazine as a step 2 drug is often safe and actually increases cardiac output by reducing afterload without depressing cardiac function. As with diuretics, the safe course is low dosing and small increments. Hydralazine is used twice a day, beginning with 25-mg doses. If larger doses are eventually employed, about 20 percent of patients will develop some symptoms of lupus (arthralgias, rash, pleurisy, leukopenia) and a positive antinuclear antibody. This is rare at doses below 200 mg/day, but it requires stopping the drug.

The more traditional step 2 approach, sympathoplegics, is also quite acceptable in geriatrics with appropriate precautions. These drugs have been widely reviewed, and only a few observations will be made here. There are several ways to group them, but most often the selection is based on avoiding patient-specific contraindications or on the opportunity to treat a coexisting condition with the same drug. All of these drugs cause some measure of sedation or exercise intolerance, symptoms that are difficult to separate from the usual high prevalence of similar complaints. Whether any of these drugs actually causes true depression is controversial, and the rumor that reserpine causes depression more commonly than other sympathoplegic drugs is simply untrue.

Beta-blockers have the longest list of distinct contraindications, some of which are relative and some of which are partly avoidable by using beta$_1$-selective drugs. Unfortunately, these drugs are expensive and may require prolonged titrations to high doses to be effective. The best reason for using beta-blockers is the opportunity to take advantage of their other indications, such as improved survival in patients recovering from a myocardial infarction (timolol or propranolol), essential tremor, stage fright, or migraine.

The only cost bargain is reserpine, which is almost free at the wholesale level. A combination tablet of hydrochlorothiazide with 0.125 mg of reserpine may be a good basic regimen for patients who need two drugs. This therapy combines low cost, one tablet, one daily dose, very little need for titration, and very low incidence of side effects, and it has been shown to be as effective as any doses of thiazide-methyldopa or thiazide-propranolol. Reserpine can cause nasal congestion, and it shares cardiodepressant properties with the beta-blockers.

High-Stepping
Occasionally older patients remain uncontrollably hypertensive and require regimens that are more expensive, more toxic, or harder to use safely. An excellent review of resistant hypertension by Gifford and Tarazi[3] should be read by any generalist who undertakes to manage these unusual patients, and advice from consultants familiar with resistant hypertension is reasonable.

The standard step 3 regimen of diuretic-sympathoplegic-hydralazine can be modified by substitutions: furosemide for thiazide, different sympathoplegics, or minoxidil instead of hydralazine. This last approach requires very cautious dosing; minoxidil is extremely potent, and both edema and angina are common consequences of reflex responses.

Two or more diuretics can be used together to block sodium reabsorption at multiple sites in the nephron—for example, combinations of furosemide with metolazone, and occasionally with spironolactone. Careful monitoring of weight, azotemia, and potassium is then essential.

On the other hand, there are experimental models of salt (volume)-sensitive hypertension in which dehydration aggravates therapy by intense renin-angiotensin activity. Patients who develop prerenal azotemia and other evidence of dehydration with unremitting hypertension might be considered for a trial of decreasing (or stopping) the diuretics while increasing therapy aimed at peripheral resistance (prazosin, clonidine, methyldopa, or direct vasodilators).

More than one sympathoplegic can be employed in the regimen: it is rational to use a beta-blocker along with either reserpine, methyldopa, clonidine, or prazosin. Some physicians still use guanethidine, usually substituted for another adrenergic blocker, but the problem of orthostatic hypotension makes this drug risky in the elderly.

---

3. R.W. Gifford, Jr., R.C. Tarazi. Resistant hypertension: Diagnosis and management. *Ann. Intern. Med.* 88:661–665, 1978.

Finally, although not necessarily last to be tried, is captopril, a completely unique agent that blocks the action of angiotensin-converting enzyme. Many physicians used this drug much earlier for patients resistant to basic therapy and did not heed the perhaps overwrought scattered reports of serious complications in patients with complex illnesses and multiple medications.

Large trials are under way of the costs and benefits of treating hypertension in the elderly. One of these, the "European Working Party on High Blood Pressure in the Elderly," should be nearing completion. The National Heart, Lung, and Blood Institute of the National Institutes of Health is launching an American look at treatment of isolated systolic hypertension. Hopefully, these studies will make it possible for physicians to feel much more secure a few years from now about this very common problem in clinical practice.

SUGGESTED READING

1. Gifford, R.W., Jr. Isolated systolic hypertension in the elderly. *J.A.M.A.* 247:781–785, 1982.
2. Gifford, R.W., Jr., Tarazi, R.C. Resistant hypertension: Diagnosis and management. *Ann. Intern. Med.* 88:661–665, 1978.
3. Kannel, W.B., Dawber, T.R., McGee, D.L. Perspectives on systolic hypertension. The Framingham study. *Circulation* 61(6):1179–1182, 1980.
4. Kirkendall, W.M., Hammond, J.J. Hypertension in the elderly. *Arch. Intern. Med.* 140:1155–1161, 1980.
5. Morisky, D.E., Levine, D.M., Green, L.W., Smith, C.R. Health education program effects on the management of hypertension in the elderly. *Arch. Intern. Med.* 142:1835–1838, 1982.
6. Simon, A.C., Safar, M.A., Levenson, J.A., et al. Systolic hypertension: Hemodynamic mechanism and choice of antihypertensive treatment. *Am. J. Cardiol.* 44:505–511, 1979.
7. Tarazi, R.C. Should you treat systolic hypertension in elderly patients? *Geriatrics,* November 1978, pp. 25–29.

Pulmonary Function and Reversible Pulmonary Dysfunction

CLINTON D. YOUNG, M.D.

Editor's note: The goals of treatment for chronic lung disease in the elderly must be clearly understood because the potential for a significant improvement in function is generally less than in younger patients, and the elderly are more susceptible to the cardiac toxicity of bronchodilators. Polypharmacy, often beneficial for the treatment of bronchospasm in younger patients, may not yield comparable or even justifiable benefits in the elderly.

The clinical evaluation of respiratory ailments in the geriatric population is complicated by three factors. First, most acutely symptomatic lung disease for which the elderly consult a physician is actually the result of chronic illness. It is often exposure-related in some way and can be traced back to inhalation of noxious airborne irritants and pathogenic organisms that tend to have a cumulative effect on the lung over time. Typical of these slow disease processes are the fibrosis and neoplastic sequelae of asbestos exposure, which take 10 to 20 years or more to appear. Even long-forgotten childhood afflictions may surface again with advancing age. It is well known that respiratory illnesses in childhood (particularly asthma and bronchitis) are risk factors for the development of chronic obstructive pulmonary disease in later life. Congenital syndromes (e.g., cystic fibrosis, protease inhibitor insufficiency, the immotile cilia syndrome) usually take their toll before the patient ages beyond 50.

Second, the changes in pulmonary function that result from aging alone mimic in some ways those of chronic lung disease. The physiologic changes from aging of weakened respiratory musculature, loss of chest wall and lung compliance, and loss of elastic recoil lead to small airways that begin to collapse earlier during expiration.

173

Third, there is a steady increase in cardiovascular disorders which cause symptoms like paroxysmal nocturnal dyspnea, dyspnea on exertion, and easy fatigue that are similar to those of lung disease.

AGING AND PULMONARY FUNCTION TESTS

Most clinically useful information comes from those indices measured by spirometry: forced vital capacity (FVC), volume exhaled in the first second (FEV_1), their ratio ($FEV_1/FVC\%$) and the maximum voluntary ventilation projected over one minute (MVV). Taking in a maximal inhalation and blowing it out as quickly and completely as possible is a relatively simple and well-tolerated maneuver, even by patients who do not feel well. General interpretation of these tests in adults is covered in many standard texts. Since lung function changes, normal values for most pulmonary function tests must be age-adjusted. Table 1 summarizes the general age-related trends.

Arterial blood gases are less helpful for assessing patients who are not acutely ill. Arterial Pco_2 stays near 40 torr, but the respiratory centers become less sensitive to changes in Pco_2. Carbon dioxide retention thus can become more of a problem in patients who have both chronic lung disease and a decreased CO_2 ventilatory drive from aging.

Objective measures of lung function are helpful for guiding therapy of both reversible and irreversible or progressive conditions. Of these, the simplest to obtain in the office is the peak expiratory flow rate (PEFR). This can be measured with a hand-held instrument and requires no elaborate interpretation. Peak expiratory flow rate is a composite assessment of patient strength, effort, and cooperation as

TABLE 1
General Trends in Pulmonary Function with Aging

Parameter	Trend with Age
Total lung capacity	No change
Residual volume	Increase
Vital capacity	Decrease
FEV_1	Decrease
Diffusion capacity	Decrease
Arterial Po_2	Decrease
Arterial-alveolar O_2 pressure difference	Increase
Arterial Pco_2	No change

well as large-airway obstruction. All these factors, influential in ameliorating or worsening lung disease, can vary from hour to hour and visit to visit. Long-term trends are therefore more significant than individual scores when PEFR data are used to guide treatment.

Other tests have occasional utility in understanding a particular patient's problems. Measurement of total lung capacity and its component volumes can help distinguish between true restriction and air trapping. The diffusion capacity of carbon dioxide is reduced in emphysema but is usually not significantly reduced in bronchitis or asthma. These tests are generally less useful and more expensive than spirometry, however.

CLINICAL SYNDROME

The syndromes of obstructive lung disease associated with dyspnea, cough, and wheeze are so common that they tend to be lumped under the generic term *chronic obstructive pulmonary disease* (COPD), obscuring the differences that can guide therapy. Limitation of air flow is caused by spasm, edema, secretions, and collapse of unstable airways; of these only pure airway collapse (with emphysema) does not benefit to some degree from drug therapy. Chronic bronchitis and emphysema are predominantly related to cigarette smoking, particularly in men. Taken together, they cause the majority of respiratory complaints in men over 40 years old and are second only to heart disease as a cause of disability in men 60 to 65 years old. Similar problems are now becoming more common in women with extensive smoking histories.

Chronic Bronchitis

Chronic bronchitis, anatomically characterized by airway edema, inflammation, and mucous gland hyperplasia, is diagnosed clinically, based on a persistent productive cough for at least three months of two consecutive years. It may stabilize and smolder for years, with acute exacerbations especially during the winter or after viral infections. Bacterial infection with *Hemophilus influenzae* or *Streptococcus pneumoniae* may produce a self-limited acute attack of bronchitis with purulent sputum or life-threatening bronchopneumonia. The patient may be overall only marginally worse after each exacerbation. Progression of the disorder causes CO_2 retention and the familiar "blue bloater" phenotype, terminating in cor pulmonale and death with mixed cardiopulmonary disease.

Acute exacerbations due to bacterial infection should be treated with broad-spectrum antibiotics (amoxicillin, doxycycline, trimetho-prim-sulfamethoxazole). If properly educated, the patient can undertake this treatment early and can in many cases avoid the need for an office visit or hospitalization. Sputum culture is useful only if there is frank pneumonia or inadequate response to therapy and need not be routinely ordered. Bronchodilators generally are of some use but usually not enough to justify high, potentially toxic doses. Sedatives and sleeping pills should be avoided because they may precipitate CO_2 narcosis, especially in older patients. Mucolytic agents (acetylcysteine with a bronchodilator) and chest physiotherapy may help the patient to clear unusually thick secretions, but rarely make a great difference. Adequate hydration is also important, but fluid overload, which might lead to congestive heart failure, should be avoided. Overly aggressive treatment with bronchodilators, steroids, and antibiotics to achieve marginal improvements in pulmonary function may well have a negative impact on the patient's quality of life.

Oxygen therapy should be guided by blood gases. The presence of cardiac disease may prevent the elderly patient from tolerating even mild levels of hypoxemia. In most instances, however, the goal is to find an oxygen dose sufficient to prevent pulmonary hypertension and polycythemia while avoiding excessive CO_2 retention. The unstable patient may benefit from a Venturi-mask/humidifier system stabilizing hemoglobin saturation at 70 to 80 percent with less risk of progressive CO_2 retention. Masks are uncomfortable, however, and nasal prongs set to deliver low flows of 1 to 2 L/min are usually a necessary concession. Since most masks require a flow of at least 4 L/min, oxygen therapy with nasal prongs is also generally less expensive.

Emphysema
The so-called pink-puffer patient with emphysema is a thin, dyspneic person working hard to maintain near normal blood gases. Productive cough is minimal, infections are less frequent, and CO_2 retention is a more ominous sign of irreversible impairment than in chronic bronchitis. Emphysema is anatomically recognized by enlargement of distal air spaces with destruction of their walls, leading to excessive floppiness and expiratory collapse of small airways.

Emphysema is a disease process aggravated though not caused by aging. The term *senile emphysema* has been used to describe enlargement of alveoli without septal destruction, but it does not produce clinical impairment unless hastened by other disorders. True emphysema results from destruction of alveolar walls by uncontrolled proteolytic enzyme activity from leukocytes responding to irritants such as cigarette smoke. "Normal" age-related loss of elastic recoil is thus augmented by an actual loss of lung tissue. Some emphysema is present at autopsy in up to 50 percent of people over 60 years of age, with a higher incidence in smokers and residents of areas with high air pollution.

The chest roentgenographic pattern of increased anteroposterior diameter, often considered an indication of emphysema, can also result from increased spinal curvature and degeneration of the intervertebral disks without evidence of lung pathology.

Treatment of emphysema in its pure form is supportive, with attention to nutrition and appropriate physical exercise to maintain general fitness. The role of bronchodilators and antibiotics is limited to the treatment of clinically evident bronchospasm and infection, and they should not be routinely prescribed. Supplemental oxygen becomes necessary in later stages when chronic hypoxemia is present.

Asthma

Wheezing and cough, common indicators of bronchospasm, may reflect asthma or bronchitis with a bronchospastic component. New-onset asthma does occur in the decades after 60, but the diagnosis and treatment are less straightforward than in most younger patients. Asthma in the elderly tends to be of the so-called intrinsic, nonallergic type. Skin tests may be positive to common aeroallergens, but exacerbations correlate poorly with exposure to the indicated antigens. Instead, a variety of nonspecific triggers are often described, including viral infection and changes in the weather. Thus, the elderly "intrinsic" asthmatic contrasts with the typical "extrinsic" asthmatic who has an onset before age 30, a family and personal history of atopy, symptoms that are seasonal or otherwise linked to allergen exposure, elevated IgE levels, and positive skin tests to allergens.

Asthma may present just as a cough, or as wheezing occurring only in special circumstances such as at night, during exertion, or with occupational exposures. Sputum eosinophilia is variably present. Because the distinction between asthma and bronchitis is apt to blur in the elderly, the correct diagnosis of asthma may be reached only by exclusion of bronchitis and cardiac disease. When this is not possible or when there are multiple medical problems, assigning clinical importance to one or the other illness may be reduced to pragmatic judgment.

The usual criterion for reversible bronchospasm is a 15 percent improvement in baseline FEV_1 or FVC or both after administration of a bronchodilator. Some asthmatics who do not improve on spirometry after a single bronchodilator dose may nonetheless still improve substantially during a one- to two-week trial of steroids and bronchodilators. Airways narrowed by tumor, edema, or loss of supporting tissue may produce wheezes that are unresponsive to bronchodilator therapy.

THERAPY FOR ASTHMA AND OBSTRUCTIVE LUNG DISEASE

Therapy for an acute attack of asthma is little different in older patients except for the limitations of cardiac tolerance to inotropic and chronotropic side effects. A history of angina or arrhythmias should be sought to help judge a tolerable peak pulse rate for tachycardia. Although a teenager could tolerate a sustained pulse rate of 140 to 150 beats per minute, older patients will rarely tolerate a tachycardia of this degree.

Theophylline (Methylxanthine) Preparations
Theophyllines should be given as one of the newer sustained-release forms (e.g., Respbid, Theo-Dur) to provide more stable blood levels and a 12-hour dosing interval. Theophylline metabolism is unpredictable in the elderly, so blood levels should be checked two to three days after dosing changes or when symptoms suggest underdosing or overdosing. Biologic half-lives of theophylline in elderly patients with normal cardiac, renal, and liver function have been shown to vary from 5.4 to 9 hours, and patients with congestive heart failure or liver disease may have an even longer theophylline half-life. The therapeutic effect is related to the blood level, which should be kept between 10 and 20 mg/dl. Administration of other drugs such as digoxin, which alters cardiac output and liver perfusion, or cimetidine, which alters liver clearance of theophylline, may affect theophylline blood levels. Simplicity of dosing schedule and prescription of as few medications as possible are particularly important in the older patient. Dosage levels should be chosen that provide reasonable comfort from day to day; it is unnecessary to make the patient wheeze-

free at the expense of side effects, excessive cost, and confusing regimens. Toxic doses may be revealed first by nausea, central nervous system stimulation, or seizures. Theo-Dur Sprinkle, a nonencapsulated sustained release theophylline preparation, has proved useful when pills are poorly tolerated.

Selective beta$_2$-adrenergic agents having minimal cardiac effects, including albuterol (British equivalent, salbutamol), metaproterenol, terbutaline, and isoetharine, should be prescribed first. Isoproterenol should not be routinely used because of its relatively high cardiac toxic potential. Many of these agents are available in metered-dose inhalers that offer the advantages of quick onset, adjustable dosing, minimal systemic side effects, and avoidance of problems with swallowing pills. Many older patients, however, have problems coordinating inhalers, resulting in unpredictable dosing, so baseline therapy with tablets will prove most satisfactory.

Whether therapy is begun first with a theophylline or an adrenergic agent is a matter of choice. In the United States, theophylline products have traditionally been used first, whereas Europe has favored adrenergic preparations. In either case, dosage of one agent should be taken to tolerance before another is added. The combination of theophylline and an adrenergic agent has been shown to be synergistic, a useful fact when neither type of drug has been well tolerated at therapeutic dosages.

Geriatric dosing for beta-adrenergic drugs is largely empirical. There is some evidence that the number of beta-agonist receptors in cell membranes declines with age, and target organs may become less responsive. Cardiac intolerance, tremor, and nervousness limit the acceptable dose. The therapeutic effect may be interfered with by beta-receptor blocking drugs administered for control of hypertension, angina, arrhythmias, or glaucoma.

Corticosteroids
Steroid therapy is commonly required for control of dyspnea in older patients. Acute exacerbations of wheezing may be met with prednisone bursts of 40 to 60 mg/day in divided doses, then tapered by 5 mg every three to five days. Prepackaged steroid packs with the tablets set out in tapered rows provide a simple, convenient way to administer bursts of steroid therapy. More severe attacks may require intravenous doses, which are often given as methylprednisolone, 250 to 1,000 mg or more per day in divided doses. Massive dosing (over 1,000 mg of methylprednisolone per day) has some advocates, but there is little evidence that it works better than lower doses.

Every effort should be made to convert to a single morning oral dose, which is tapered slowly (5 mg every two to three weeks) and then empirically changed to an alternate-day regimen or discontinued altogether. Some patients, however, may require long-term single-daily-dose maintenance steroid therapy. Metered-dose aerosol steroids may facilitate withdrawal from oral steroids but present some of the same problems that the elderly have with inhalers described earlier. They may also cause oral yeast infection unless the mouth is rinsed with water after each dose.

Because chronic steroid therapy may be necessary in elderly asthmatics, some will fall victim to side effects of steroids, such as cataracts, glucose intolerance, and osteoporosis. These effects are sufficiently debilitating to require some compromise in attempts to control symptoms tightly with the chronic use of steroids.

Anticholinergics
Atropine is occasionally useful by the aerosal route for relief of bronchospasm, but in effective doses the side effects of atropine (tachycardia, urine retention) are poorly tolerated by many patients. Newer preparations with fewer side effects are forthcoming.

Cromolyn Sodium
Cromolyn sodium is an inhaled powder useful primarily in allergic "extrinsic" asthma. It can be tried before steroids in the difficult stabilized asthmatic, but it rarely offers significant benefit in the elderly "intrinsic" asthmatic. It is useful only for chronic therapy and does not provide immediate relief.

General Measures
Education of the patient crucially affects his compliance and the ultimate success of outpatient care. Sessions should be brief, clear, and repeated as necessary; written instructions are mandatory if the patient is forgetful or dependent on others. Prevention of further exacerbations may be aided by commonsense avoidance of nonspecific irritants and tobacco. An occasional geriatric patient may obtain some relief against aeroallergens from allergy shots if these can be shown to have a role in his situation. Here again, avoidance of the offending allergen is the better approach if possible. Frank discussion with the patient or family may reveal that there is no one at home to dust, or that a cat is the patient's only regular companion.

OTHER RESPIRATORY PROBLEMS

Bronchogenic Carcinoma

Successful therapy of lung cancer depends on location, extent, cell type, and luck. Many feel that the elderly patient should be offered an aggressive attempt at cure, if feasible. Mutilating or debilitating surgery for a patient with multiple organ system senescence, however, is not appropriate.

Pulmonary Embolism

Pulmonary embolism is a very common acute problem in elderly patients in whom immobility and cardiovascular disorders are frequent. The same risk factors may delay recognition of symptoms or obscure the diagnosis. Agitation and tachypnea may be the only clues. As in other age groups, most emboli are from the pelvis and deep leg veins. Minidose heparin, 5,000 units subcutaneously every 12 hours, helps prevent embolism in patients undergoing thoracic, abdominal, or gynecologic surgery. It has not helped in patients undergoing prosthetic orthopedic surgery and hip procedures, presumably because there is too much release of tissue clotting factors. Minidose heparin may also be of prophylactic benefit in medical illnesses requiring immobilization, such as acute myocardial infarction or severe congestive heart failure.

Full-dose heparin remains the treatment of choice for pulmonary embolism and is managed in the same way as for younger patients. The incidence of bleeding in women over 60 is almost 50 percent, so there is real justification for establishing the diagnosis as definitively as possible, using lung scans and pulmonary angiograms as needed.

Abnormal Patterns of Breathing

Cheyne-Stokes breathing, a regular cyclic pattern in which the breathing rate slows to the point of apnea and then progressively increases before slowing again, is caused by a slow respiratory center response to changes in PCO_2 with overshooting in either direction. It is commonly associated with diffuse central nervous system disease, including cerebrovascular disorders and low cardiac output. Treatment should be directed toward underlying problems; the respiratory pattern itself is rarely harmful.

Sleep-Associated Breathing Disturbances

Sleep apnea syndromes resulting from disorders of central respiratory control and intermittent upper airway obstruction have recently been recognized. Men between 40 and 60 years are at greatest risk for obstructive apnea. Elderly patients with COPD are another high-risk group because their respiratory centers have become more tolerant of an elevated P_{CO_2}, and borderline hypoxia is present even when the patient is awake and breathing. Complaints of inadequate nocturnal sleep, daytime hypersomnolence, and loud snoring are clues to the diagnosis. Polysomnographic recordings of air flow, electroencephalography, and respiratory effort provide objective verification. Treatment is based on stimulant drugs to correct the central component and tracheostomy, weight loss, and other measures to remove or bypass the upper airway obstruction.

Aspiration Pneumonia

Elderly patients are at great risk for hazards of aspiration as a result of decreased alertness, poor mobility, decreased cough reflex, poor or absent dentition, and inattentive or hurried feeding by assistants. Careful recording of respiratory rates in these patients is often a surprisingly effective way to detect problems early, even before fever, leukocytosis, or purulent sputum appear.

SUGGESTED READING

1. American Thoracic Society. Definitions and classifications of chronic bronchitis, asthma, emphysema. *Am. Rev. Respir. Dis.* 85:762–768, 1962.
2. Burr, M.L., Charles, T.J., Roy, K., Seaton, A. Asthma in the elderly: An epidemiological survey. *Br. Med. J.* 1:1041–1044, 1979.
3. Knudson, R.J., Clark, D.F., Kennedy, T.C., Knudson, D.E. Effect of aging alone on mechanical properties of the normal adult human lung. *J. Appl. Physiol.* 43(6):1054–1062, 1977.
4. Plummer, A.L. Asthma: Special challenge in the elderly. *Geriatrics* 36(6):87–91, 1981.
5. Rossman, I. (Ed.). *Clinical Geriatrics,* 2nd ed. Philadelphia: J. B. Lippincott, 1979.

5

NEUROLOGIC
AND PSYCHIATRIC
DISORDERS

Depression in the Elderly

RAOUF F. BADAWI, M.D.

Editor's note: One of the most gratifying experiences for a geriatric physician is the uncovering of depression in its various forms. The demented and possibly depressed patient represents a special challenge in diagnosis. The pleasure to be gained from the successful treatment of the elderly depressed patient compares favorably with the most dramatic successes in clinical medicine.

Depression may be the most important psychiatric condition of late life, and its early recognition can save the patient much needless misery and unnecessary investigations. An elderly patient whom I recently saw in psychiatric consultation had severe ischemic heart disease for which she had seen two cardiologists. Although both recognized that she had "emotional problems," neither referred her for psychiatric evaluation. Her general internist eventually referred her after she became floridly disorganized. Small doses of doxepin resulted in a gratifying improvement, and she has been euthymic since. When she emerged from her depression, her cardiac status improved with a diminution in the frequency of her anginal attacks, and she was soon discharged from the hospital.

Every age has its own frustrations and sufferings in addition to those it shares with all ages. Those of old age seem so obvious that it is often said by the uninformed that depression and suicide in the elderly are readily understood. This is a misconception held by younger people who are unable to put themselves in the place of the old. The elderly do not, as a rule, find it easy to understand the depression and suicides of their contemporaries. The mistaken belief that mental illness in old age is incurable dies hard. We now have the means of managing depression in the elderly.

The risk of depression does increase with age. The exact prevalence of depression in the elderly remains essentially unknown but has been placed as high as 14 percent. In order to avoid overlooking depression, let us then follow the dictum that in the elderly it is important to rule out rather than to rule in depression.

DEFINING DEPRESSION

Depression has been operationally defined as an emotional expression of the state of hopelessness. The clinician must identify the patient's underlying sense of hopelessness, pessimism, and despair to alert himself to the probable presence of a depressive disorder.

The word *depression* can be used to denote any of three different entities. It may refer to (1) a feeling, tone, or prevailing mood; (2) a syndrome (cluster of signs and symptoms); or, (3) a group of disorders—the depressive disorders as defined by the *Diagnostic and Statistical Manual of Mental Disorders (Third Edition)* (the book of criteria for psychiatric diagnoses).[1] In its latest classification of emotional illnesses, the American Psychiatric Association variously classified depression under the following headings:

1. Major depressive disorder, singular episode versus recurrent
2. Bipolar affective disorder, manic, depressed, or mixed
3. Specific affective disorder, cyclothymic disorder, and dysthymic disorders
4. Atypical depressive disorders
5. Adjustment disorders with depressed mood
6. Bereavement

Thus, it is important to realize not only that depressions are a heterogeneous group of disorders, but that the management of the patient depends on accurate understanding of the psychopathology and dynamics involved in the depressive process.

Depression can be either a primary or a secondary disorder. If it is primary, it can be either unipolar or bipolar, the latter diagnosis being made on the basis of the history of previous manic or hypomanic states. When clear precipitating associated factors are present that can explain the patient's despondency, such as alcohol abuse, drug addiction, physical illness, or another psychiatric illness, the depression is a secondary affective illness.

---

1. Washington, D.C.: American Psychiatric Association, 1980.

The typical depressive psychosis is readily identifiable. Its presentation includes deflation of mood, loss of the capacity to love, loss of interest in the external world, inhibition of activity, deflation of self-esteem, and self-accusation. What sets it apart from other depressions is a need for punishment, which may be accompanied by delusional projections, and the presence of vegetative symptoms, the most relevant of which are terminal insomnia, anorexia, and mood variations of the endogenous type.

DIAGNOSIS OF DEPRESSION

The diagnosis of depressive disorders in the elderly is frequently not quite so obvious and often taxes our clinical acumen for several reasons. Transient depressive moods are more frequent in the elderly, who may be more prone to philosophical introspection. Hypochondriacal preoccupations among the elderly are well known and can mask an underlying illness. Depression can be interpreted by the patient and others as an appropriate response to an underlying physical illness or life situation. Agitation, rather than retardation, is more frequently seen in geriatric patients and is often treated by physicians with antipsychotics which, when prescribed alone, will aggravate the depression. The elderly frequently live alone and are isolated from the relatives or other caring persons who could provide the physician with adequate historical information. Also, paranoid delusions and lability of affect are characteristic of early dementia, and their presence may well be interpreted in an organic basis rather than as a reflection of an underlying depressive illness.

The conditions presenting special diagnostic challenges in the elderly include depressive pseudodementia, depression complicating a preexisting dementia, masked depression, drug-induced depression, physical illness associated with depression, and grief reactions.

Depressive Pseudodementia
A patient whose depressive illness has produced symptoms that mimic a dementing process may not present as much difficulty in diagnosis as the patient in whom dementia and a major depressive disorder coexist. In depressive pseudodementia, memory impairment and regressive personality change are less prominent, orientation is preserved, and withdrawal may be more severe. Thus the patient may

understand what is said to him but may refuse to answer because of irritability (the organically demented patient who is not depressed will almost invariably try to answer and respond, although his answers may be nonsensical). Frontal lobe release signs will be absent, and the patient may have a better integrated electroencephalogram with preservation of basic rhythms. If the patient's cooperation can be solicited, psychological tests can help to clarify the diagnosis.

Depresssion Complicating Dementia
In patients with depression complicating dementia, there may be a rapid onset of regressive symptoms or a personality change that cannot be accounted for on an organic basis. Biologic symptoms of depression, specifically anorexia and terminal insomnia, are present. Thought content and delusional beliefs characterized by self-accusatory statements or expressions of hopelessness and despair are present also. Patients may have a family history or previous history of depression.

There will remain a number of cases in which it is still almost impossible to reach a definitive diagnosis. An amobarbital or diazepam interview will frequently be conclusive. The depressed patient will produce depressive themes that reflect his depressed thought content. By contrast, the demented patient's confusion and disorientation become more pronounced.

Masked Depression
The elderly are more likely to recognize the cognitive, biologic, and somatic symptoms of depression than they are the affective component of their condition. They may come to the physician's office complaining of vague and undefined symptoms for which an organic basis is lacking, or the exaggeration of the symptoms of a preexisting physical disorder without a clear-cut physical deterioration commensurate with their subjective sense of distress. Complaints of pains and aches, loss of energy, fatigability, lassitude, loss of interest, libidinal indifference, and insomnia are common. They may vigorously deny subjective feelings of depression, but anhedonia should alert the physician to the affective nature of their disturbance.

Of greater diagnostic difficulty are those elderly patients who exhibit personality change toward increased irritability, alcohol abuse, or antisocial activity. Again, the physician should suspect the possible presence of a treatable underlying affective illness expressing itself in that manner instead of immediately attributing these symptoms to the presence of an organic cerebral process.

DIFFERENTIAL DIAGNOSIS

Physical illness also can present as depression. In those elderly patients who have a preexisting history of depressive illness, an important exhaustive investigation may be inappropriately withheld. Because of a history of depression, metastatic cancer of the liver in one of my patients was missed by two of her physicians. Among the physical conditions that are associated with major depression, one should consider malignancies, especially cancer of the head of the pancreas; endocrinopathies, especially hyperthyroidism and hypothyroidism; Parkinson's disease; and rheumatoid arthritis.

Many drugs in common usage can induce depression. Among these are alcohol; phenacetin; benzodiazepines; barbiturates; antipsychotics in general; antiarthritic agents like phenylbutazone and indomethacin; some antibiotics; anticonvulsants like carbamazepine; the antihypertensives, such as alpha-methyldopa, reserpine, propranolol, hydralazine, and clonidine; the antiparkinsonian agents, such as amantadine and L-dopa; the cardiac drugs, such as digitalis and procainamide; and adrenocorticosteroids.

Grief reactions, whether acute or chronic, can usually be managed without medication. It has been estimated that the mortality rate for the recently bereaved elderly far exceeds that of their peer group, perhaps reflecting the unconsious wish for reunion with the deceased. Prompt treatment of severe grief reactions in the elderly is therefore of paramount importance.

TREATMENT

The cornerstone of successful treatment is accurate diagnosis. To avoid treating a symptom rather than a patient, antidepressants should generally be used as just one parameter in overall management rather than as an end in themselves. The general principles of managing depressive illness with antidepressants apply in the elderly in much the same manner as they apply in younger age groups.

The family's active participation in the treatment process is often crucial, since the precipitating events of the elderly person's depression frequently center around feelings of alienation, uselessness, and abandonment. It is important for family members to involve themselves with the patient in a warmly active, understanding, accepting way.

In treating the elderly, the therapist himself should play an active role in the treatment process. A touch or a hand on the shoulder can and usually does communicate immeasurably more than words. Reverse transference reactions—when the patient views the therapist as his own child—should be accepted and appreciated. Ventilation should be encouraged and the patient's concerns respected in a receptive and direct way.

Social support programs that can meet the patient's specific needs can be identified and utilized, especially when the elderly have no concerned family nearby. These programs may, indeed, be more important than medication or the therapist himself.

When prescribing antidepressants for the elderly patient, the physician must keep in mind several principles. There is significant individual variability in the metabolism of these agents, so as a general rule the elderly should be started with small doses, which may be slowly increased to obtain optimum results. Table 1 lists some of the differences in actions and an approximate guide to the cost of the various tricyclics that might be considered. Serum levels of tricyclics should be used frequently as indicators of appropriate dosage and medication compliance, since many elderly patients have memory disturbances and forget to take their medication. Drug interactions affecting the metabolism and actions of the tricyclic antidepressants are common. For example, since depression may be accompanied by

TABLE 1
Properties of Commonly Used Antidepressants

Drug Name	Usual (HS) Initial Dose (mg)	Sedative Effect[a]	Anticholinergic Effects[a]	Cost for 1 Month[b]
Amitriptyline (Elavil, Endep)	25–50	5+	6+	3+
Doxepin (Sinequan, Adapin)	25–50	6+	3+	3+
Imipramine (Tofranil)	25–50	3+	4+	4+ 1+ (generic)
Nortriptyline (Aventyl, Pamelor)	25–50	2+	3+	2+
Desipramine (Norpramin, Pertofrane)	25–50	2+	1+	3+
Protriptyline (Vivactil)	10–30	1+	2+	2+

[a]1+ = least side effects; 6+ = greatest side effects.
[b]1+ = ~$5; 2+ = ~$10; 3+ = ~$15; 4+ = ~$20.

psychosis, interactions and adverse effects from antipsychotics must be remembered. A history of glaucoma and prostatic hypertrophy is not an absolute contraindication to tricyclic antidepressants, but patients with these problems should be managed in conjunction with appropriate specialists.

Cardiac toxicity from tricyclic antidepressants results from a dose-related quinidine-like activity on cardiac conduction. It is therefore important to monitor cardiac response to tricyclic antidepressants in vulnerable populations like the elderly by serial electrocardiograms, looking for a prolonged QRS duration and increased frequency of arrhythmias. Prolonged conduction constitutes a relative contraindication to the use of tricyclic antidepressants because of the risks of precipitating partial or complete heart block with profound bradycardia.

In patients who are unresponsive to tricyclic antidepressants, or when their use is contraindicated, electroconvulsive therapy should be considered. The coexistence of depression and dementia is not an absolute contraindication to electroconvulsive therapy.

SUGGESTED READING

1. Blazer, D., Williams, C.D. Epidemiology of dementia and depression in our elderly population. *Am. J. Psychol.* 137:439–444, 1980.
2. Lazor, I., Karasw, T.B. Evaluation and management of depression in the elderly. *Geriatrics* 35:47–53, 1980.
3. Snow, S., Wells, C.E. Case studies in neuropsychiatry diagnosis and treatment of coexistent dementia and depression. *Clin. Psychol.* 42:439–441, 1978.
4. Thompson, T.L., Moran, M.G., Nies, A.S. Psychotropic drug use in the elderly. *N. Engl. J. Med.* 308:194–199, 1983.
5. Wells, C.E. Pseudodementia. *Am. J. Psychol.* 136:895–900, 1979.

Dementia, Delirium, Depression, and Alzheimer's Disease

PAUL BECK, M.D., and
ALAN HALPERIN, M.D.

Editor's note: Delirium or dementia should never be assumed to be irreversible without a thorough workup. For the physician familiar with the reversible causes of delirium or dementia, a good history and physical examination, and a few laboratory and radiographic tests will suffice. When no reversible etiology is found, the physician must help the patient and family cope with the many problems that invariably occur in demented patients.

Deterioration of mental functioning in an elderly person poses dilemmas for family and caregivers. Forgetfulness, poor judgment, emotional lability, personality change, and confusion are disturbing to family, friends, and physicians, and it is difficult to inquire about the nature of changes in mental function without challenging the older person's integrity and independence. Although it is tempting to attribute changes to aging, "senility," or "organic brain syndrome," the nature of the intellectual or behavioral problem must be adequately characterized to ascertain whether the cause is reversible and to determine how therapeutic or supportive interventions can minimize the loss of independent functioning, even when the cause is irreversible.

DEFINITIONS

The first approach to an intellectual or behavioral problem in an elderly patient is the characterization of its clinical features, looking for evidence of dementia, delirium, or depression (recently redefined in the *Diagnostic and Statistical Manual of Mental Disorders (Third Edition) (DSM-III)*.[1] Although these behavioral syndromes often co-

---

1. Washington, D.C.: American Psychiatric Association, 1980.

192

exist in the same patient (either as an aggravating factor or as a consequence of the primary problem), the clinical features of one syndrome usually predominate. Identification of the predominant syndrome will suggest the probable causes of the mental dysfunction.

Dementia

Dementia in *DSM-III* encompasses a variety of cognitive disorders that were previously known as "organic brain syndromes," "senile dementia," and "presenile dementia." Dementia is now defined as (1) loss of intellectual abilitites of sufficient severity to interfere with social or occupational functioning; (2) memory impairment; (3) at least one of the following: *(a)* impairment of abstract thinking, *(b)* impairment of judgment or, *(c)* disturbances of higher cortical function (such as agnosia or apraxia), or *(d)* personality changes; and (4) no clouding of the state of consciousness. Dementia usually has an insidious onset and a relatively stable and progressive course.

Approximately 5 to 10 percent of people older than 65 years of age and 20 percent of those older than 80 are clinically demented, as are up to 50 percent of the patients in nursing homes. It is estimated that 15 percent of all patients with dementia have a reversible cause and that another 20 to 25 percent can be improved with medical intervention. Patients less than 65 years of age have a greater frequency of reversible causes than do older ones.

Delirium

Delirium is defined in *DSM-III* as (1) clouding of consciousness with a reduced capacity to shift, focus, and sustain attention to environmental stimuli; (2) at least two of the following: *(a)* perceptual disturbance (misinterpretations, illusions, or hallucinations), *(b)* speech at times incoherent, *(c)* disturbance of the sleep-wakefulness cycle (insomnia or daytime drowsiness), or *(d)* altered psychomotor activity; (3) disorientation and memory impairment; and (4) clinical features that develop over a short period of time (usually hours to days), with fluctuation over the course of a day. Terms previously used to describe delirium include "acute brain syndrome," "metabolic encephalopathy," "toxic psychosis," "toxic encephalopathy," or "acute confusional state."

Depression

Depression is defined as (1) a dysphoric mood (feeling depressed, sad, blue, hopeless, low, down in the dumps, irritable) or loss of interest or pleasure in all or almost all usual activities or pastimes;

(2) at least four of the following: *(a)* appetite poor or excessive and/ or significant weight loss or gain, *(b)* psychomotor agitation or retardation, *(c)* insomnia or hypersomnia, *(d)* decrease in sexual drive, *(e)* loss of energy (or fatigue), *(f)* feelings of worthlessness, self-reproach, or excessive or inappropriate guilt, *(g)* complaints or evidence of diminished ability to think or concentrate (slowed thinking or indecisiveness), *(h)* recurrent thoughts of death or suicide attempt; and (3) absence of delusions, hallucinations, or bizarre behavior when not depressed.

The coexistence of depression, dementia, or delirium in the same elderly patient can occur, and it is not unusual for a patient to become depressed during the early stages of dementia, particularly when there is still an awareness of the progressive cognitive deficits. Similarly, primary depression often produces a loss of cognitive function in the elderly (sometimes called pseudodementia) that is difficult to distinguish clinically from true dementia.

CLINICAL EVALUATION

The history and physical examination provide important data that are crucial for characterizing an elderly patient's intellectual or behavioral problem. A careful history obtained from close family members may help assess the severity and progression of the behavioral or intellectual changes of which the patient may be unaware. For example, Alzheimer's disease causes a gradual and progressive decline of intellectual function, while patients with multiinfarct dementia frequently have a stepwise decline in intellectual functioning. Patients or their families may be able to remember specific times when intellectual and cognitive function began to deteriorate. Acute intellectual changes may be superimposed on a chronic level of dysfunction, as in the case of adverse drug and alcohol effects. Many common drugs that are well tolerated by younger patients can cause delirium or depression or may exacerbate dementia in the elderly (see Table 1).

Chronic subdural hematomas and subarachnoid hemorrhages can cause reversible dementia. The presence of urinary incontinence and gait disturbances raises the possibility of normal pressure hydrocephalus. In addition, patients should be questioned about the history of treated or inadequately treated syphilis. A family history of dementia, gait disturbance, or focal neurologic signs should be obtained

TABLE 1
Common Medications Causing Delirium in the Aged

Disorder	Medication	Common Examples
Cardiovascular conditions	Antiarrhythmics	Procainamide, propranolol, quinidine
	Antihypertensives	Clonidine, methyldopa, reserpine
	Cardiac glycosides	Digitalis
	Coronary vasodilators	Nitrates
Gastrointestinal conditions	Antidiarrheals	Atropine, belladonna, homatropine, hyoscyamine, scopolamine
	Antinauseants	Cyclizine, homatropine-barbiturate preparations, phenothiazines
	Antispasmodics	Methanthelene, propantheline
Musculoskeletal conditions	Antiinflammatory agents	Corticosteroids, indomethacin, phenylbutazone, salicylates
	Muscle relaxants	Carisoprodol, diazepam
Neurologic-psychiatric conditions	Anticonvulsants	Barbiturates, carbamazepine, diazepam, phenytoin
	Antiparkinsonian agents	Amantadine, benztropine, levodopa, trihexyphenidyl
	Hypnotics and sedatives	Barbiturates, belladonna alkaloids, bromides, chloral hydrate, ethchlorvynol, glutethimide, methaqualone
	Psychotropics	Benzodiazepines, hydroxyzines, lithium salts, meprobamate, monoamine oxidase inhibitors, neuroleptics, tricyclic antidepressants
Respiratory-allergic conditions	Antihistamines	Brompheniramine, chlorpheniramine, cyproheptadine, diphenhydramine, tripelennamine
	Antitussives	Opiates, synthetic narcotics
	Decongestants and expectorants	Phenylephrine, phenylpropanolamine, potassium preparations

(continued)

TABLE 1 *(continued)*

Disorder	Medication	Common Examples
Miscellaneous conditions	Analgesics	Dextropropoxyphene, opiates, phenacetin, salicylates, synthetic narcotics
	Anesthetics	Lidocaine, methohexital, methoxyflurane
	Antidiabetic agents	Insulin, oral hypoglycemics
	Antineoplastics	Corticosteroids, mitomycin, procarbazine
	Antituberculosis agents	Isoniazid, rifampin

Source: Liston, E.H., Delirium in the aged. *Psychiatr. Clin. North Am.* 5:49–66, 1982.

to rule out Huntington's disease and give genetic counseling. A history of previous psychiatric disorders increases the likelihood of depression (pseudodementia) as the cause of a cognitive disorder in an older patient. A detailed review of systems is important to ensure that no superimposed systemic diseases are contributing to the patient's intellectual or behavioral impairment.

A detailed, thorough physical examination is needed to determine the patient's ability to interact with his or her environment and to rule out any systemic diseases that may potentially cause delirium or reversible dementia. The examination begins with vital signs to rule out fever or hypotension as acute causes of brain dysfunction, and a quick screen of mental status to ascertain the level of the intellectual function. The mental status examination should include the following:

1. Level of consciousness, affect
2. Orientation
3. Short-term memory: Ask the patient to repeat forwards five numbers and to recall objects
4. Long-term memory: Ask the patient about historical events (consistent with the patient's education)
5. Intellectual functioning: Ask the patient to perform simple calculations and interpret proverbs

Next, a detailed neurologic examination is essential. Frontal lobe signs such as the grasp reflex, oral responses, palmomental reflex, and glabella tap reflex are signs of diffuse cerebral dysfunction that are frequently present in dementia. A detailed review of the cranial nerves should include a search for papilledema, visual field defects, disturbances of extraocular movements, pupillary reactivity (tertiary syphilis), and hearing loss. Abnormal movements, such as tremors (Parkinson's disease) and tardive dyskinesia, and the gait should be observed. A small shuffling and unstable gait may represent normal pressure hydrocephalus; ataxic gait suggests cerebellar disease from alcoholism, tumors, strokes, or hypothyroidism; a shuffling and rigid gait is found in Parkinson's disease; a slapping, wide-based ataxic gait suggests tabes dorsalis or subacute combined degeneration. A sensory examination should be performed to rule out the dorsal and lateral column disease of vitamin B_{12} deficiency.

CAUSES OF MENTAL DYSFUNCTION

Delirium

The reported incidence of delirium is 15 to 30 percent on general medical and surgical wards, 10 to 50 percent on psychiatric wards, and about 40 percent on neurologic wards. The delirious elderly patient may be either stuporous or agitated, with the former more easily overlooked; dysphasia, abnormal movements, impaired coordination, urinary incontinence, focal neurologic signs, and autonomic system dysfunction tend to occur in older patients with delirium.

Of the myriad of disorders that cause delirium in the elderly (Table 2), most are caused by impaired oxygenation of brain tissue, retention of metabolic waste products (e.g., CO_2 or organic acids), fever, electrolyte imbalance, or medications and drugs. The elderly also seem to be more susceptible to delirium during accidental hyperthermia (heat stroke), hypothermia, vitamin deficiencies, alcohol ingestion, infections, and various endocrine disorders. Factors predisposing to delirium in the aged include sleep disorders, hearing loss, impaired vision, and unfamiliarity with caregivers or the physical environment, although none of these reliably predicts the development of delirium in an individual elderly person. Correction or improvement of the underlying pathologic process frequently leads to clearing of the sensorium and restores patients to their predelirium level of intellectual functioning.

Because drug use is highly prevalent among the elderly, the number and types of medications (see Table 1) should be determined for each patient evaluated for intellectual or behavioral dysfunction. Predisposing factors to drug-induced delirium in the elderly include (1) pharmacokinetic factors (diminished renal elimination of drugs and/or metabolites, decreased drug metabolism in liver leading to

TABLE 2
Disorders Causing Delirium in the Aged

Disorder	Examples
Central Nervous System Disease	
Neoplasm	Primary intracranial neoplasm, metastatic neoplasm—bronchogenic carcinoma, breast carcinoma
Cerebrovascular disease	Arteriosclerosis, cerebral infarction, subarachnoid hemorrhage, transient ischemic attacks, hypertensive encephalopathy, vasculitis (lupus), cranial arteritis, disseminated intravascular coagulation
Infection	Neurosyphilis, brain abscess, tuberculosis, meningoencephalitis (bacterial, viral, fungal), septic emboli (subacute bacterial endocarditis)
Head trauma	Chronic subdural hematoma, extradural hematoma, cerebral contusion, concussion
Ictal and postictal states	Idiopathic seizures, space-occupying lesion, posttraumatic lesions, electroconvulsive therapy
Cardiovascular Disease	
Decreased cardiac output	Congestive heart failure, cardiac arrhythmias, aortic stenosis, myocardial infarction
Hypotension	Orthostatic hypotension, vasovagal syncope, hypovolemia
Metabolic Disorders	
Hypoxemia	Respiratory insufficiency, anemia, carbon monoxide poisoning
Electrolyte disturbance	Kidney disease, adrenal disease, diabetes mellitus, diuretics, edematous states, inappropriate secretion of antidiuretic hormone, dehydration, starvation
Acidosis	Diabetes mellitus, kidney disease, pulmonary disease, chronic diarrhea
Alkalosis	Hyperadrenalcorticism, pulmonary disease, psychogenic hyperventilation
Hepatic disease	Acute hepatic failure, cirrhosis, chronic portahepatic encephalopathy
Uremia	Chronic glomerulonephritis, chronic pyelonephritis, acute renal failure, obstructive uropathy
Endocrinopathies	Hypothyroidism, thyrotoxicosis, "apathetic" hyperthyroidism, hypoglycemia, hyperglycemia, hypoparathyroidism, hyperparathyroidism, hypoadrenalcorticism, hyperadrenalcorticism

(continued)

TABLE 2 *(continued)*

Disorder	Examples
Deficiency states	Hypovitaminosis—thiamine, nicotinic acid, vitamin B_{12}, folate deficiency, iron deficiency
Other Disorders	
Trauma	Burns, surgery, multiple injuries, fractures (fat embolism)
Sensory deprivation	Cataracts, glaucoma, otosclerosis, darkness ("sundown syndrome")
Exogenous toxins	Medications, alcohol, withdrawal syndromes, heavy metals, solvents, insecticides, pesticides, carbon monoxide
Temperature regulation	Exposure and accidental hypothermia, heat stroke, febrile illnesses

Source: Liston, E.H., Delirium in the aged. *Psychiatr. Clin. North Am.* 5:49–66, 1982.

prolonged drug half-life, altered volume of drug distribution, or reduced serum albumin concentration leading to increased amounts of circulating unbound drug); (2) abrupt discontinuation of a drug (including ethanol, sedatives, tranquilizers), leading to drug withdrawal syndrome; and (3) multiple drug use, which includes drugs prescribed by physicians for coexisting organic or functional diseases, over-the-counter medications, and ethanol (up to 10 percent of the elderly are alcoholic). Fortunately, most drug-induced delirium can be reversed by reducing or stopping the offending agent.

Reversible Dementia
Of the causes of dementia and their frequencies (shown in Table 3), up to one-third have potentially reversible causes, and the remainder may have some response to therapeutic interventions.

Pseudodementia Pseudodementia is a variant of depressive illness that causes cognitive changes highly suggestive of a primary dementia. Because pseudodementia frequently responds to tricyclic antidepressant drugs (60 to 70 percent) or to electroconvulsive therapy, it is important to identify those depressed individuals who comprise 4 to 6 percent of all demented elderly patients. Unlike the truly demented individual, the patient with pseudodementia usually shows a relatively well-defined onset and rapid progression of cognitive dysfunction; he makes little effort to answer questions ("I don't know")

TABLE 3
Causes of Dementia

Category	Percentage of Total Dementias	Distinctive Characteristics
Irreversible Causes		
Alzheimer's disease	54	CT: atrophy, enlarged ventricles, progressive decline
Multiinfarct dementia	8	CT: numerous old infarcts, stepwise progression
Huntington's disease	5	Family history
Potentially Reversible Causes		
Normal pressure hydrocephalus	6	Gait disturbance, urinary incontinence CT: enlarged ventricles, no atrophy
Dementia secondary to alcohol	5	Signs of chronic alcoholism
Drugs	3	See text (p. 202)
Intracranial masses	5	Focal neurologic findings
Depression	4	See Table 4 (p. 201)
Miscellaneous: metabolic disorders, intracranial disorders, CNS infections, systemic illnesses, chemicals, nutritional deficiencies, trauma, dehydration, etc.	9	See text (pp. 202–203)

Source: Halperin, A.K., and Beck, P., Dementia. In Fletcher, R., Dornbran, L., Hoole, A., and Pickard, G., *Ambulatory Care Manual.* In press.

or to perform requested tasks. He frequently demonstrates pervasive affective changes with loss of social skills, minimizes other skills and abilities, and is often distressed over his cognitive and memory losses despite the lack of effort to cope with deficits. Frequently there is a prior history of psychopathology in the patient with pseudodementia. Table 4 describes the differential features of pseudodementia and true dementia.

Tricyclic antidepressants should be used, though with caution, in elderly patients with pseudodementia. Nortriptyline and desipramine tend to have lesser anticholinergic side effects and may be better tolerated. When used, they should be started in a low dose, 25 mg/day, and the maximum dose should rarely exceed 75 mg/day to minimize the risk of cardiac arrhythmias.

TABLE 4

Clinical Features of Pseudodementia and True Dementia

Clinical Feature	Pseudo-dementia	Dementia
Duration of symptoms before physician consulted	Short	Long
Onset can be dated with some precision	Usual	Unusual
Family aware of dysfunction and severity	Usual	Variable[a] (rare in early stages, usual in late stages)
Rapid progression of symptoms	Usual	Unusual
History of prior psychopathology	Usual	Unusual
Patient's complaints of cognitive loss	Emphasized	Variable[a] (minimized in late stages)
Patient's description of cognitive loss	Detailed	Vague
Patient's disability	Emphasized	Variable[a] (concealed in late stages)
Patient's valuation of accomplishments	Minimized	Variable[a]
Patient's efforts in attempting to perform tasks	Small	Great
Patient's efforts to cope with dysfunction	Minimal	Maximal
Patient's emotional reaction	Great distress	Variable[a] (unconcerned in late stages)
Patient's affect	Depressed	Labile, blunted, or depressed
Loss of social skills	Early	Late
Behavior congruent with severity of cognitive loss	Unusual	Usual
Attention and concentration	Often good	Often poor
"Don't know" answers	Usual	Unusual
"Near miss" answers	Unusual	Variable[a] (usual in late stages)
Memory loss for recent versus remote events	About equal	Greater
Specific memory gaps ("patchy memory loss")	Usual	Unusual
Performance on tasks of similar difficulty	Variable	Consistent

Source: Reprinted with permission from Small, G.W., Liston, E.H., Jarvik, L.F., Diagnosis and treatment of dementia in the aged. In Geriatric Medicine. *West. J. Med.* 135:469–481, 1981; and adapted from Wells, C.E., The differential diagnosis of psychiatric disorders in the elderly. In Cole, J.O., and Barrett, J.E. (Eds.), *Psychopathology in the Aged.* New York: Raven Press, 1980.

[a]Wells lists the characteristics of the later stages of dementia. These manifestations, however, can be variable early in the course of dementia and are helpful in the differential diagnosis only if they are in the direction seen in later stages of dementia.

Normal Pressure Hydrocephalus Normal pressure hydrocephalus, thought to be caused by deficient resorption of cerebral spinal fluid, is characterized by progressive dementia, gait disturbances, and urinary incontinence. The computed tomography (CT) scan shows mild ventricular enlargement without cortical atrophy; radionuclide cisternography, long-term pressure recording, and the cerebrospinal fluid infusion test can confirm the diagnosis, but their use is controversial. Normal pressure hydrocephalus is usually an idiopathic disorder, although it may be secondary to central nervous system diseases such as previous subarachnoid hemorrhage, meningitis, or tumors. There are conflicting opinions regarding criteria for the diagnosis of normal pressure hydrocephalus, the natural history of the disease, and the likelihood of a successful result with ventriculoatrial or ventriculoperitoneal shunting. Patients with the classic triad of dementia, a prominent gait disturbance, and urinary incontinence, and who have the diagnosis confirmed by CT scan, have approximately a 50 percent chance of improving; there is less improvement if any of these criteria are absent. Improvement is variable in degree and may be short-lived; only a few patients have had a complete remission lasting for years. Furthermore, serious complications from shunts occur in about 35 percent of patients and include subdural hematomas, intracerebral hemorrhage, shunt malfunction, seizures, and nonhemorrhagic strokes.

Dementia Caused by Drugs Drugs can cause dementia as well as delirium. The most troublesome drugs are antihypertensives (especially reserpine, clonidine, and methyldopa) and neurotropic drugs with central anticholinergic activity (including antiparkinsonian drugs, tricyclic antidepressants, monoamine oxidase inhibitors, and other antidepressant agents). Because of the reduced central nervous system (CNS) cholinergic activity observed in patients with senile dementia of Alzheimer's type (SDAT), it appears likely that drugs with anticholinergic effects may unmask some patients with early SDAT. Reducing the dose or discontinuing the drugs and investigating alternative treatment are necessary when evaluating possible drug-induced dementia in elderly patients.

Miscellaneous Disorders Miscellaneous disorders account for a significant number of dementias, although no single etiology is very common. These disorders include endocrine diseases such as hyperthyroidism, hypothyroidism, Addison's disease, Cushing's disease, steroid administration, hypoglycemia, hypercalcemia, and hypopi-tuitarism; metabolic and electrolyte disturbances such as hepatic en-cephalopathy, hyponatremia, and uremia; nutritional deficiencies such as Wernicke-Korsakoff syndrome found in alcoholics, anemias as-sociated with vitamin B_{12} or folic acid deficiency, and pellagra; certain cerebral infections such as tuberculous and fungal meningitis, brain abscess, and neurosyphilis; and dehydration from diuretics, poor fluid intake, or loss of body fluids.

Irreversible Dementias

Senile dementia of Alzheimer's type was first noted by Alzheimer in 1907 as a type of presenile degenerative dementia. Until the 1960s the dominant view was that arteriosclerotic vascular disease caused senile dementia. Current evidence indicates that ischemic disease does not cause SDAT, and the majority of patients with senile dementia have a degenerative process identical to the histologic changes present in the presenile form of the disease. Senile dementia of Alzheimer's type now refers to the occurrence of this disease entity at any age.

Morphologically, in late-stage SDAT there is gross atrophy of the cerebral cortex and dilation of the cerebral ventricles. Microscopi-cally, the brains of deceased advanced-stage SDAT patients dem-onstrate neuritic degeneration in the hippocampus and in the frontal, occipital, and parietal cortex; the predominant lesions are amyloid-containing plaques in extraneuronal spaces and neurofibrillary tan-gles—that is, densely packed protein microfibrils in the neuronal cytoplasm. Neither of these microscopic lesions occurs in infarcted brain.

Biochemically, affected areas of the brain are deficient in choline acetyltransferase (CAT); CAT enzyme activity is inversely correlated with the amount of senile plaque and premortem clinical measure-ments of dementia. It has recently been shown that the main sources of CNS cholinergic innervation are the axons that originate in (1) the nucleus basalis of Meynert (projecting into the frontal, prefrontal, and parietal cortex) and (2) in the medial septal nucleus and the diagonal band of Broca (innervating the occipital cortex and hip-pocampus). Cholinesterase inhibitors and cholinergic agonists im-prove memory function, in a manner remarkably analogous to the response in Parkinson's disease, and enhancement of CNS acetyl-choline secretion may be beneficial in the early stages of SDAT.

Clinically, the dementia associated with Alzheimer's disease usually is a progressive disease that evolves through several phases. In the early phase, subtle changes of memory loss and somatic complaints are common. In the middle phase, impairments in judgment, orientation, intellect, and memory become more prominent. The ability to comprehend, assimilate, and integrate new information is impaired, and attention to social amenities is decreased. In the late phase, the patient's personality and identity can be totally lost. The factors influencing the progression from one phase to another are unknown, and the rate of progression is variable. In the later stages of the disease, life expectancy is decreased—the average survival is six years less for demented individuals than for age-matched controls. Senile dementia of Alzheimer's type is the fourth leading cause of death in the United States and now accounts for over half of the diagnoses of dementia.

The ability of drugs to improve cognitive function in SDAT patients is controversial. A combination of dihydrogenated ergot alkaloids, Hydergine, which exerts its effects through enhanced metabolic action, has been the most extensively studied, with conflicting results. Dihydrogenated ergot alkaloids may be of some long-term benefit in the treatment of some demented patients, but it is not known which patients will respond. The initial dose of dihydrogenated ergot alkaloids should be 1 mg three times per day, and this regimen should be followed for at least two months before being discontinued. The results with papaverine, a vasodilator, are also controversial, and the use of lecithin, choline, and physostigmine (in an effort to increase deficient amounts of acetylcholine in the brain) has not yet demonstrated any consistent improvement in memory or cognitive function.

Multiinfarct dementia (MID) may be distinguished from SDAT clinically and morphologically. Patients with MID have had numerous cerebral infarctions that are visible by CT scan, usually involving more than 50 grams of brain tissue. They usually have an abrupt onset, a stepwise progression of their dementia with a fluctuating course, hypertension, and focal neurologic signs and symptoms. Although the damage produced by multiple infarctions cannot be reversed, further deterioration may be retarded by vigorous treatment of associated medical problems such as hypertension, diabetes, valvular heart disease, and cerebrovascular disease. Dihydrogenated ergot alkaloids have been reported to bring about variable improvement of mental function. Patients with arteriosclerotic cerebrovascular disease live approximately ten years less than age-matched controls.

DIAGNOSTIC STRATEGIES

In some cases the etiology of the dementia may be obvious from the history and physical examination alone—for example, late-stage Alzheimer's disease, dementia following multiple strokes, Huntington's disease, drugs, depression, hyperthyroidism, or hypothyroidism. In cases where the diagnosis is not obvious after the history and physical examination, however, the following laboratory tests are recommended:

- complete blood count
- serologic tests for syphilis
- standard screening chemistry tests (e.g., SMA-12)
- thyroid function tests
- serum B_{12} and folate levels
- urinalysis
- chest x-ray

If none of the above tests is diagnostic, further neurologic testing is indicated. Subdural hematomas, intracranial tumors, normal pressure hydrocephalus, MID, and Alzheimer's disease can be diagnosed with a CT scan. An electroencephalogram is rarely helpful in the workup of dementia. A lumbar puncture need be performed only when tertiary syphilis, other central nervous system infections, or an otherwise undetected neoplasm is suspected. The dementia workup is often best done on an outpatient basis because changes in environment such as hospitalization can exacerbate symptoms.

SUPPORTIVE INTERVENTIONS

Dementia should not be viewed as hopeless. Although there is no specific treatment for most causes of dementia, there are many supportive measures that can help stabilize and improve the functional capacity of these patients.

1. Health care personnel should optimize communication with the demented person by speaking slowly, simply, and sincerely.

2. Changes in the environment should be minimized because mental deterioration frequently accompanies a change in location (i.e., avoid hospitalization or admission to a nursing home).

3. The routine use of sedatives and psychotropic drugs should be avoided unless severe agitation is present. In this case, haloperidol (Haldol) in low doses from 0.5 to 1 mg daily may be helpful. If nocturnal wandering or sleep disturbance is a problem, a short-acting

benzodiazepine such as oxazepam (Serax) may be helpful. All drugs must be used with caution.

4. Correction of sensory impairments such as visual and hearing deficits can help maximize function.

5. Family support groups for patients with Alzheimer's disease are effective in enabling families to have more realistic expectations of patients with this disorder and fewer feelings of guilt and anger.

6. Social services such as visiting health nurses, homemaker aides, home-delivered meals, physical therapy, respite care, senior citizens' centers, and day care centers for the elderly can be an invaluable resource to the patient and family.

7. All coexistent medical conditions should be aggressively treated.

SUGGESTED READING

1. Black, P. Idiopathic normal pressure hydrocephalus: Results in shunting in 62 patients. *J. Neurosurg.* 52:371–377, 1980.
2. *Diagnostic and Statistical Manual of Mental Disorders,* 3rd ed. Washington, D.C.: American Psychiatric Association, 1980.
3. Liston, E.H. Delirium in the aged. *Psychiatr. Clin. North Am.* 5:49–66, 1982.
4. McDonald, R.J. Hydergine: A review of 26 clinical studies. *Pharmakopsychiatry* 12:1–15, 1979.
5. Richardson, K. Hope and flexibility: Your keys to helping OBS patients. *Nursing* 82:65–69, 1982.
6. Schneck, M.K., Reisberg, B., Ferris, S.H. An overview of current concepts of Alzheimer's disease. *Am. J. Psychiatry* 139:166–173, 1982.
7. Spar, J.E. Dementia in the aged. *Psychiatr. Clin. North Am.* 5:67–86, 1982.
8. Wells, C.E. Pseudodementia. *Am. J. Psychiatry* 136:895–900, 1979.

Cerebral Vascular Disease

SEYMOUR EISENBERG, M.D.

Editor's note: Preventing strokes is preferable to even the most skillful management of a stroke after it has occurred. In addition to attention to long-range risk factors for atherosclerosis, the physician who cares for elderly patients must be concerned with factors listed here that can acutely precipitate a stroke in a susceptible patient.

In the last 50 years the incidence of stroke has declined significantly; this seems true wherever accurate data are available. Measurable decline was actually apparent before the development and widespread use of antihypertensive agents, but the more recent 5 percent per year decline is almost certainly due to the better detection and treatment of hypertension. Nevertheless, stroke or cerebral vascular accident (CVA) remains the third leading cause of death among the elderly and, along with dementia, is probably the greatest fear of persons entering this phase of their life.

Definite risk factors for cerebral vascular disease have been identified by the Framingham study and other longitudinal studies; long-standing and poorly controlled hypertension and diabetes mellitus are clearly associated with an increase in the incidence and severity of cerebral vascular disease. Age per se becomes an overriding risk factor after 65.

To approach the problem of stroke prevention in a meaningful way, one must have a clear perception of the dual nature of the task—that is, the long-term prevention of atherosclerosis in general and ultimately the somewhat different problem of the prevention of the acute clinical event, the stroke. Belated institution of measures to decrease atherosclerosis is of uncertain benefit; in elderly persons there is often not enough time to undo that which took years to develop. Identifying high-risk individuals with improper health hab-

207

its at an early age and instituting dietary, activity, and pharmacologic measures to forestall atherogenesis is a high priority of preventive medicine that is receiving an encouraging amount of attention.

Of equal or greater importance to the present generation of geriatric patients are the identification and management of the stroke-prone patient. The vascular disease is probably relatively irreversible; whether regression of atheromata can be achieved is a debatable issue. On the other hand, there are clearly measures that can avoid the precipitation of a devastating cerebral infarction—the ultimate failure. I shall focus primarily on how one can identify the stroke-prone individual and what can be done to prevent or delay the acute event.

PREVENTION OF CEREBRAL ATHEROSCLEROSIS

Several long-term longitudinal studies have established generally accepted atherogenic risk factors. Control of these factors promises a major decrease in the incidence of this disease. A general awareness of the problems of fat and cholesterol ingestion, a sedentary life-style, and a high salt intake has led to some important changes in eating habits and activity levels, and there should be an increasingly apparent impact on cardiovascular disease as these changes gather momentum. In addition, diminished tobacco use and improved management of diabetes mellitus may yield benefits. The significant decline in strokes and in fatal heart attacks that has already occurred is eloquent testimony to these trends. It is encouraging to speculate that future generations of people entering their seventies will be more vigorous, more active, and more involved in their own health care and that the disabling and enfeebling effects of cerebral and coronary atherosclerosis will be at least delayed.

PREVENTION OF THE ACUTE VASCULAR EVENT

The stroke-prone individual can be recognized in most instances without difficulty. Table 1 lists the characteristics that are likely to be found. Treatment after a stroke is not at all satisfactory, so primary care physicians must be alert to the imminence of a stroke in order to initiate appropriate therapy and avoid abrupt iatrogenic perturbations which might in themselves be provocative of an acute event.

Hypertension
Hypertension is not only important in the atherogenic process but also is an acute provocative factor in the person with cerebral ath-

TABLE 1

Characteristics of the Stroke-Prone Patient

Age >65 years old
Moderate obesity
Cigarette smoker
Moderate to heavy drinker
Past history of transient ischemic attacks
Past history of hypertension/diabetes
Congestive heart failure
Ischemic heart disease
Peripheral vascular disease
Atrial fibrillation
Carotid artery disease/bruit
Elevated serum cholesterol/uric acid
Left ventricular hypertrophy
Serum hemoglobin >16.5

erosclerosis; the mechanism whereby hypertension precipitates occlusion is not completely clear except for cerebral hemorrhage that is generally thought to be associated with severe hypertension. The Veterans Administration study of the treatment of hypertension had to be abruptly halted in patients with diastolic pressures higher than 114 mm Hg because of the remarkable incidence of strokes in untreated patients. The data in elderly subjects with mild to moderate hypertension (diastolic pressure 90 to 114 mm Hg are not as dramatic but are accumulating and convincing.

Caution is mandatory in the treatment of elderly hypertensive patients because of their basic vulnerability to adverse reactions. For example, they are particularly vulnerable to orthostatic hypotension because their vascular responses to volume changes are attenuated. The volume depletion following the use of diuretics may cause a sudden drop in cerebral vascular perfusion that can actually provoke the very stroke one is attempting to prevent. The elderly are particularly susceptible to the sedative and depressive effects of antihypertensive agents.

Education of patients to help them understand the goals of treatment—the prevention of organ damage, and particularly the prevention of strokes and congestive heart failure—is essential. It must be recognized in the decision to treat that many patients who are treated would have suffered no ill effects from their mild hypertension; the majority of such patients would not have a stroke. Even this disclaimer must be honestly presented in the interest of properly informing the patient of the nature of this disorder. Studies of cerebral blood flow in hypertensive patients do not support the widely held view that hypertension of some degree is necessary to achieve proper perfusion. It is true, however, that the elderly do not autoregulate their cerebral vascular resistance as efficiently as do younger people, and abrupt lowering of the blood pressure may lead to a sudden decrease in flow that can cause thrombotic occlusion.

Erythremia (Relative and Absolute Polycythemia)
Studies from my laboratory indicated that the hematocrit and blood viscosity were increased in persons with recent strokes. Data from the Framingham study showed a threefold increase in strokes in persons with hemoglobin concentration greater than 16.5, as compared with those whose hemoglobin concentration was less than this figure. Blood viscosity increases abruptly when the hematocrit exceeds 52 percent, so it would seem prudent to do intermittent phlebotomies to control erythremia in stroke-prone individuals, although there has not been a controlled study to demonstrate this protection.

Cigarette Smoking
Heavy cigarette smoking is widely accepted as a risk factor in atherogenesis, particularly in coronary artery disease, but there is no reason why the cerebral circulation should be spared. Just as smoking may play a role in acute coronary events and sudden death, so might it be implicated in a provocative role in strokes and transient ischemic attacks, probably through similar pathogenetic mechanisms.

Heart Disease
Patients with congestive heart failure are at great risk of stroke, perhaps because of secondary alterations in cerebral blood flow. The dramatic increase in hematocrit, serum fibrinogen concentration, and blood viscosity that occurs during aggressive diuresis, all related to a decline in plasma volume, may account for the reported increased incidence of stroke. The institution of anticoagulant therapy—low-dose heparin, at least—may be warranted during this active treatment period, particularly if a patient has had previous strokes, transient ischemic attacks (TIAs), diabetes mellitus, or other risk factors.

Myocardial Infarction
The increased incidence of stroke in persons with acute myocardial infarction could be related to hypotension, inactivity, mural thrombi, or to a putative hypercoagulable state. The diagnosis may be further obscured by the electrographic changes associated with strokes. In

addition, stroke patients may suffer a myocardial infarction during their convalescence.

Diabetes and Serum Lipids

Elevated lipid levels may predispose to intravascular coagulation, and it is probable that glycosylated erythrocytes in the poorly controlled diabetic are more apt to aggregate, leading to disturbed flow through small vessels. Control of both blood sugar and blood lipids probably decreases the likelihood of stroke.

Dehydration

Strokes are more likely to occur during the course of other acute illnesses, particularly those associated with contraction of the extracellular and plasma volume. This impression is based on my personal observation and experience in an acute care center over a number of years.

Neoplasia

A variety of neoplasms are associated with an increased risk for intravascular thromboses, including stroke, and preventive measures might be considered depending on the patient's general clinical state and circumstances.

Previous Cerebral Events

The group at highest risk for stroke are persons who have suffered previous CVAs or TIAs. The presence of obviously serious atheromatous disease of the cerebral vasculature has become overt in these patients, whereas it may only be presumed or suspected in others. One cannot assume that a single diseased vessel in the cerebral vasculature has developed a thrombus or has been transiently compromised; nor does degree of recovery reveal a great deal about the condition of other cerebral vessels. The incidence of reinfarction is substantial under the best circumstances and is almost to be anticipated if hypertension and other risk factors are uncorrected. Transient ischemic attacks, when there is a bruit in the neck, may or may not be associated with more distal intracranial vascular lesions. Surgery for such lesions in the carotid system is advocated in some centers; others now use antiplatelet aggregating agents as the mainstay of treatment in this circumstance. The management of TIAs in elderly patients is best summarized in the following way.

1. Treat vertebrobasilar disease with either anticoagulants or platelet inhibitors. If the patient is unsteady and subject to falls, or if

compliance and follow-up are a problem, anticoagulants might be too hazardous.

2. If amaurosis fugax is part of the ischemic syndrome, if a bruit is heard at the carotid bifurcation, or if atheromatous emboli were identified in the ipsilateral retina, surgery should be strongly considered.

3. For the vast number of nonspecific dizzy spell problems and vertigo or asymptomatic bruits in elderly patients, aggressive invasive workup is not warranted; antiplatelet aggregating agents are probably the most prudent treatment modality.

Platelet Aggregation
The role of platelet aggregation in the genesis of cerebral infarction and in TIAs is not clear. The efficacy of antiplatelet aggregating agents is uncertain and continues under study at the present time; it is likely that agents will be developed that affect this system favorably. Although the diminished incidence of stroke in Greenland Eskimos has been imputed to prostaglandin alterations induced by their diet of cold-water fish, convincing data are not yet available.

MANAGEMENT OF THE PATIENT WITH AN ACUTE STROKE

Treatment of Progressing Stroke
Patients with a stroke that is significantly worsening in the first 24 hours are said to have a "progressing stroke" if intracranial bleeding has been excluded. Improved mortality and morbidity results have been reported when heparin in a full dosage schedule is employed early in these circumstances, followed by warfarin (Coumadin) therapy for several weeks. If hypertension is not satisfactorily controlled, however, one should be reluctant to use anticoagulants.

Management of the Completed Stroke
The primary goal in management of the completed stroke is to exclude treatable disease. An adequate, detailed history and physical examination, often complicated by alterations in the patient's consciousness or the presence of aphasia, should include a detailed chronological account of the development of the neurologic deficit. Thus, a thrombotic event occurring during sleep can be distinguished from the progressive and dramatic presentation of a cerebral hemorrhage or from an acute cerebral embolus in the young to middle-

aged person with mitral valve disease and atrial fibrillation. The history should also include the patient's general state of health—hypertension and its treatment, cardiovascular disease—as well as any history of heart failure, murmurs, rheumatic fever, arrhythmias, fever, chest pain, or past history of syphilis. The physical examination should include taking blood pressure in both arms and a careful search for hypertensive or diabetic retinopathy, bruits in the neck, perforation of the nasal septum, rales in the chest, cardiomegaly, abnormalities of cardiac rhythm, or heart murmurs. Splenomegaly or petechiae should raise the possibility of bacterial endocarditis: femoral bruits and attenuated distal pulses would be evidence of a severe generalized atherosclerotic process.

Laboratory examination should include a hemogram to rule out anemia or polycythemia, a serologic test for syphilis, blood cultures if the patient is anemic or febrile, serum lipids, blood sugar, serum creatinine, electrolytes, and serum proteins. Though expensive, a computed tomography scan in all patients with an acute stroke is probably reasonable and cost-effective. Spinal fluid examination should be performed unless there is a contraindication to lumbar puncture.

Initially, care should be directed mostly toward maintaining an airway, normalizing blood pressure, and avoidance of aspiration, congestive heart failure, dehydration, or polycythemia. If the blood pressure is exceedingly high, the possibility of hypertensive encephalopathy must be seriously considered, and the blood pressure rapidly returned toward normal. Control of heart rate to maximize cardiac output is needed when there is significant bradycardia or tachycardia. Oxygen should be used only when there is significant hypoxemia; otherwise, oxygen has vasoconstrictor properties and is possibly harmful.

Vasodilator therapy is usually unsuccessful and may be harmful because either normal or ischemic tissue could be deprived of blood through a paradoxical "steal syndrome." Inhalations of carbon dioxide (5–7%) increase total cerebral blood flow, but results of such treatment have been largely disappointing. Papaverine and other drugs with putative vasodilatory properties are of little value, and their use is discouraged. The circumstances prevailing at the injury site—local hypoxia, carbon dioxide and lactate accumulation—favor maximal vasodilatation. It is unlikely that further dilatation of these vessels can be effected.

REHABILITATION AND LONG-TERM GOALS

The primary goal of management, to return the patient to as completely functional and independent an existence as possible, requires the immediate institution of an active treatment program by an interdisciplinary team of professionals. Prevention of contractures and disuse atrophy is critical during the acute-care period, with passive motion and exercises at the bedside. The first few weeks are critical in regard to recovery of function; any degree of reversibility that exists at this point must be fully exploited. Thereafter, training is equally intense but is directed more toward maximal self-care, substituting the unaffected for the impaired. The team should include a psychiatrist, physical therapist, occupational therapist, speech therapist, and social worker. Ultimately, decisions will have to be made regarding the patient's degree of impairment, capacity for self-care and independent living, and potential for rehabilitation.

The converse of all this active, multidisciplinary intervention, the attitude of hopelessness and pessimism which makes the only goal that of disposition and custodial care, is almost certain to lead to tragic consequences, with maximal disability and dependence.

SUGGESTED READING

1. Eisenberg, S. Blood viscosity and fibrinogen concentration following cerebral infarction. *Circulation* 33, 34 (Suppl. 11):10–14, 1966.
2. Garraway, W.M., Whisenant, J.P., Furlen, A.J., et al. The declining incidence of stroke. *N. Engl. J. Med.* 300:449–452, 1979
3. Kannel, W.B., Blaisdell, D.W., Gifford, R., et al. Risk factors in stroke due to cerebral infarction. A statement prepared by a subcommittee of the Council on Cerebrovascular Disease of the American Heart Association. *Stroke* 2:423–438, 1971.
4. Leonberg, S.C., Elliott, F.A. Prevention of recurrent stroke. *Stroke* 12:731–735, 1981.
5. Millikan, C.H., McDowell, F.H. Treatment of progressing stroke. *Stroke* 12(4):397–408, 1981.

Anticonvulsant Therapy in the Elderly

PETER GAL, PHARM.D., and
JACK D. McCUE, M.D.

Editor's note: Prophylactic anticonvulsant treatment of patients with cerebrovascular disease is difficult to justify until a seizure has actually occurred. Once treatment is begun, the physician must be alert to central nervous system toxicity. Anticonvulsants should be discontinued in patients with seizures that follow a stroke after a suitable seizure-free interval.

The literature concerned with the indications for the initiation of anticonvulsant therapy and for subsequent discontinuation of treatment is limited and often anecdotal. Using what is available, however, this chapter will focus on a few of the practical aspects of seizure management in the elderly that must be considered by primary care practitioners: (1) the treatment of seizures following strokes; (2) special considerations in the use of anticonvulsant agents in the elderly; (3) the indications for discontinuation of anticonvulsants.

STROKES AND SEIZURES

Cerebrovascular disease, a rare cause of seizures in young people, is the single most common cause of seizures in the elderly. Up to 30 percent of first seizures in patients over 69 years of age are attributed to cerebrovascular disease, and patients with known cerebrovascular disease have a 10 to 30 percent risk of subsequently developing seizures. Some factors that have been associated with a higher risk of seizures include an abnormal electroencephalogram (EEG), indicating a potential seizure focus following a stroke; embolic rather than thrombotic strokes; and infarctions located in the cerebral cortex. Initial seizures may occur up to many months after the stroke, although the majority occur within one week of the acute illness. These rather limited observations, however, are of little help in the man-

215

agement of most patients; studies that confirm and expand the list are needed. We believe that, in general, a less than 30 percent overall risk of seizure warrants close monitoring, but it does not justify prophylactic anticonvulsant use.

Whether anticonvulsant therapy is begun after a first seizure probably affects future events; thus it is unclear what the incidence of second seizures is in patients not treated with anticonvulsants after the first seizure. In one report, seizure recurrence among patients who had already had a seizure after a stroke was 31 percent (most of these patients were receiving anticonvulsants).[1] Recurrent seizures were more likely to be encountered in patients with head trauma, multiple seizures, status epilepticus, and a generalized spike-wave EEG pattern.

Current data do not permit the definition of a group of stroke patients at a high enough risk to justify routine use of anticonvulsants. Once a seizure has occurred, anticonvulsant therapy is, of course, indicated; this group of patients, even when treated, is at a greater risk of recurrence of seizures.

ANTICONVULSANTS IN ELDERLY PATIENTS

The use of anticonvulsants must take into consideration their greater toxicity in elderly patients. The potential for central nervous system toxicity, cardiovascular side effects, and drug interactions is increased in elderly patients, who may have multiple underlying illnesses, reduced organ reserves, and are often taking multiple drugs. Patients with cerebrovascular disease and other types of organic brain disease are more likely to suffer from central nervous system toxicity in the form of impaired mental function, agitation, and involuntary movement disorders.

Drug choice depends on the type of seizure, whether the risk of toxicity of a particular drug is greater for a certain patient, the effect of anticonvulsants on concurrent diseases and other drugs, and cost. Most seizures in the elderly are either generalized tonic-clonic seizures or complex partial seizures, so the drugs most likely to be used are phenytoin, phenobarbital, and carbamazepine. Generally, the use of a single agent rather than multiple drugs is safest in this medically complex group of patients. Plasma levels must be monitored to ensure

---

1. W.A. Hauser, V.E. Anderson, R.B. Loewenson, S.M. McRoberts. Seizure recurrence after a first unprovoked seizure. *N. Engl. J. Med.* 307:522–528, 1982.

the optimal dose adjustments for seizure prevention with the least toxicity.

Phenytoin

The most commonly used anticonvulsant, phenytoin (Dilantin), remains surprisingly difficult to dose. The wide interpatient variability in the rate of drug elimination, the nonlinear pharmacokinetics of phenytoin, and a high degree of protein binding that is altered by many drugs and disease states make this a hard drug to use, despite many years of experience with it. Although it is generally not considered a major antiarrhythmic drug, except perhaps for the treatment of digitalis-induced arrhythmias, phenytoin also has antiarrhythmic effects that occur at the same plasma concentrations needed for seizure control.

The central nervous system toxicity of phenytoin is particularly troublesome in the elderly. Sedation, disorientation, confusion, ataxia, and visual disturbances occur at toxic levels, but even at lower levels intellectual function is impaired, especially in patients with underlying brain damage. Chronic toxicity has been associated with a progressive and irreversible cerebellar degeneration.

When administered intravenously at too fast a rate, phenytoin can cause hypotension. Younger patients can tolerate intravenous doses at rates of up to 50 mg/min, but the elderly may tolerate only 10–20 mg/min.

In one study phenytoin was reported to depress both humoral and cellular immune mechanisms,[2] and another study showed an increased frequency of upper respiratory infections after patients were started on phenytoin.[3] The latter investigators associated this phenomenon with depressed IgA concentrations in serum and in nasal secretions, although alternate explanations are tenable. In similar studies with phenobarbital and carbamazepine, no increase in infections was observed.

Dose One should attempt to achieve plasma phenytoin levels of 10–20 μg/ml with a single daily dose, as in younger patients. Intravenous infusions should be slow, less than 20 mg/min, to avoid serious hypotension. Intramuscular phenytoin should not be used because

2. E.H. Reynolds, Chronic antiepileptic toxicity: A review. *Epilepsia* 16:319–353, 1975.
3. N.E. Gilhus, J.A. Aarli. Immunoglobulin concentrations in nasal secretions and frequency of respiratory disease in epileptic patients. In R. Canger, F. Angeleri, J.K. Penry (Eds.), *Epileptology: XIth Epilepsy International Symposium* (New York: Raven Press, 1980), pp. 479–481.

absorption is erratic and considerable muscle damage occurs. Absorption of phenytoin suspension through nasogastric tubes is impaired in patients also receiving enteral feedings; crushed phenytoin Infatabs appear to avoid this problem.

Phenobarbital

Often disregarded in the choice of anticonvulsants because of fear of excessive sedation or paradoxical excitation, phenobarbital is an underused agent for the treatment of seizures in the elderly. The general impression of the frequency and severity of central nervous system toxicity is based on largely anecdotal data and is not borne out by our experience. Tolerance to sedation often develops within a few weeks, and administering the daily dose at bedtime not only avoids most sedation but may help elderly insomniacs (and their roommates) to sleep better.

Unlike the increased problems seen with phenytoin in patients with brain disease, barbiturates are thought by some investigators to have beneficial effects on the hypoxic and ischemic brain, possibly minimizing further damage. One might well consider phenobarbital, therefore, as the preferred drug for many stroke patients who have had a seizure.

Respiratory depression is not a problem with ordinary doses. Combinations of phenobarbital and benzodiazepines or alcohol, however, may depress the often already abnormal respiratory centers of the elderly. Addiction or intentional abuse of phenobarbital is, as a rule, not a serious issue in the elderly; accidental or iatrogenic withdrawal syndromes, especially in view of the elderly person's often erratic compliance with drug regimens, pose a greater risk.

Dose The long half-life of phenobarbital (two to five days) allows once-a-day dosing. When the drug is given as a single bedtime dose, the goal should be a therapeutic plasma concentration of 15–40 µg/ml. Liver enzyme induction occurs over the first month of therapy, so the required dose of phenobarbital and possibly other drugs taken concurrently will slowly increase.

Carbamazepine

The psychomotor depression that can complicate the use of phenytoin and phenobarbital appears to be absent with carbamazepine (Tegretol). Some neurologists believe, in fact, that is has beneficial psychotropic effects, particularly in brain-damaged patients, while others attribute this observation to improved seizure control and discontinuation of other mentally depressing anticonvulsants. Carbamazepine may be superior to other anticonvulsants for controlling complex partial seizures.

Patients treated with higher doses of carbamazepine, especially those receiving concurrent thiazide diuretics and those with congestive heart failure, may develop the syndrome of inappropriate secretion of antidiuretic hormone (SIADH), characterized by dilutional hyponatremia. Interestingly, phenytoin may actually correct this problem, and when phenytoin and carbamazepine are given concurrently, discontinuation of phenytoin may allow it to emerge.

Aplastic anemia is a rare complication of carbamazepine therapy, occurring primarily in patients treated for trigeminal neuralgia. A transient drop in the white blood cell count to 3,000 to 4,000 cells/ mm^3 is not unusual, however, and does not require discontinuation of carbamazepine. In general, frequent white blood cell counts for the first six months of therapy are prudent. Because elderly Caucasian women have a higher incidence of aplastic anemia than the general population, they may deserve closer monitoring. Overall, while the toxicity of carbamazepine is different, it is not more severe than that of phenytoin or phenobarbital.

Dose Initial dosing of carbamazepine requires starting with small amounts (e.g., 100 to 200 mg every 12 hours) and then making subsequent adjustments slowly to minimize gastrointestinal side effects. Ultimate dose requirements should be targeted to the lowest blood levels between 4 and 12 μg/ml that control seizures without toxicity. Nystagmus often occurs at subtherapeutic levels and cannot be used as an indicator of toxicity. Carbamazepine is more expensive than phenytoin or phenobarbital.

DISCONTINUATION OF ANTICONVULSANTS

Unlike younger patients, elderly patients, out of fear, respect, or timidity, may not press their physician for discontinuation of anticonvulsants. Their physician must determine for them, especially for those whose mental status is impaired by a psychiatric or dementing illness, whether anticonvulsants can be safely stopped. Unlike children with idiopathic epilepsy who can discontinue anticonvulsants after two to four seizure-free years, the elderly person who develops idiopathic epilepsy usually does not remain seizure-free without treatment. The elderly patient with an abnormal EEG and no underlying structural cause for seizure should, therefore, probably remain on anticonvulsants for life.

Seizures occurring within the first week following a stroke, on the other hand, need not usually be treated indefinitely. Unfortunately, the optimum duration of therapy needed after a single episode of stroke-related seizures is unknown. One seizure-free year following a stroke-related seizure would probably justify attempting discontinuation of anticonvulsants.

Nursing home patients may have been given anticonvulsants without adequate documentation of need. Many are on subtherapeutic doses, moreover, and can safely have them discontinued. Routine prophylactic treatment of elderly patients receiving analeptic drugs, such as phenothiazines, who have had nondescript syncopal attacks, or those with cerebrovascular disease without a history of seizures, is not indicated.

SUGGESTED READING

1. Annegers, J.F., Hauser, W.A., Elveback, L.R. Remission of seizures and relapse in patients with epilepsy. *Epilepsia* 20:719–737, 1979.
2. Chadwick, D., Reynolds, E.H., Marsden, C.D. Anticonvulsant-induced dyskinesias: A comparison with dyskinesias induced by neuroleptics. *J. Neurol. Neurosurg. Psychiatry* 39:1210–1218, 1979.
3. Dickinson, E.S. Seizure disorders in the elderly. *Pri. Care* 9:135–142, 1982.
4. Gilhus, N.E., Aarli, J.A. Imunoglobulin concentrations in nasal secretions and frequency of respiratory disease in epileptic patients. In Canger, R., Angeleri, F., Penry, J.K. (Eds.), *Epileptology: XIth Epilepsy International Symposium*. New York: Raven Press, 1980.
5. Hauser, W.A., Anderson, V.E., Loewenson, R.B., McRoberts, S.M. Seizure recurrence after a first unprovoked seizure. *N. Engl. J. Med.* 307:522–528, 1982.
6. Hildick-Smith, M. Epilepsy. In Caird, F.I. (Ed.), *Neurologic Disorders in the Elderly*. Littleton, Mass.: John Wright-PSG, 1982.
7. Moseley, J.L., Penry, I.K. Antiepileptic medication in chronic care facilities. *Public Health Reports* 90:140–143, 1975.
8. Reynolds, E.H. Chronic antiepileptic toxicity: A review. *Epilepsia* 16:319–353, 1975.
9. Reynolds, E.H., Shorron, S.D. Monotherapy or polytherapy for epilepsy? *Epilepsia* 22:1–20, 1981.
10. Rivinus, T.M. Psychiatric effects of the anticonvulsant regimens. *J. Clin. Psychopharmacol.* 2:165–192, 1982.

Parkinsonism

COLIN D. HALL, M.D.

Editor's note: *The effective treatment of parkinsonism, nearly exclusively a problem of the elderly, is now possible in many previously intractable cases. Familiarity with treatment options and with confusing manifestations of drug toxicity is essential for the primary care practitioner who attempts the challenge of devising and monitoring a drug regimen for parkinsonism.*

CLINICAL FEATURES

Moderate or severe parkinsonism is easy to recognize. The patient has an unchanging, expressionless facies—rarely smiling or even blinking. There is lack of body movement, and the patient will sit rigidly in a chair with legs uncrossed, arms resting on the chair arms, and head bent forward. He will attempt to rise by rocking his body backward and forward several times and then trying to throw himself up, often unsuccessfully. When walking he will be stooped forward, his steps will be short and shuffling, and he will have none of the usual associated arm swinging that accompanies walking. In bed, he will be unable to roll around to alter his position and unable to rise unassisted. There is frequently a resting tremor of the limbs and head. Above all, there is a marked delay in initiation of any sort of motor activity.

This clinical picture is the result of a series of physical abnormalities, discussed in the following sections.

Tremor

Tremor is often the most noticeable clinical sign of parkinsonism but is in fact usually the least incapacitating. It is not present during sleep but appears at periods of relative rest. Tremor usually starts in the hand with alternating flexion and extension of the thumb across the

221

palm, a "pill-rolling" motion, and commonly spreads with time to involve the arm and leg on the same side, the head, and then the opposite limbs. It is often clearly seen in the extended tongue. The tremor has a rate of three to five oscillations per second. It is usually suppressed by use of the limb but returns a few moments after the limb is rested. In about 10 percent of patients there is also an "end-point" tremor during movement, similar to that found in cerebellar disease.

Rigidity

Tone in the limbs is increased, with the increase being perceptible through all motions of passive flexion, extension, and rotation of a limb. The descriptive term "lead-pipe" rigidity is used, the continuous resistance being similar to that found on bending a lead bar. If the tremor is noticeable through the movement, the effect is similar to that of moving a bar through a ratchet, and the term "cog-wheel" rigidity may be used.

Bradykinesia

Bradykinesia is the most incapacitating feature of parkinsonism. Even with great conscious effort, it is difficult or impossible to initiate the sequence of muscle actions that result in motor activity. The patient becomes "frozen" within his own body. To add to his frustration, he will find at times that he can carry out motions that have been impossible for months or years, only to lose the ability again immediately.

Loss of Postural Control

Movements are carried out *en bloc* without the customary adjusting movements that allow one to keep one's body in position. Falling is a real hazard. When the parkinsonian patient stands with his heels together, the slightest push can cause him to totter and fall in any direction.

DIAGNOSTIC FEATURES

The disease usually progresses insidiously over several years, and those close to the patient may not appreciate its presence until it is brought to their attention. In the early stages it may present a very difficult diagnostic problem, mimicking early hemiparesis, depression, or other conditions. Some specific features may be helpful in reaching the correct diagnosis.

Facial Expression

Abnormalities of facial expression are the most helpful sign. There is a generalized, unhappy-looking droop to the face, without the asymmetry found in hemiplegia. There is little spontaneous blinking, but if the patient is asked not to blink and then a finger is lightly tapped on the bridge of the nose, he will continue to blink with each tap, not showing the normal spontaneous suppression of this response. This is called a positive glabellar response, or Myerson's sign. Spontaneous smiling is rare, and when it occurs, it appears strained and somehow humorless. An unaffected smile rarely accompanies parkinsonism, whatever the sufferer's underlying emotional state.

Blepharospasm

When the patient's eyes are gently closed, usually after a second or so a rhythmic fluttering of the eyelids will appear and will continue until the eyes are reopened. This is almost always seen in untreated parkinsonism and is a very helpful clinical sign.

Sialorrhea

There is a change in sweating, with the production of a thick, tenacious, rather greasy sebum, particularly over the brow. This is often accompanied by a scaly dermatitis.

Voice Changes

The voice loses power and range in parkinsonism. A frequent early sign is not being able to continue singing in the church choir. Eventually syllables may be rapidly and continuously run together, with paucity of tongue and lip movement, and this may result in totally unintelligible speech.

Handwriting

Handwriting tends to become smaller and more cramped, often with some evidence of tremor in the lines. These changes are more noticeable at the end of lines and eventually at the end of words. Words may run together on the page and become a series of illegible scratches.

Gait

Watching the patient walk is particularly helpful. Early in the disease, the more affected side may show a paucity or absence of arm swing on walking. With progression, neither arm will swing, and they will be held adducted with the elbows somewhat flexed across the body. There is almost always some degree of kyphosis, and torticollis may be a feature. Initiation of walking from a standing position is increasingly difficult and is usually accomplished by leaning the center of gravity forward to start off. It may then become very difficult to stop, and the patient may be forced almost to run forward with small steps in order to keep up with the upper body, resulting in a "festinating" gait. Attempts to turn are particularly difficult; the whole body comes around *en bloc* and lacks the normal fluidity of motion.

Strength
There is no specific loss of muscle strength, although the proximal limb muscles will usually be rather easy to overcome.

Reflexes
The deep tendon reflexes are generally unaffected in parkinsonism, although it is not uncommon to find them diffusely rather brisk or rather difficult to elicit. The plantar responses are flexor.

Oculogyric Crises
With the decline of postencephalitic parkinsonism, oculogyric crises are now rare. The features are similar to those developing in some patients as an idiosyncratic reaction to phenothiazines. There is severe spasmodic retrocollis, sometimes with opisthotonos, and the eyes roll back uncontrollably in the head. The patient has an associated feeling of panic. The attacks may last from minutes to days and recur without obvious precipitant or warning.

Intellectual Changes
Traditionally, it was said that parkinsonism was not accompanied by changes in mentation, but it has become obvious that it may frequently be accompanied by some degree of intellectual deterioration and even by frank dementia.

ETIOLOGY

Parkinsonism is a syndrome—a constellation of clinical features rather than a single disease.

Idiopathic Parkinsonism (Paralysis Agitans)
Most patients who develop parkinsonism fall into the category of idiopathic parkinsonism, where no etiologic or precipitating factor can be found. Males and females are affected equally. The age of onset is usually the sixth or seventh decade, but it can affect any age

group, even juveniles. There is a higher incidence in other family members, but no clear genetic or contagious factor is apparent.

Postencephalitic Parkinsonism

Following the pandemic of von Economo's encephalitis lethargica in 1918–1920, a significant number of suvivors showed evidence of florid parkinsonism as an immediate or late sequela. Further outbreaks of this presumed viral infection accounted for some other cases, but there is no evidence that it is responsible for recently acquired cases of parkinsonism.

Drug-Induced Parkinsonism

The phenothiazines and butyrophenones are responsible for a large number of cases of parkinsonism. These medications block the action of dopamine in the brain by preventing the uptake on postsynaptic nerve terminals. The effect is dose-related and thus may appear within days of starting high-dosage therapy. It is reversible, but the symptoms may take weeks to abate, particularly after depot injections of phenothiazine.

Metoclopramide, which has a structure similar to phenothiazines, may also cause parkinsonian features. Methyldopa infrequently causes parkinsonism, presumably by competitive inhibition of dopamine. Reserpine may produce mild features of parkinsonism by reducing dopamine production in the brain.

Parkinsonism as a Feature of Other Diseases

Severe, usually degenerative diseases of the brain may result in features of parkinsonism. These features are usually relatively inconsequential in the overall neurologic illness. While treatment with potentially toxic antiparkinsonian medication should not be undertaken lightly, at times significant improvement in the patient's well-being can be achieved.

Atherosclerotic Parkinsonism

Single, or much more commonly, recurring episodes of cerebrovascular disease may result in a picture almost indistinguishable from parkinsonism. This is particularly likely following multiple small infarcts, frequently associated with hypertension or diabetes. Generally, tremor is not a feature, and there may be accompanying hyperreflexia, extensor plantar responses, pseudobulbar palsy, or focal brain deficits. If the diagnosis is in question, a trial with L-dopa is justified, but it is rarely successful in atherosclerotic disease.

Alzheimer's Disease, Senile Dementia, and
Degenerative Cortical Diseases
Alzheimer's disease, senile dementia, and other degenerative cortical diseases are frequently accompanied by mild to moderate parkinsonism. Dementia generally dominates the clinical picture, and treatment rarely causes a significant improvement in the patient's well-being.

Progressive Supranuclear Palsy
Progressive supranuclear palsy, an uncommon disease, is often mistaken for idiopathic parkinsonism in the elderly. It is manifested as a clinical triad of defects in conjugate gaze, progressive dementia, and parkinsonism, any of which can predominate in the early stages. It is not unusual for all cases of parkinsonism to be accompanied by difficulty in upward gaze, but the striking defect in these patients is the inability to move the eyes laterally. The whole head has to be turned, and there is often an accompanying retrocollis or torticollis, requiring the patient to turn the whole body to look to the side. Vertical gaze is also impaired. Rigidity and bradykinesia may be prominent. The dementia is generally progressive and may become severe. The motor abnormalities rarely respond to L-dopa; anticholinergic medication may be more effective.

Shy-Drager Syndrome
In the Shy-Drager syndrome, a rare disease, parkinsonian features are combined with dysautonomia. There is usually failure of pupillary response to light, urinary incontinence, impotence in the male, disturbance of sweating. and profound postural hypotension. The parkinsonism is of secondary importance.

Other Disorders
Parkinsonian features, mild or prominent, may be part of the clinical picture following a variety of brain insults, including posttraumatic and postencephalitic states, severe metabolic insults such as profound hypoglycemia, anoxia or hyponatremia, exposure to carbon monoxide, syphilis, and brain tumor invading the basal ganglia. Some parkinsonian features are generally present in significant hepatic or renal encephalopathy.

EVALUATION

Parkinsonism remains a clinical diagnosis. Laboratory studies are undertaken only if there are focal corticospinal tract findings such as extensor plantar responses and unilateral hyperreflexia or weakness, sensory loss, a particularly rapid progression, or some other warning that other diseases may be present.

DIFFERENTIAL DIAGNOSIS

Benign Essential Tremor

Benign essential tremor is frequently misdiagnosed and unsuccessfully treated as parkinsonism. The tremor is most prominent during movement and can often best be demonstrated by asking the patient to drink from a cup. There is often a similar history in first- or second-generation relatives of advanced years. There is no associated bradykinesia or alteration in tone, and a warm spontaneous smile from the patient is an excellent differential diagnostic feature. The tremor is often completely or partially abolished for some hours by moderate amounts of alcohol, and this can be used as a clinical test. L-dopa and anticholinergics are unsuccessful, but propranolol, 60 to 120 mg/day in divided doses, may be beneficial.

Depression

Severe involutional depression may at times be mistaken for parkinsonism, and vice versa. There is some evidence that depression may accompany parkinsonism at an incidence higher than that seen in other equally debilitating diseases, perhaps as a result of the alteration in biogenic amine levels in the brain.

Drug Ingestion

Chronic overuse of sedative drugs in the elderly may produce reversible parkinsonian features.

Frontal Lobe Tumor

Occasionally benign or malignant tumors invading or compressing the frontal lobes may present a picture compatible with early idiopathic parkinsonism. This condition should be considered if headache, seizures, or rapid personality changes are part of the clinical picture.

Hypothyroidism

Myxedema, with a paucity of facial expression and overall bradykinesia, may be confused with parkinsonism.

PATHOGENESIS

The major pathologic changes in parkinsonism are loss of the dark-staining melanin-containing cells of the substantia nigra in the mid-brain and loss of cells in the nuclei of the basal ganglia. Dopamine is produced in the cells of the substantia nigra and is transported along axons to the basal ganglia; after it is liberated, it suppresses cells that are stimulated by acetylcholine. The loss of dopamine or its inhibition by phenothiazines leads to an uncontrolled stimulatory effect by acetylcholine, and thus to the symptoms and signs of parkinsonism.

TREATMENT

Decisions regarding treatment must be based on the degree of incapacitation of the patient. There is no evidence that early treatment prevents the natural progression of the disease. Unfortunately, L-dopa, the most effective therapy, has significant toxic side effects. Also useful are the anticholinergic medications, amantadine, and the dopamine analogue bromocriptine.

L-*Dopa*

Dopamine does not cross the blood-brain barrier, so its administration does not significantly elevate brain dopamine levels. The precursor, L-dopa, readily crosses into the brain and is decarboxylated to active dopamine. This is the most effective medication for the relief of all aspects of parkinsonism; it does not, however, ameliorate the intellectual changes. It is particularly effective in relieving bradykinesia. Administration should be gradual and titrated to clinical response. A reasonable schedule is to start with 250 mg twice a day and add 250 mg every third day. The dosage is increased until there is a good clinical response or unacceptable side effects appear. It is most effective if it is titrated through the day, and should be taken at 2- or 3-hour intervals while awake. If there is no therapeutic effect after giving 8 g/day, the drug should be discontinued.

Side effects of L-dopa are discussed in the following paragraphs.

Dyskinetic Movement Disorders   These disorders are the major factor limiting dosage. They are related to dosage level and duration and generally do not occur until several months after treatment starts. They may then appear at doses that were previously well tolerated. Almost any movement disorder may develop, but orofacial dyskinesias, writhing movements of the head and neck, and dystonic posturing of the limbs are the most common.

Nausea and Vomiting   This side effect is usually seen early. It is reduced by taking the medication with food, either with meals or a small snack; reducing the dosage and then reincreasing it more gradually may help.

Gastrointestinal Hemorrhage L-Dopa is an irritant to the upper gastrointestinal tract, and caution must be used if there is a history of peptic ulcer disease. Administration with antacids may help prevent these side effects in susceptible patients.

Postural Hypotension This may occur at any stage of treatment and may be severe. Elastic stockings may help, but severe symptoms generally require a reduction in dosage.

Cardiac Arrhythmia Although this condition is not a contraindication to L-dopa usage, careful monitoring, probably in hospital, is required with initiation of therapy in patients with significant cardiac arrhythmias.

Exacerbation of Narrow-Angle Glaucoma This condition excludes the use of L-dopa for Parkinson's disease.

Alteration of Taste and Darkening of Urine These minor side effects do not require alteration of medication.

Psychological Changes These changes are generally related to levels of dosage and rate of administration. Depression has been reported as a result of rapid administration. More commonly the patient may have persistent, usually frightening hallucinations, and some patients develop overt psychosis with manic features. An early warning of these states may be vivid nightmares and alteration in the sleep cycle, and this should be an indication for some reduction in dosage.

On-Off Phenomena After a therapeutic regimen has been well established and has been successful for months or years, the patient may develop periods, lasting minutes to hours, throughout the day when the beneficial effects of L-dopa will suddenly be lost. At these times the patient may be suddenly frozen in a particular posture, or he may be quite unable to perform tasks that were readily accomplished only minutes before.

Adverse Drug Reactions Vitamin B_6, even in the doses found in foods like fortified breakfast cereals, may result in negation of the therapeutic effects of L-dopa. Monoamine oxidase inhibitors should not be used in conjunction with L-dopa. Some patients find that their condition deteriorates for a period after eating meat, perhaps as a result of competition for uptake across the blood-brain barrier by amino acids and L-dopa.

L-Dopa plus a Peripheral Decarboxylase Inhibitor

The combination of L-dopa and a peripheral decarboxylase inhibitor prevents conversion of L-dopa to dopamine outside the brain, allowing smaller doses of L-dopa to be administered with the same brain levels. Although this combination reduces the side effects of nausea and vomiting and perhaps hypotension, it does not reduce, and may even exacerbate, psychogenic effects, dyskinesias, and the on-off phenomenon. The combination may reduce the need for frequent dosage, but it has the disadvantage of using two different medications, L-dopa and the decarboxylase inhibitor, carbidopa, which are available only in fixed-dosage tablets.

Bromocriptine
With a formula and action very similar to dopamine, bromocriptine has the same psychogenic side effects but may be less likely to produce dyskinesia. Although its full role has not yet been evaluated, it may be most effective as an adjunct to L-dopa, in divided doses of up to 15 mg/day.

Amantadine
Amantadine has moderate antiparkinsonian effects, generally lasting only a few weeks or months. Dosage is 100 mg twice a day. Side effects are unusual but include drowsiness, nightmares, hallucinations, and confusion. Long-term use may produce livedo reticularis.

Anticholinergics
Anticholinergic drugs have a mild but significant effect on relieving parkinsonian symptoms. There is no clear advantage to any single agent, and patients who fail to respond to one may be helped by another. These drugs include trihexyphenidyl (Artane), which is given two to three times per day, 2 to 5 mg per dose. Predictable anticholinergic side effects include urine retention, dry mouth, constipation, and occasionally psychogenic effects, particularly visual hallucinations.

Antihistamines
Antihistamines may be of some value because of their mild anticholinergic properties. The most commonly used is diphenhydramine (Benadryl), 25 to 50 mg one to three times per day. The side effect of drowsiness may also make it useful as a night sedative.

THERAPEUTIC REGIMEN

There is no single "correct" way to treat parkinsonism. A "cookbook" approach must be avoided, and treatment must be carefully individualized for each patient if optimal results are to be obtained. Particularly when therapy is initiated and in the later stages when drug-induced side effects become a limiting factor, the patient should be seen often and the effects of small changes in dosage and timing should be evaluated. The following sections provide a structure for rational treatment.

Initiation of Medication

Mild and nonlimiting features need not be treated, but the patient should be followed to ensure that an insidious progression does not lead to unrecognized incapacity. If the features are secondary to some other condition such as Alzheimer's disease or diffuse cerebrovascular disease, a decision must be made as to whether the potential benefits of medication outweigh the potential side effects. If the patient is known to be taking medication that may induce parkinsonism, this should be withdrawn for several weeks and the effect evaluated before commencing therapy.

When the decision to treat has been made, if symptoms are mild, an initial course of amantadine or anticholinergic medication may be given and the results evaluated over several weeks, or L-dopa may be started immediately. If tremor alone is the problem, a trial of anticholinergic medication is worthwhile. If the disease is moderate or severe, L-dopa should be used initially as described earlier. The initial concomitant use of the decarboxylase inhibitor carbidopa is recommended by some, but I reserve this for those patients who develop significant gastrointestinal or hypotensive side effects. If carbidopa is added, the L-dopa requirement will be reduced by approximately 75 percent.

Maintenance Therapy

Generally, the dosage should be increased until there is significant relief but not all parkinsonian features have disappeared. If side effects of L-dopa occur, the physician should try reducing the dosage and then gradually increasing it again to find the optimal level. The patient will usually know when a level of dyskinesia that is acceptable to balance the beneficial effects of therapy has been reached. If the tolerated dose is regarded as therapeutically suboptimal, amantadine should be added. If this is ineffective or loses its effect, anticholinergics should then be added. Finally, it may also be worth adding bromocriptine in divided doses of up to 15 mg/day.

Treatment of Side Effects

Individual experimentation is the key to treating side effects. Dyskinesias are treated by reducing medication. The patient may know when movement disorders will be most severe and can try reducing the dosage immediately before they occur. The on-off phenomenon may be alleviated by taking smaller amounts of medication at shorter intervals to reduce the peaks and troughs of dopamine levels. Hallucinations may be resolved by reducing the dosage of any of the medications that could cause this side effect by trial and error. Unfortunately, hallucinosis may also be a feature of the underlying disease and may not regress completely with medication withdrawal. While the same is true of psychosis, frank psychosis must be treated by hospitalizing the patient, completely withdrawing medication, and then gradually reinstituting it to appropriate doses.

Drug Holiday

Eventually, a point is generally reached where medication appears to have lost its efficacy or where side effects are unacceptable. It may then be beneficial to hospitalize the patient, withdraw all medication for five days to a week, and then gradually reinstitute it over a week or two. There will be initial marked symptomatic deterioration, but with reinstitution of L-dopa there may be significant improvement over the prewithdrawal state—sometimes with a smaller total drug dose.

Surgical Treatment

There is now rarely, if ever, an indication for surgical ablation of the ventrolateral thalamus, an operation which is effective in reducing tremor and rigidity but which has only limited benefit in treating bradykinesia.

Supportive Therapy

The occupational therapist may be of significant benefit in providing adaptive equipment. Some patients find physical therapy helpful, although it is difficult to confirm its physical or psychological benefits. Speech disorders that do not respond to L-dopa are generally not helped by speech therapy, but at times an alternative means of communication such as a communication board may be valuable. Patient support groups have been organized under the auspices of the Parkinson's Disease Foundation, and these may be of help to the family in sharing the psychological burden as well as providing ideas for alleviating physical handicap.

PROGNOSIS

The course of the disease is very variable. Some patients will show only mild symptoms that barely progress over several years, and others will follow a progressive downhill course which, despite all intervention, will result in institutionalization within a very few years. Many patients seem to respond well to therapy for several years, only to have a rapid and terminal deterioration over a few months. The patient who suddenly deteriorates should also be carefully evaluated for other superimposed disease.

Despite the limitations, parkinsonism is the first of the "degenerative" neurologic diseases to respond to medication, and we can offer these patients and their families a significant measure of hope and relief. It is the physician's responsibility to devote the necessary time, skill, and effort for optimal treatment.

SUGGESTED READING

1. Bauer, R.B., McHenry, J.T. Comparison of amantidine, placebo and levodopa in Parkinson's Disease. *Neurology* 24:715–720, 1974.
2. Clinical therapeutic rounds: Individualization of drug therapy for the parkinsonian patient. *J.A.M.A.* 233:1198–1201, 1975.
3. Duvoisin, R.C. *Parkinson's Disease: A Guide for Patient and Family.* New York: Raven Press, 1978.
4. Klanans, H.L., Glantz, R.H. Ten years of L-dopa in parkinsonism. *Guidelines to Neurosciences* 4:1, 1980.
5. Mental symptoms and parkinsonism (editorial). *Br. Med. J.* 2:67, 1973.
6. Teychenne, P.F., Bergorud, D., Racy, A., et al. Bromocriptine: Low dose therapy in Parkinson's Disease. *Neurology* 32:577–583, 1982.

Vertigo and Balance Disorders in the Elderly Patient

W. PAUL BIGGERS, M.D., and
J. PATTERSON BROWDER, M.D.

Editor's note: Complaints of dizziness are universal in elderly patients. Most are managed well with reassurance, commonsense advice, and occasionally a prescription. Physicians must keep in mind the serious causes of vertigo that are common, especially those of vascular etiology, which require special vigilance or specific therapy.

Dizziness, vertigo and disturbance in balance are among the top ten complaints voiced by patients consulting primary care physicians, and they are even more common among elderly patients. Disorders of equilibrium can result in falls with serious orthopedic complications, head injuries, or both. Unfortunately, too often the patient leaves the hospital only to fall again because attention was focused on the fall rather than on its cause. Disequilibrium may herald serious disease, including posterior fossa tumors, basilar artery insufficiency, and impending stroke. Care of the elderly patient demands a thorough familiarity with the multitude of causes of disturbance in balance, and an ability to separate peripheral vestibular causes from central ones and to recognize when the cause is a potentially life-threatening condition.

APPROACH TO THE DIAGNOSIS OF DISEQUILIBRIUM

Like most complex problems in medicine, the vexing problem of diagnosing the etiology of loss of balance and/or syncope is best approached methodically, concentrating on the most likely diagnoses while at the same time constantly bearing in mind those disorders which, though rare, could be serious and life-threatening.

It must be emphasized at the outset that the symptoms of periodic disequilibrium in the older patient should alert the physician to the possibility of perfusion problems in the distribution of the basilar

234

artery. There are no pain fibers in the inner ear. Unfortunately, tinnitus and disequilibrium are the inner ear's only way to express inadequate oxygenation of its neuroepithelium. When disequilibrium has a circulatory etiology, more catastrophic basilar artery insufficiency symptoms may ensue in the future. Especially worrisome are episodes of dizziness that are associated with amaurosis fugax and episodic loss of consciousness (drop attacks); this history should alert the physician that a thorough cerebrovascular evaluation is needed.

An elevated blood pressure may be the first clue that dizziness is the sign of a serious disorder. Headaches and dizziness can be the prodrome of a hypertensive crisis or can herald an impending stroke. If the patient presents with focal neurologic signs, consideration should be given to cerebrovascular insufficiency or a space-occupying intracranial mass. Wallenberg's syndrome, caused by insufficiency of the posterior inferior cerebellar artery, is the most common of the brain stem vascular syndromes. It consists of (1) vertigo with nystagmus *away from* the side of the lesion, (2) ataxia with falling *toward* the side of the lesion, (3) loss of pain and temperature sensation in the ipsilateral face and contralateral body, (4) dysphagia secondary to ipsilateral paralysis of the palate and vocal cord, and (5) ipsilateral Horner's syndrome.

More commonly, the patient with disequilibrium presents with no associated signs or symptoms. One must then consider disorders of the systems that contribute to the sense of balance and the maintenance of balance: (1) the vestibular system (the vestibular portion of the inner ear and the eighth nerve with the vestibular nuclei in the pons), (2) the ocular system, and (3) the proprioceptive/exteroceptive system. Input from all three of these systems is coordinated and modulated by the cerebellum prior to ascension of the signal to higher cortical centers of consciousness for interpretation.

The history including a thorough otologic, ophthalmologic, and neurologic history, and the physical examination must be thorough in order to provide a baseline from which rational investigation of the patient with a disorder of disequilibrium can proceed. Very often, investigation along these lines will point to a clear source of the patient's complaint, such as otitis media or an abrupt change in visual acuity. The old axiom of asking that most important question, "What drugs are you taking?" still holds true. The gamut runs from A to Z—from the unexpected sensitivity to antihypertensive drugs to an allergic reaction to zinc. Particular attention should be focused on the most recent drugs added to a patient's regimen, especially those with a central nervous system effect such as sedatives or psychotropic agents. Over-the-counter drugs, which the patient may neglect to mention, should not be overlooked.

Disequilibrium that is unassociated with neurologic or ophthalmologic disorders may be very difficult to diagnose and treat. Occult vascular disease, either in the neck or intracranially, is of particular concern in older patients. Emotional disturbance, however, is rarely a cause of disequilibrium in the elderly patient. Just as in other organ systems, a diagnosis of psychological etiology should be a diagnosis by exclusion. There is no substitute for clinical experience in dealing with patients with these complaints, and careful clinical judgment must guide the physician as to how far to pursue an occult cause of dizziness in the absence of confirming signs.

TESTING FOR DISORDERS OF EQUILIBRIUM

The accurate diagnosis of disorders of equilibrium has been facilitated greatly in recent years by "site-of-lesion testing." Before discussing specific disorders, it will be helpful to review briefly those tests currently available and to explain the basic pathophysiology involved in some of the more important tests.

Electronystagmography
Electronystagmography (ENG) takes advantage of the fact that the eye is a dipole whose cornea-retinal potential can induce a change in an electrical field that can be measured and that depends on the direction of movement. Since much of the vestibular system is devoted to maintenance of the field of last gaze, disorders of the vestibular system may be reflected in ocular signs, especially nystagmus, as well as by disorders of conjugate eye movement. Spontaneous nystagmus is always pathologic although not always serious. Since both light and visual fixation can suppress minimal spontaneous nystagmus, it may be recognizable only when the patient's eyes are closed by using ENG. Electronystagmography can also test the ability of the eyes to track a moving object in a smoothly coordinated fashion, as well as detecting nystagmus evoked in head position and evaluating nystagmus evoked by a visual stimulus (optokinetic testing) for asymmetry. Finally, each vestibular system can also be quantitatively tested using caloric stimulation.

Auditory Brain-Stem-Evoked Potentials
Recent advances in computer analysis of data have allowed the development of techniques to study the progression of neural infor-

mation from the cochlea through the brain stem to the auditory cortex beyond. This technique, referred to as *brain-stem-evoked response audiometry* (BERA) or the auditory brain stem response (ABR), is particularly useful in studying lesions of the vestibular portion of the eighth nerve and lesions of the brain stem, particularly the medial longitudinal fasciculus. The test consists of a rapid series of auditory clicks that produce a set of neural impulses whose progress from synapse to synapse toward the auditory cortex can be recorded. The latency between various synapse points is measured and compared with the opposite side. Acoustic neuromas produce a significant ipsilateral delay in the progression of neural impulses, and multiple sclerosis, as might be predicted, produces extreme increases in latency.

Stapedial Reflex and Reflex Decay

The stapedial reflex protects the inner ear from excessively loud noise by a sudden contraction of the stapedius muscle that "bowstrings" the ossicular chain. In most individuals the stapedial reflex is elicited at about 70 dB above their threshold for the detection of sound, but in individuals with retrocochlear disease, the stapedial reflex may be absent or may rapidly decay. This test is a reliable predictor of retrocochlear disease in that more than 70 percent of surgically proved acoustic neuromas and other cerebellar pontine angle tumors will demonstrate stapedial reflex abnormality.

Full Battery Audiometry

Full battery audiometry should be obtained in every patient with attacks of paroxysmal vertigo. It is also indicated in the patient with *unilateral* sensorineural hearing loss to rule out an acoustic neuroma. The full battery includes pure tone and speech threshold determinations, speech discrimination scores in quiet and in noise, and stapedial reflex responses.

Special Radiologic Studies

Special radiologic studies, such as computerized tomography employing air-contrast techniques, can demonstrate very small lesions in the cerebellar pontine angle region that may be responsible for vertigo and disequilibrium. Although this and other radiographic techniques have become an important part of the workup of patients with disequilibrium, they should not be the first line of testing and should be employed only when indicated by other, less expensive, noninvasive testing techniques, including ENG and audiometry.

DIFFERENTIAL DIAGNOSIS OF DISEQUILIBRIUM

Vertigo has been described as a hallucination of movement. When the baseline physical examination and history fail to uncover an obvious cause of the symptoms, it is necessary to return to the history and concentrate on the patient's complaint of disequilibrium to see if the complaint is really one of true vertigo rather than unsteadiness. One technique that has proved helpful is to ask the patient to describe an attack, but explain that the words "dizziness" or "vertigo" must not be used. This approach often yields more detailed information by avoiding the vagueness inherent in the terms commonly used to describe attacks of disequilibrium. Most patients with vertigo will complain of a sensation of movement in space, accompanied by nausea. Many patients will also describe an associated otologic complaint such as hearing loss, tinnitus, or a feeling of fullness in the ear. Vertigo is usually an intense, dramatic symptom that is more severe than disequilibrium arising from the central nervous system. The environment seems to spin around those with vertigo, while patients with more central lesions feel that they are "turning around on the inside" or are simply "unbalanced."

Another good question to ask is, "What are the duration and pattern of your symptoms?" Vertigo is characteristically episodic, lasting only a few seconds to minutes. Disequilibrium that is described as continuous is almost certainly not true vertigo, usually arising centrally to the inner ear. Although typical attacks of true vertigo are relatively short in duration, patients may have a residual "queasy" feeling lasting from a few hours to days after the episode. Another question is, "How does moving your head affect your symptoms?" Head movement almost always aggravates true vertigo but has very little effect on other forms of disequilibrium.

The association of nystagmus and past pointing during the acute phase of an episode are the two most reliable physical signs that accompany true vertigo. They are often subclinical and are not seen by the physician, although ENG can be employed to bring out nystagmus. Because lesions of the inner ear that produce vertigo and nystagmus are virtually always unilateral and paralytic, the nystagmus usually points away from the involved ear. True vertigo usually indicates a lesion of the inner ear, the vestibular nerve, or, more rarely, the vestibular nuclei; vertigo rarely is caused by disease outside the peripheral vestibular system.

As a general rule, any patient with true vertigo deserves a thorough workup, an otologic examination, and testing by an otolaryngologist, particularly when the vertigo is associated with a hearing complaint. The clinical setting in which one encounters the patient in many ways determines the timing of referral, the depth of examination, and what testing should be done before making an appropriate referral. Two settings must be distinguished, vertigo with acute onset and chronic vertigo.

Acute Onset of Severe Vertigo
The physician should carefully question the patient for a history of head trauma with possible temporal bone fracture and perilymph fistula. Perilymph fistula can result also from forceful coughing, sneezing, straining, or lifting. If the tympanic membrane is intact, the diagnosis of fistula is quite difficult. Usually fistulas develop at the oval or round windows, with perilymph leaking imperceptibly into the middle ear space. A fistula tes can be performed with a pneumatic otoscope or a Politzer bag to create positive pressure within the external auditory canal. If the test is positive, the eyes undergo a forced deviation away from the stimulated ear, followed by a few beats of nystagmus (Hennebert's sign). The fistula test unfortunately is often falsely negative. If an emergency audiogram indicates significant cochlear pathology, the patient with a history suggesting fistula should undergo middle ear exploration as soon as possible in order to attempt to identify and repair the fistula; prompt surgery lessens the possibility of permanent cochlear damage.

When head trauma, drug intoxication, and significant cardiovascular disease with impending stroke have been ruled out, and there are no focal neurologic signs, symptomatic therapy is appropriate. Diazepam is an effective suppressant of the vestibular system, but the dosage required to control vertigo may cause the patient to be quite sedated; often the patient welcomes the relief of sleep. Therapy may be initiated with intravenous titration and then maintained by oral administration of the drug. Prompt follow-up examination by an otolaryngologist should be arranged.

Chronic Vertigo
A drug history, blood pressure determination, and cardiovascular examination along with an otoneurologic history form a baseline for further diagnostic studies in patients with chronic vertigo. In patients with persistent complaints of vertigo and an associated hearing complaint, the physician should consider middle ear disorders. Baro-

trauma (a result of descent in inadequately pressurized aircraft, producing acute negative pressure in the middle ear space, often with hemorrhage) and otitis media can often produce a mild labyrinthitis with true vertigo, tinnitus, and a conductive hearing loss. Therapy consists of reassurance, systemic and topical decongestants, and appropriate antibiotic therapy directed at *Streptococcus pneumoniae, Hemophilus influenzae,* and anaerobes. It should be noted that in the elderly patient, especially men, decongestant drugs with sympathomimetic effects may produce symptoms of lower urinary tract obstruction. In the chronically draining ear, with or without cholesteatoma, vertigo is an ominous sign. Thus, vertigo associated with a foul-smelling ear discharge demands thorough investigation. Rarely, one can see otorrhea and vertigo as a result of severe external otitis. In this case, symptoms should clear promptly with appropriate topical acidified antibiotic therapy following gentle irrigation with 1.5% acetic acid at body temperature to remove excessive epithelial debris.

Otosclerosis
Otosclerosis can occasionally be associated with mild vertigo or unsteadiness; it often begins in the second decade of life but becomes clinically important in the fifth and sixth decades. Vertigo in the presence of otosclerosis usually indicates involvement of the inner ear with the disease.

Meniere's Disease
Typical Meniere's disease consists of episodic vertigo, fluctuating sensorineural hearing loss, and roaring tinnitus, often associated with a feeling of fullness in the ear. The fluctuating sensorineural hearing loss is less obvious to the patient than are the vertiginous episodes because the disease is usually unilateral. In classic Meniere's disease, tinnitus will often intensify prior to the onset of a vertiginous episode by minutes to hours. Symptoms can last for several hours and are often severely incapacitating, recurring every few days in the most severe cases to once or twice a year in the least severe episodes.

Many patients with Meniere's disease will give a history of excessive salt intake 24 to 48 hours preceding the more severe episodes. Other factors contributing to the emergence of Meniere's disease include diabetes mellitus, hyperlipidemic states, and syphilitic osteitis of the temporal bone. It is said that the more thorough the investigation of the patient, the less often will the diagnosis of "idiopathic" Meniere's disease be made. A dramatic response to a trial of salt restriction and mild oral diuretic therapy, with or without vasodilators, is helpful in establishing the diagnosis of Meniere's disease.

Positional Vertigo

The symptoms of positional vertigo are usually mild and can be tolerated for long periods before the patient seeks medical advice. Hearing symptoms are not present, and vertigo almost never occurs unless the patient changes head position. Two types of positional vertigo are identified: (1) benign positional vertigo, typically occurring when the patient turns over in bed at night or rolls over to get out of bed; (2) Paroxysmal positional vertigo, which can be elicited by moving the patient rapidly from a sitting position to a supine position while forcibly turning the head to one side (Dix-Hallpike maneuver).

Paroxysmal positional vertigo is typically characterized by rotatory nystagmus with a latent period before onset and fatigue in the intensity of nystagmus when the maneuver is repeated. The patient also experiences feelings of true vertigo during the maneuver. This maneuver must be performed with caution in the elderly patient, especially in those felt to be susceptible to vertebral artery insufficiency and potential basilar stroke.

Both benign positional vertigo and paroxysmal positional vertigo are self-limited diseases, and 90 percent of cases resolve within six months to a year after onset; the patient usually requires only reassurance that there is no serious underlying illness and should be advised to move slowly in changing positions.

Cervical Vertigo

Cervical arthritis and "whiplash" injuries to the neck can cause vertigo brought about by certain movements of the neck. In some instances the presence of cervical vertigo can be substantiated by ENG, and referral to a specialist is indicated when this diagnosis is suspected. Treatment of cervical vertigo in the acute phase consists of muscle relaxants and immobilization of the neck by means of a soft cervical collar for approximately one month and thereafter as needed. The patient should be warned that cervical vertigo following neck injury may persist up to two years.

Multiple Sclerosis

Vertigo is one of the more common presentations of multiple sclerosis. An episodic but unpredictable pattern of vertigo-associated eye findings, especially temporal retinal pallor and internuclear ophthalmoplegia, requires a thorough investigation, including BERA. The BERA will have greatly prolonged latency between the wave forms due to demyelinization of the medial longitudinal fasciculus. Multiple sclerosis rarely begins after age 60, but exacerbations and intensification of symptoms often occur in the fifth decade.

Vestibular Neuronitis
Vestibular neuronitis (also called viral labyrinthitis) is a severe form of vertigo that often occurs following a mild upper respiratory tract infection. Neurologic and audiometric evaluations are entirely within normal limits. A severe unilateral vestibular paresis, however, is demonstrable on caloric testing by ENG. Treatment is symptomatic, and the disease is self-limited but may require several weeks for recovery.

THERAPY

Treatment of vertigo in the geriatric patient must be carefully individualized. An excellent rule of thumb is that in the initial management, one should *stop the drugs.* Disorders of equilibrium and light-headedness are among the more common side effects listed for many classes of commonly prescribed drugs. Therapy for the vertiginous patient can be divided into two general categories: specific and symptomatic.

Specific Therapy
Specific therapy includes various surgical procedures. The endolymphatic subarachnoid shunt popularized by Dr. William House and subsequent modifications of this procedure have proved to be effective in 60 to 70 percent of patients with intractable, carefully documented cases of Meniere's disease. Great emphasis is placed on the early detection of acoustic neuroma, because modern neurootologic techniques allow for tumor removal with sparing of the ipsilateral seventh cranial nerve and ipsilateral, useful auditory function. Large acoustic neuromas have a significant mortality and morbidity rate, especially in the geriatric patient population. Other examples of specific therapeutic intervention include antibiotics for bacterial or syphilitic labyrinthitis, anticoagulation for vertebrobasilar insufficiency, and appropriate drug and/or pacemaker therapy for cardiac arrhythmia. Obviously therapy should be directed at a specific underlying disorder that has been well documented whenever possible. Unfortunately, in the majority of cases in the geriatric population, specific therapy is not available and the physician must rely on symptomatic treatment.

Symptomatic Therapy

Many different classes of drugs have been used to treat disequilibrium and vertigo. Unfortunately, the effectiveness of each of these drugs has been determined by empirical observation, and it is difficult to predict for each individual patient which drug or combination of drugs will prove to be efficacious. Several classes of drugs are routinely utilized, and each merits a few comments.

Tranquilizers have been used effectively to suppress the sensation of motion. Diazepam has been shown to decrease the output from the vestibular nuclei, possibly by suppressing the reticular facilitory system. This drug seems to affect crossed vestibular and cerebellar-vestibular inhibitory transmission. Excessive sedation with decreased alertness, along with some risk of drug dependence, are especially troublesome side effects in geriatric patients.

The phenothiazine drugs (chlorpromazine and its derivative prochlorperazine) are effective in suppressing nausea and vomiting. This effect is thought to occur through their direct action on the chemoreceptive trigger zones in the brain stem. Trimethobenzamide is an antihistamine with strong antiemetic activity; it does not have the bothersome extrapyramidal and excessive sedative effects of the phenothiazines.

Several additional types of antihistamines (meclizine, cyclizine, dimenhydrinate, and promethazine) have been useful in treating milder forms of disequilibrium and vertigo. They each have some degree of sedation and produce varying degrees of dryness of the mucous membranes.

Anticholinergic drugs, including scopolamine and atropine through their parasympatholytic activity, are effective in relieving the autonomic symptoms associated with vertigo. Unfortunately they produce marked dryness of the mucous membranes and have well-known unpleasant side effects, although the new transdermal preparations appear to be much better tolerated.

The butyrophenone tranquilizers (droperidol and haloperidol) have antiemetic properties along with dopaminergic blocking properties, with potential extrapyramidal side effects and significant sedation properties. The combination of droperidol and fentanyl (a narcotic) is available commercially as Innovar. Innovar has been used by otologic surgeons because of its significant antivertiginous and antiemetic effects in the immediate postoperative period. We use droperidol, with or without fentanyl, for patients with severe vertigo, and administer the drug intramuscularly in a carefully monitored hospital setting.

Prolonged severe vertigo is certainly one of the most distressing symptoms that a patient can experience and that the physician must attempt to alleviate. We prefer diazepam initially because it has less troublesome side effects than the phenothiazines or the butyrophenones. The initial dose of 10 mg is given intravenously slowly and is followed by 5 to 10 mg given orally every 6 hours. If nausea and vomiting are prominent symptoms, an antiemetic drug (preferably trimethobenzamide) is used concomitantly. Drugs with sedation properties that may significantly alter the status of consciousness are of course contraindicated in any patient in whom one suspects a progressing ischemic process in the central nervous system.

Chronically recurring vertigo poses a different therapeutic problem, especially for the independent-living geriatric patient. The antihistamine antivertiginous drugs seem to be most useful in this situation.

Other Therapy

Vasodilator therapy has given unpredictable results, and the potential for postural hypotension and other side effects requires close monitoring and cautious utilization of these drugs in the geriatric patient. Many patients seem to benefit from the elimination of excess caffeine and nicotine intake. In our experience, reduction of salt intake along with chlorothiazide diuretic therapy five days per week with potassium supplementation is useful in the conservative management of Meniere's disease, and reduces the risk of potassium depletion. Sodium restriction and diuretics may reduce perilymphatic fluid pressure and allow for the expansion of the endolymphatic space, dissipating endolymphatic pressure, but this explanation is still conjectural.

Cervical collars have proved effective in the therapy of cervical vertigo. They should be worn by the patient for at least six weeks. Elderly patients with persistent disequilibrium should be encouraged to use walkers and canes for added support to prevent falls.

SUGGESTED READING

1. Busis, S.N. Diagnostic evaluation of the patient presenting with vertigo. *Otolaryngol. Clin. North Am.* 6:3, 1973.
2. Gacek, R.R. The vestibular system. In English, G.M. (Ed.), *Otolaryngology*, 4th ed. Philadelphia: Harper and Row, 1976.
3. McCabe, B.F. Vestibular physiology: Its clinical application. In Paparella, M.M., Shumrick, D.A. (Eds.), *Otolaryngology*. Philadelphia: W.B. Saunders, 1980.

4. Rubin, W., Busis, S.N., Brooker, K.H. Otoneuroiogic examination. In English, G.M. (Ed.), *Otolaryngology*, 4th ed. Philadelphia: Harper and Row, 1976.
5. Rubin, W., Norris, C. Electronystagmography (ENG) technique and significance. *Laryngoscope* 76:961–963, 1966.

6

ENDOCRINE
DISORDERS

The Endocrinology of Aging

JAMES R. CARTER, M.D.

Editor's note: *The only major changes observed in endocrine function with normal aging are cessation of ovarian function at the menopause and postmenopausal calcium loss leading to osteoporosis; other changes are generally compensated for by the intricate feedback mechanisms of the endocrine system. More extreme alterations in endocrine function have been observed in inactive, institutionalized, or hospitalized elderly patients, so future studies should clearly distinguish between healthy, active aging persons and those with debilities or chronic illness.*

The old idea that the endocrine system might in some way be the cause of aging has largely disappeared as more information has become available. Considerable interest concerning the way aging affects hormones, however, has led to recent insights into the endocrine and metabolic changes that occur as a part of the normal aging process.

Because of the rather dramatic events surrounding the menopause, it has unfortunately been taken by many people as the paradigm for glandular changes with aging; in fact, it is the exception rather than the rule. The only other dramatic event occurring in the elderly is the appearance of postmenopausal osteoporosis in women. Aside from these two events, one is impressed with the relatively minor changes that occur in other endocrine systems during aging. This is true, however, only if one studies a healthy, ambulatory population of the elderly, which is not an easy study population to reach in large numbers. A number of misconceptions have been fostered by studies that compared healthy young people with institutionalized older individuals. These misconceptions are gradually being corrected as investigators realize the importance of selecting their older study subjects with care.

The complexity of the endocrine system requires a careful look at a number of loci that might change with aging. Hypothalamic control of the pituitary, pituitary control of endocrine glands, hormonal secretion by the endocrine gland, binding of hormones in the circulation (for thyroid and steroid hormones), hormone degradation rates, response of the appropriate end organ(s) to the hormone, and feedback control of the hypothalamus and pituitary are all sites where changes might occur. Nonetheless, in view of the importance of the endocrine system for smooth functioning of the organism as a whole, one might predict teleologically that the changes observed would be relatively minor.

METABOLISM

On the average, weight changes little with aging. This is not true of body composition, however. From the fourth decade on, lean body mass declines by approximately 6 percent per decade. This change is most notable in muscle mass, which in men declines about 40 percent from the third to the eighth decade of life; a lesser decline is seen in women largely because of the relatively smaller muscle mass in young women compared to men. Putting together these observations, it is clear that there is a marked increase in both the absolute and the relative amounts of adipose tissue with aging. Understanding these changes in body composition is important in interpreting some of the data to be discussed.

Energy requirements (assumed to be equivalent to caloric intake) clearly decline with age. In a Baltimore study,[1] average daily intake for men declined from 2,700 kcal per day in the third decade to 2,100 kcal in the seventh to eighth decade. In a similar study from Scotland,[2] the figures were 3,000 and 2,050 kcal, respectively. The Baltimore group estimated that one-third of this decline was due to a decline in metabolic needs and two-thirds of decreased physical activity. In women the change is less striking, average figures being 2,200 kcal and 1,900 kcal in the Baltimore study for the young and the elderly, respectively.

1. R.B. McGandy, C.H. Barrows, Jr., A. Spanias, et al. Nutrient intake and energy expenditure in men of different ages. *J. Gerontol.* 21:581–587, 1966.
2. H.N. Munro. An introduction to nutritional aspects of protein metabolism. In H.N. Munro and J.B. Allison (Eds.), *Mammalian Protein Metabolism*, vol. 2. (New York: Academic Press, 1964), pp. 3–39.

It has been known for a long time that basal metabolic rate declines steadily with age, the decrease averaging about 25 percent by the time the ninth decade is reached. This has been interpreted as a general slowing down of the "metabolic machinery" of body cells. It has recently been pointed out, however, that this decline exactly parallels that of lean body mass. A more acceptable interpretation, then, is that total active metabolic mass declines with age (adipose tissue generally having a low respiratory rate), but that metabolic activitiy per cell remains relatively constant throughout life.

Changes in glucose metabolism with age have been extensively studied, and although there is general agreement on the facts, there is disagreement on the interpretation of those facts. On the average, fasting blood glucose changes little with age. Response to glucose challenge, however, clearly deteriorates. Using a 75-g or 100-g oral glucose challenge, there is an increase in the 2-hour postchallenge blood glucose of about 10 mg/dl per decade over the age of 40. This has been variously interpreted as reflecting a "normal" aging change or, conversely, as a progressive increase in the prevalence of diabetes with age. The vigorous debate over this point has contained all the elements of academic foolishness. If one accepts the fact that *clinically significant* diabetes rarely if ever occurs in the absence of fasting hyperglycemia, the answer becomes obvious: we should stop doing generally worthless glucose tolerance tests (except for research purposes) in the elderly and rely on the presence of symptoms and the demonstration of fasting hyperglycemia (serum glucose >130 mg/dl) to diagnose diabetes mellitus.

The mechanism for this deterioration in glucose tolerance is gradually being elucidated. Insulin responses to glucose challenge do not change significantly with age; thus, the body's response to insulin must be reduced. DeFronzo and his colleagues at Yale have recently shown this in a more direct fashion using the elegant "insulin clamp" technique.[3] For a given level of circulating insulin (experimentally induced), less glucose is metabolized by the elderly than by the young. This has been interpreted as reflecting relative insulin insensitivity in the elderly. However, the Yale group has overlooked an equally plausible interpretation, similar to that applied to basal metabolic rate changes. The observed reduction in glucose metabolism may simply be another manifestation of reduced "metabolic mass" in the elderly;

3. R.A. DeFronzo. Glucose intolerance and aging. *Diabetes* 28:1095–1101, 1979.

clear demonstration that cellular sensitivity to insulin is reduced has not yet been provided.

THYROID FUNCTION

Early studies in elderly patients demonstrated that circulating levels of thyroxine (T_4) and triiodothyronine (T_3) are reduced when compared with those of younger persons. However, it now appears that these results were biased by the inclusion of older patients who were institutionalized, hospitalized, or both. More recent studies utilizing only healthy, ambulatory older individuals show little if any change in circulating levels of the thyroid hormones. The response of the pituitary (i.e., release of thyroid-stimulating hormone, TSH) to the stimulating factor from the hypothalamus (thyrotropin-releasing hormone, TRH) has been variably reported but is probably somewhat depressed in the elderly. However, thyroid response to TSH appears intact. Of interest is the fact that degradation of circulating thyroid hormones is clearly diminished in the elderly; the rate of disappearance of T_4 is reduced by approximately 50 percent (i.e., the T½ is twice as long). Since the level of T_4 is unchanged, this implies a compensatory reduction in the rate of secretion of T_4 by the thyroid, which has now been confirmed by direct measurement of secretory rates in older subjects. This is an example of the fine regulation possible within the endocrine system because of the multiple feedback loops. A concomitant of the change in T_4 secretory rate is that replacement doses of thyroxine for hypothyroidism should be less in the elderly than in the young, and this has been confirmed by Davis and his colleagues in Buffalo.[4]

ADRENALS

As might be expected for such a critical hormone as cortisol, levels of the hormone and response to stress are well maintained in the elderly. This has been shown clearly in studies of old and young patients undergoing elective surgery, and by testing with metyrapone. As with thyroxine, metabolism of cortisol declines by some 30 percent in the elderly, and this is nicely balanced by an appropriate reduction in cortisol secretion from the adrenal cortex. Thus, while urinary

---

4. F.B. Davis, R.S. LaMartia, S.W. Spaulding, P.J. Davis. Conventional therapy over-treats elderly hypothyroid patients (abstract). *Proc. Endocrine Soc.* 39:83, 1980.

excretion of cortisol and its metabolites declines with age, serum levels are unchanged.

Renin and aldosterone responses are less well preserved with aging. Although basal concentrations remain normal, there is a clearly documented decrease in response to the volume contraction stresses of sodium depletion or prolonged upright posture. This implies that elderly patients may be less effective in conserving sodium in the face of dehydration than their younger counterparts.

MINERAL HOMEOSTASIS

It has been known for a long time that, beginning at the time of the menopause, women enter a period of negative calcium balance that frequently terminates in clinically significant osteoporosis. While some calcium loss occurs in older men, it is of much lesser magnitude and rarely of clinical significance. The two major manifestations of this change in women are loss of height due to compression fractures of the vertebrae, and fractures of the hip. Fractures of all types occur at a rate of about 700,000 per year among postmenopausal women, and there are 50,000 deaths annually related specifically to hip fractures. Loss of mineral from the appendicular skeleton (measured at the wrist) begins at age 50, proceeds rapidly from then until age 65, and then progresses more slowly from 65 years on. Total loss eventually exceeds 30 percent of bone mass. Even more surprising are the results of studies done on the axial skeleton (spine). Here, loss of bone mass begins in the thirties and proceeds at a steady pace through the seventh decade of life, eventually reaching an average loss of 45 percent of bone mineral.

Recent studies have clarified to some extent the mechanisms involved in postmenopausal osteoporosis. Estrogen clearly inhibits rates of bone resorption, and in its absence bone loss is accelerated. Calcium absorption from the gut also declines after age 50 in women, so that larger calcium intake is required to maintain balance. This appears to be due at least in part to a decrease in the concentration of circulating 1,25-dihydroxy vitamin D, the most active metabolite of vitamin D and the form believed primarily responsible for increasing calcium absorption from the gastrointestinal tract. To worsen matters, these metabolic events occur at a time when dietary calcium intake is generally declining in the female population. Balance studies suggest that 800 mg of dietary calcium a day is required to maintain balance in healthy young women; this figure is estimated to *increase* to 1,200 to 1,500 mg per day in elderly women. Yet dietary studies indicate that, on the average, women over 60 in the United States consume only 400 mg of calcium per day in the diet.

The ability of estrogen therapy, begun at the time of the menopause, to at least delay if not prevent the development of postmenopausal osteoporosis is well established. Concern about its routine use has centered around the probable increase of uterine cancer seen in women on long-term postmenopausal estrogen therapy. It should be noted that many of the studies demonstrating this finding have used supraphysiologic doses of estrogen. A very recent study from the Mayo Clinic group[5] has shown a striking reduction in spinal compression fractures in women on a combination of calcium, estrogen, and fluoride (no additive effect of vitamin D could be shown) as compared to a control group, with groups on estrogen alone or on calcium and fluoride alone falling in between.

It appears that postmenopausal osteoporosis represents one area where we can practice significant preventive medicine. All women entering the menopause should be advised to remain physically active (inactivity clearly accelerates bone resorption) and to add 1 gram per day of calcium to their diet, either as a quart of milk or 4 Os-Cal tablets a day. For all women amenable to regular medical follow-up (i.e., annual Papanicolaou smear and early reporting of vaginal bleeding), I would recommend modest doses of estrogens (Premarin, 0.625 mg, or ethinyl estradiol, 20 µg daily) three weeks out of four, except in the presence of a strong family history of uterine cancer. Because of the frequent adverse side effects, fluoride should probably be reserved for those women who already have established and symptomatic osteoporosis. At present, there is no convincing evidence for adding vitamin D to the above regimen (for a careful statement of a somewhat more conservative view on estrogens, see the chapter on the menopause).

GONADAL FUNCTION

At the time of menopause, ovarian follicular function ceases. There is gradual cessation of estrogen secretion and plasma levels of estrogens decline, although estrone declines the least and becomes the

---

5. B.L. Riggs, E. Seeman, S.F. Hodgson, et al. Effect of the fluoride/calcium regimen on vertebral fracture occurrence in postmenopausal osteoporosis. *N. Engl. J. Med.* 306:446–450, 1982.

predominant form of circulating estrogen. At this point almost all estrogen comes from the adrenal, especially from the peripheral conversion of androstenedione to estrone. Of interest is the fact that the ovary continues to provide about half of the androgens circulating in the postmenopausal woman.

In response to declining levels of sex hormones, both luteinizing hormone (LH) and follicle-stimulating hormone (FSH) secretions from the pituitary increase (lack of negative feedback), and FSH secretion becomes pulsatile, similar to LH secretion in the premenopausal woman. The function of this change in the secretory pattern of FSH is unknown.

Initial studies in elderly men showed a gradual but significant decline in testosterone levels after the age of 45 to 50. Again, however, these findings were probably biased by the inclusion of institutionalized patients. Recent studies from Scandinavia on healthy ambulatory males failed to show this decline with age. However, LH and FSH levels rise gradually with age, and the pituitary response to the hypothalamic-releasing factor LH-RH increases. That Leydig cell mass in the testis declines is suggested by diminished testosterone secretion following exogenous human chorionic gonadotropin (HCG). Thus, in the healthy aging male, testicular function gradually declines, but this is adequately compensated for by an increased secretion of the pituitary trophic hormones, with the result that circulating levels of testosterone remain relatively constant. Sexual function, the result of a complex interaction of many factors, is maintained in healthy men and women well into the eighth and ninth decades, although in general, intercourse occurs less frequently than in the young. Sexual activity in the elderly has only recently become the subject for serious study, and much remains to be learned.

THE PITUITARY

Several aspects of pituitary function have been covered in the preceding sections. Response of growth hormone to a variety of secretory stimuli clearly decreases with age; the significance of this change is unclear. Prolactin secretion declines in postmenopausal women but increases in older men, so that by age 60 concentrations found in men equal or exceed those found in women. Again, the significance of this change, if any, is unknown.

Changes in posterior pituitary function are interesting and may have practical implications. Somewhat surprisingly, vasopressin secretion in response to hypertonic stimuli increases in the elderly, and suppression of vasopressin secretion by inhibitors such as alcohol is less than in the young. At the same time, the ability of the kidney to respond to vasopressin (endogenous or exogenous) declines with age. Thus, the elderly can neither concentrate nor dilute their urine as readily as their younger counterparts. It is apparent that careful attention must be paid to fluid intake and output in a sick elderly patient, since such a person would be prone to either fluid overload (water intoxication) or rapid dehydration depending on the circumstances.

SUGGESTED READING

1. Andres, R. Aging and diabetes. *Med. Clin. North Am.* 55:835–846, 1971.
2. Davis, F.B., et al. Conventional therapy overtreats elderly hypothyroid patients. *Proc. Endocrine Soc.* 1980, p. 83.
3. Davis, P.J., Davis, F.B. Hyperthyroidism in patients over the age of 60 years. *Medicine* 53:161–181, 1974.
4. DeFronzo, R.A. Glucose intolerance and aging. *Diabetes* 28:1095, 1979.
5. Harman, S.M., Tsitouras, P.O. Reproductive hormones in aging men. *J. Clin. Endocrinol. Metab.* 51:35–40, 1980.
6. McGandy, R.B., Barrows, C.H., Jr., Spanias, A., et al. Nutrient intake and energy expenditure in men of different ages. *J. Gerontol.* 21:851–857, 1966.
7. Munro, H.N. Nutrition and aging. *Br. Med. Bull.* 37:83–88, 1981.
8. Munro, H.N. An introduction to nutritional aspects of protein metabolism. In Munro, H.N., and Allison, J.B. (Eds.), *Mammalian Protein Metabolism,* vol. 2. New York: Academic Press, 1964, pp. 3–39.
9. Riggs, B.L., Seeman, E., Hodgson, S.F., et al. Effect of the fluoride/calcium regimen on vertebral fracture occurrence in postmenopausal osteoporosis. *N. Engl. J. Med.* 306:446, 1982.

Diabetes Mellitus

ROBERT E. SEVIER, M.D.

Editor's note: The diagnosis and skillful management of diabetes mellitus in the elderly is one of the greatest challenges in primary care medicine. Diagnostic standards, therapeutic guidelines, and all aspects of clinical management must take into account both biologic and psychosocial aging. Serious complications, acute or chronic, may already be apparent at initial presentation, and vigilance must be maintained by both patient and physician to ensure satisfactory medical care and the prevention of serious sequelae.

As the number of Americans over 65 years of age approaches 45 million or 15 percent of the population by the turn of the century, it can be projected that as many as 2.75 million of these will have diabetes. Among this group diabetes is the third leading cause of death by disease, the leading cause of new cases of blindness, and the leading cause of amputations. With proper advice and care, however, most elderly diabetics can enjoy a relatively normal and symptom-free existence and can expect a reasonably normal survival. The incidence of newly diagnosed diabetes increases steadily by decade after age 40, reaching a peak of 6.5 percent between 65 and 74 years of age and declining to 5.8 percent after age 75, with few cases discovered after age 90.

Diabetes is best classified according to the recommendations of the National Diabetes Data Group, published in 1979 and since widely accepted throughout the world (Table 1). Type I or insulin-dependent diabetes consists of those who absolutely require insulin to avoid ketoacidosis and certain death. This group accounts for some 10 percent of diabetics among the elderly and is divided about equally between those who have been diagnosed earlier in life and have survived and those who are diagnosed in their later years. Type II

TABLE 1

Classification of Diabetes Mellitus and Other Categories of Glucose Intolerance

Diabetes mellitus (DM)
  Insulin-dependent type (IDDM) or type I
  Non-insulin-dependent type (NIDDM) or type II
    1. Nonobese NIDDM
    2. Obese NIDDM
  Other types
    1. Pancreatic disease
    2. Hormonal
    3. Drug- or chemical-induced
    4. Insulin receptor abnormalities
    5. Certain genetic syndromes
    6. Others
Impaired glucose tolerance (IGT)
Gestational diabetes (GDM)
Previous abnormality of glucose tolerance (Prev AGT)
Potential abnormality of glucose tolerance (Pot AGT)

Source: Adapted from National Diabetes Data Group. Classification and diagnosis of diabetes mellitus and other categories of glucose intolerance. *Diabetes* 28:1039–1057, 1979.

or non-insulin-dependent diabetes consists of those who under usual circumstances do not require insulin to avoid ketoacidosis and to survive. This group accounts for some 80 percent of elderly diabetics, most of whom will have been diagnosed by age 70 and about three-fourths of whom will be obese. Other types of diabetes, as defined in Table 1, are likewise generally not insulin-requiring and account for the remaining 10 percent of elderly diabetics. Patients with either type II or "other" types of diabetes may require insulin at times of major stress, illness, injury, or surgery, and insulin is sometimes used electively in these patients in an effort to improve their clinical management.

DIAGNOSIS

The diagnosis of diabetes in the elderly is made difficult by the natural deterioration in glucose tolerance with aging, which reflects primarily an impaired ability to respond to a glucose challenge. While fasting glucose values increase only 1 to 2 percent with aging, values 2 hours after a standard glucose challenge rise approximately 10 percent for each decade after age 40. Possible contributory factors include physical inactivity, degeneration of the pancreatic islets, decreased insulin secretion, decreased dietary intake, decreased resting metabolic rate, decreased lean body mass, and insulin antagonism or insensitivity. The bulk of evidence from numerous properly designed studies suggests that only the last two factors are likely significant and that the two are intimately related.

Considering these physiologic changes of aging, some recommend that diabetes be diagnosed in the older individual only when there is distinct abnormality of the fasting blood sugar (plasma glucose >140 mg/dl). The broader recommendation of the National Diabetes Data Group (Table 2) is that the diagnosis of diabetes be considered certain in persons who (1) show classic signs or symptoms and unequivocal elevation of plasma glucose; (2) show fasting plasma glucose levels of 140 mg/dl or greater on more than one occasion; or (3) show fasting plasma glucose levels of less than 140 mg/dl but plasma glucose levels of 200 mg/dl or greater both at 2 hours and at some other point between zero time and 2 hours after a standard glucose challenge, again on more than one occasion. For precise application of these criteria, the patient should have ingested no less than 150 g of carbohydrate daily for three days before testing and should receive a 75-g dextrose challenge. While this approach will clearly avoid erroneous diagnosis in nondiabetics, a substantial number of patients who will thus be relegated to the category of "impaired glucose tolerance" (Table 1) will be clinically symptomatic or will evolve complications diagnostic of diabetes, or both. These patients merit close

TABLE 2

Diagnostic Criteria for Diabetes Mellitus in Nonpregnant Adults

Any of the following are considered diagnostic:
1. Presence of classic symptomatology, such as polyuria, polydipsia, ketonuria, and rapid weight loss, together with unequivocal elevation of plasma glucose.
2. Fasting plasma glucose[a] ≥140 mg/dl on more than one occasion.
3. Fasting plasma glucose[a] <140/mg/dl but sustained hyperglycemia during the standard oral glucose tolerance test[b] on more than one occasion. Both the 2-hour value and some other value between zero time and 2 hours must be ≥200 mg/dl.

Source: Adapted from National Diabetes Data Group. Classification and diagnosis of diabetes mellitus and other categories of glucose intolerance. *Diabetes* 28:1039–1057, 1979.
[a]If venous whole blood or capillary whole blood determinations are used, appropriate adjustment of diagnostic values will be required.
[b]See text.

clinical surveillance and perhaps deserve management similar to that employed in frank diabetes, especially if 2-hour postprandial plasma glucose values on ordinary diet are higher than 160 mg/dl.

Finally, there has been a recent suggestion that elevated levels of glycosylated hemoglobin (HbA_{1c}) be considered diagnostic of diabetes independent of specific blood sugar criteria. Since the glycosylation of lens protein appears to be a factor in the development and advancement of cataracts in diabetes, and since there is increasing evidence that glycosylation of other proteins may play a role in microvascular complications of diabetes, individuals with glycosylated hemoglobin levels consistently above 9 percent clearly deserve close surveillance.

CLINICAL PRESENTATION

Many, if not most, elderly diabetics lack classic symptoms and may go undiagnosed until they develop some complication of the disease. An increase in the renal threshold for glucose, together with a natural decline in the glomerular filtration rate with aging, may preclude polyuria and resultant polydipsia despite striking hyperglycemia. Even when present, polyuria, nocturia, and urinary frequency may be ignored by the man with prostatism or the woman with weakened pelvic supports or may develop so insidiously as to generate little concern. Less common and nonspecific symptoms such as nausea, anorexia, and fatigue should be sought and special regard given to patients with generalized pruritus, fungal intertrigo, balanitis, vulvovaginitis, paronychiae, foot ulcers, urinary tract infection, and other unhealing cutaneous wounds or infections. Other presenting symptoms may include rapid deterioration of visual acuity resulting from osmolar changes in the lens due to hyperglycemia or from advancing cataracts or retinal disease, or manifestations of neuropathy (e.g., pain, extraocular muscle palsy or other evidence of mononeuritis, paresthesias, orthostatic hypotension, impotence, or nocturnal diarrhea). Finally, diabetes may be discovered during hospitalization for a vascular event such as myocardial infarction, cerebrovascular accident, or peripheral vascular occlusion with or without gangrene. Diabetes in the elderly patient rarely presents initially as coma, especially not as ketoacidosis, and the presence of coma or ketoacidosis mandates a careful search for some otherwise obscure precipitating condition.

MANAGEMENT

Maintaining near-normal blood sugar levels is both desirable and obtainable in most cases of diabetes; when such a goal can be safely met in the elderly diabetic, the advancement of complications of the disease, especially lenticular cataracts, may be slowed. An appropriate goal, then, would be to keep fasting plasma glucose consistently less than 150 mg/dl and 2-hour postprandial glucose levels less than 200 mg/dl. This may prove difficult or impossible in the obese individual who is uncooperative with respect to diet or in the patient with organic brain syndrome or other factors that compromise optimal management; on the other hand, even tighter control may be possible in the highly motivated patient. The avoidance of severe hypoglycemia is equally important, however, since this may result in injury, cerebrovascular accident, or myocardial infarction in this age group. Thus the goals and methods of therapy must be individualized, with attention given to the patient's mental status, overall clinical condition, concurrent acute and chronic disease, living arrangements, socioeconomic factors, personal and cultural habits, and specific physical impairments such as decreased vision or severe arthritis that might prevent satisfactory self-care.

Essential elements of diabetes management in the elderly include diet, exercise, insulin or oral hypoglycemic agents when appropriate, education, and specific treatment of infections or other concurrent conditions, particularly those that also constitute major cardiovascular risk factors. The combination of diabetes and hypertension is recognized as being especially lethal, and aggressive treatment of hypertension is mandatory. Except where there is a clear contraindication, both pneumococcal and influenzal immunization should be given according to standard guidelines. Special attention must be paid to the influence that other medications might have on the diabetes and to the possibility of interaction between these drugs and insulin or oral hypoglycemic agents: corticosteroids, thiazides, furosemide, estrogens, and chloramphenicol may foster hyperglycemia, whereas beta-blockers, phenylbutazone and its derivatives, probenecid, salicylates, sulfisoxazole, and bishydroxycoumarin may potentiate hypoglycemia.

Residence in any institutional setting or the presence of another responsible adult in the home generally facilitates management of the elderly diabetic. For those who live alone, an occasional home visit by the physician or by a public health nurse or other skilled worker from various community agencies can provide valuable insight into patient care problems while giving emotional and educational support as well as direct assistance in care. Because the elderly may deny the existence of their diabetes, education and ongoing reeducation of the patient about the disease are critical. This should begin with the physician and his office or hospital staff, and again the efforts of visiting health care professionals can be most valuable. Participation in the programs of local diabetes associations should be encouraged, not only for the obvious educational benefit but also for the emotional support and reassurance such programs provide.

Because of the high renal threshold for glucose in most elderly patients, routine monitoring of urines may be of limited usefulness on a daily basis. At times of stress or illness, however, extreme hyperglycemia may develop and may be reflected in the urine, indicating a need for temporary alteration of management. The role of home glucose monitoring in the elderly, attractive because of the limitations of urine testing, is as yet uncertain, but such monitoring may prove useful in the occasional labile insulin-requiring older diabetic. Furthermore, home glucose monitoring may be useful in motivating selected patients to achieve tighter control.

Diet

Many older patients with type II diabetes can be managed by diet alone or, where indicated, by diet in combination with weight reduction. Ideal weight can be estimated by allowing 100 pounds in the female and 106 pounds in the male for the first 5 feet of height, adding for each additional inch of height 5 or 6 pounds in females or males, respectively. A 10-percent adjustment may be appropriate if the frame is considered small or large. When weight loss is desired, dietary allowance should be 10 calories per pound of ideal (not actual) body weight, whereas the patient at or near ideal weight may be allowed 15 calories per pound. These caloric allowances may require reduction as age advances beyond 60 years or when physical problems preclude a reasonable level of physical activity.

Generally the standard diets of the American Diabetes Association suffice; at any given calorie level these diets call for 50 to 60 percent of calories as carbohydrate, predominantly in complex form, 15 to 20 percent as protein, and the remainder as fat, with an emphasis on unsaturated fats. The use of high-carbohydrate, high-fiber diets has proved quite satisfactory in type II diabetes and may be of particular value in older patients with a tendency toward constipation and decreased bowel function. Dietary intake should be divided among no fewer than three meals per day, with a small bedtime feeding added in those receiving insulin or oral hypoglycemic agents and perhaps also small midmorning and midafternoon feedings in those receiving insulin.

Oral Hypoglycemic Agents

The oral hypoglycemic agents available in this country, the sulfonylureas, have been the subject of considerable controversy since the 1970 report of the University Group Diabetes Program (UGDP).[1] However, opinion among many diabetologists has swung again toward favorable consideration of these agents in type II diabetes when diet and weight reduction fail to ensure adequate control. Renewed interest in the sulfonylureas stems in part from the fact that many of the UGDP conclusions have not been borne out by subsequent studies, but probably more from increased understanding of the mechanism of action of these agents. It was initially thought that sulfonylureas simply stimulated additional insulin release from intact pancreatic islets; although this mechanism is clearly operative in the first several weeks of therapy, it now appears that the more important and longer-lasting mechanism of action is in extrapancreatic tissues where hepatic glucose output is diminished, muscle glucose transport facilitated, and insulin receptor numbers increased.

Sulfonylureas available in this country include tolbutamide (Orinase), tolazamide (Tolinase), acetohexamide (Dymelor), and chlorpropamide (Diabinese). The principal differences among these agents lie in their patterns of metabolism and excretion and in their pharmacologic half-lives. Tolbutamide is principally inactivated by the liver, with the inactive metabolite excreted in the urine; it has an effective half-life of 3 to 5 hours. While it must be used with caution in the presence of impaired liver function, its short half-life minimizes the risk of prolonged hypoglycemia, especially nocturnal, and thus makes it perhaps the agent of choice in the elderly diabetic. The remaining three agents are modified in the liver to yield active metabolites, which in turn are excreted in the urine; thus they tend to have longer half-lives and must be used with extreme caution in the

---

1. C.L. Meinert, G.L. Knatterud, T.E. Prout, C.R. Klimt. A study of the effects of hypoglycemic agents on vascular complications in patients with adult-onset diabetes. *Diabetes* 19(Suppl.):789–830, 1970.

presence of impaired renal function. Tolazamide and acetohexamide have half-lives of 7 to 10 and 10 to 12 hours, respectively, while chlorpropamide is much more tightly protein-bound, yielding an effective half-life of 24 to 36 hours. Chlorpropamide has the additional potential for interacting unfavorably with alcohol, with a resultant disulfiram-like effect, and for producing hyponatremia due to an antidiuretic hormone-like effect on the renal tubules. For all these reasons, the use of chlorpropamide in the elderly is perhaps best discouraged.

Toxic effects of the sulfonylureas fortunately tend to be relatively minor and uncommon; they include anorexia, nausea, other gastrointestinal effects, headache, pruritus and skin reactions, hepatic reaction with cholestasis, and suppression of hematopoietic elements.

Two new sulfonylurea compounds, glybenclamide and glipizide, will likely soon be available in this country. Experience in the laboratory and in other countries suggests that the principal advantage of these drugs lies in a greater potency per unit of dosage.

Although the practice of combining insulin and sulfonylureas, particularly in the obese patient in whom the use of insulin has become necessary, has some basis in theory and some enthusiastic advocates, there is little reason to consider this approach in the majority of situations.

Insulin

The principles of insulin use in the older diabetic are similar to those in the young. The hazards of forgotten doses or of faulty technique in drawing up and administering insulin are obviously greater in the elderly. Hospitalization is recommended for the institution of insulin therapy and for instruction of the patient, and starting doses should be small with dosage adjustments made slowly and in small increments.

Frequently it is possible to achieve satisfactory control with a single daily injection of an intermediate-acting insulin such as NPH or Lente. When it is necessary to combine regular insulin with the intermediate insulin to achieve better daytime control without increased risk of nocturnal hypoglycemia, it must be remembered that the effect of the regular insulin will be largely lost if the mixture remains in the syringe for more than 5 minutes before injection, such as when the insulins are mixed in advance by a family member or the visiting nurse. A stabilized premixed insulin consisting of 70% NPH and 30% regular has recently been marketed and may prove of value.

When acceptable fasting plasma glucose values cannot be achieved without evening or nocturnal hypoglycemia, the dose of intermediate insulin may be split, with two-thirds to three-fourths given before breakfast and the remainder given before the evening meal or later, even as late as bedtime. The use of a single daily dose of Ultralente insulin to provide a continuous low and essentially "peakless" basal insulin concentration combined with supplemental regular insulin at mealtimes may also prove effective. The proper education of each patient with respect to the pattern of action of his particular insulin as well as to the recognition and treatment of hypoglycemia is absolutely essential, as is the provision of appropriate between-meal or bedtime feedings.

Surgery, trauma, severe illness, or major stress may mandate the temporary use of insulin in those not ordinarily insulin-dependent. The approach is similar to that just outlined, except that often larger and more frequent doses of regular insulin may be required. There are as many approaches to perioperative management of insulin as there are diabetologists, but the use of a constant infusion of regular insulin at 0.05 units per kilogram per hour, together with frequent monitoring of plasma glucose perhaps deserves special mention.

The new highly purified insulins appear to offer no particular advantage to the older diabetic except when there is clearly immunologic insulin resistance, lipoatrophy or lipodystrophy at injection sites, or when intermittent use of insulin is anticipated, as for coverage of a surgical procedure.

Exercise
Exercise enhances the peripheral utilization of glucose by both insulin-dependent and non-insulin-dependent tissues. In insulin-dependent tissues, such as muscle and liver, this phenomenon is mediated in part through an increase in insulin receptors or an enhancement of receptor affinity for insulin or both, thus effectively reducing the peripheral insulin resistance characteristic of type II diabetes. In addition, exercise suppresses both endogenous pancreatic insulin release and hepatic glucose production and output. In the diabetic taking exogenous insulin, exercise enhances insulin absorption from the injection site, and this factor combined with the physiologic effects of exercise can lead to profound lowering of plasma glucose, necessitating the intake of supplemental calories during exercise if clinical hypoglycemia is to be avoided. In the type II diabetic, however, especially if the patient is managed with diet alone, favorable lowering

of glucose during exercise can be expected without serious risk of hypoglycemia. In addition to these beneficial effects, regular exercise results in a reduction of plasma very-low-density lipoprotein (VLDL) levels while increasing high-density lipoprotein (HDL) levels, in turn perhaps retarding advancement of the atherosclerotic process. Given the striking association of diabetes with cardiovascular disease, a regular exercise program for the older diabetic seems prudent. Finally, in the elderly exercise has the added advantages of increasing the general sense of well-being and independence, combating depression, improving bowel and sleep patterns, and perhaps benefiting other chronic diseases.

While running or other extremely vigorous exercise regimens may be undesirable in the elderly, walking at a brisk pace, swimming, aquatic exercise, golf, bicycling, the use of a stationary bicycle, and formal exercise groups especially designed for this age group are usually safe and effective. In all such programs, proper emphasis must be placed on foot care, the avoidance of excessive cardiovascular stress, and the protection of joints involved by degenerative arthritis or other disease. The physician should be specific in his prescription for exercise and should reinforce the importance of this aspect of treatment by proper questioning at each visit.

Approach to the Individual Patient
The patient who is initially found to be diabetic on presenting with another acute or critical illness or injury will generally require urgent management, often to include insulin. Rarely the elderly diabetic will present in ketoacidosis or a hyperglycemic hyperosmolar nonketotic state, both of which likewise require insulin and other aggressive measures. Less acute situations characterized by extreme hyperglycemia (fasting plasma glucose >300 mg/dl, postprandial plasma glucose >450 mg/dl) or by significant ketonuria may require insulin for satisfactory initial management, but it can often be discontinued later.

Most elderly diabetics are discovered incidentally or present with relatively minor symptoms and lesser degrees of hyperglycemia. Once the diagnosis has been confirmed, therapy should begin with the institution of proper diet and an exercise regimen together with patient education. If significant glycosuria is present, urine testing should be done twice daily, on arising in the morning and before the evening meal, employing the double-voided technique for specimen collection and a reliable semiquantitative method of testing. Fasting and 2-hour postprandial plasma or capillary glucose values should be obtained at two- to three-week intervals.

If after six to eight weeks glycosuria has cleared, symptoms have improved or resolved, and fasting glucose is less than 160 mg/dl (venous) or 140 mg/dl (capillary) and postprandial values are less than 200 mg/dl (venous) or 175 mg/dl (capillary), the same treatment should be continued indefinitely with surveillance at three-month intervals unless indicated more frequently by other problems or by clinical change. If glucose values have not reached these levels but weight loss has been satisfactory and both symptoms and glycosuria have largely abated, again the same regimen may be continued. However, if progress has not been satisfactory despite patient compliance, consideration should be given at this time to the addition of a sulfonylurea, preferably tolbutamide for reasons indicated earlier. The starting dose should be 250 to 500 mg given before breakfast, with the dosage slowly increased at three-week intervals to a maximum of 1,500 mg if necessary. If postprandial glucose values reach satisfactory levels but fasting levels remain excessive, the dosage may be split with a portion given before the evening meal; using split doses, the total may be gradually increased if necessary to 2,500 mg. Larger doses are unlikely to be of further benefit and may lead to toxicity.

If tolbutamide is initially ineffective or if a "secondary failure" occurs after its extended use, a trial of tolazamide or acetohexamide may prove successful. These agents should be started at doses of 250 mg daily before breakfast and the dosage gradually increased if necessary. Occasionally divided doses will be necessary to ensure satisfactory fasting glucose levels, but care must be taken to detect and avoid nocturnal hypoglycemia. With divided doses, ordinarily two-thirds should be given in the morning and one-third before the evening meal, with the maximum daily dose limited to 1,500 mg of either agent.

Patients treated with sulfonylureas should be followed at three-month intervals unless there are specific indications for more frequent visits. After six months of established satisfactory control, especially if there has been concomitant weight loss, an attempt should be made to reduce doses or to withdraw these agents altogether; often it will be found that control by diet alone is again possible.

When blood glucose values cannot be adequately controlled by diet or by a combination of diet and sulfonylureas, consideration should be given to the institution of insulin therapy. When the patient's overall condition permits the safe use of insulin, it is perhaps most wisely begun in the hospital. NPH or Lente insulin should be started at 15 units each morning, with the dose gradually increased at intervals of several days. If late afternoon and evening blood glucose levels are controlled but fasting hyperglycemia persists (goal values as earlier), the dose may be split, with one-third or less given either before the evening meal or near bedtime. When midday hyperglycemia persists despite satisfactory fasting and evening glucose values, regular insulin in amounts of 5 to 15 units may be combined with the morning dose. Occasionally it may prove necessary or desirable to combine regular insulin with the intermediate insulin given before the evening meal as well, but under no circumstances should regular insulin be given at bedtime as part of routine management.

ACUTE COMPLICATIONS

Hypoglycemia

Although they occur less commonly than in younger patients, hypoglycemic attacks may be devastating to the elderly by precipitating injury, cerebrovascular accident, or myocardial infarction. Accordingly, the elderly diabetic taking either insulin or a sulfonylurea must be repeatedly educated (along with his or her spouse or living companion) about the pharmacologic properties of the agent used, the importance of regular and adequate food intake, and the early recognition and management of hypoglycemia. Any episode of neurologic symptoms, including sudden agitation or confusion, should be considered a manifestation of hypoglycemia until proved otherwise. Injectable glucagon may be provided for emergency use, although early contact with a rescue squad or other skilled medical personnel is usually more satisfactory. Observation and treatment of the elderly patient following severe hypoglycemia should extend longer than in the younger diabetic; hypoglycemia associated with chlorpropamide, because of that drug's long half-life, may necessitate hospitalization and 24 to 72 hours of intravenous glucose administration.

Ketoacidosis

Ketoacidosis is uncommon in the elderly, even in an insulin-dependent individual. Accordingly, the appearance of ketoacidosis should prompt a thorough search for some serious precipitating event such as myocardial infarction, cerebrovascular accident, sepsis, or other major infection, and proper management requires aggressive attention to both the ketoacidosis and the underlying condition. Not surprisingly, mortality may run as high as 30 percent. Principles of management of ketoacidosis are similar to those in the younger diabetic, although fluid replacement generally must proceed more slowly because of decreased cardiovascular tolerance, especially if there has been antecedent heart disease or renal insufficiency. Protocols utilizing continuous low-dose intravenous insulin infusion or small hourly intramuscular insulin doses appear to be safe for use in the older diabetic.

Hyperosmolar Nonketotic Coma

Hyperosmolar nonketotic coma is almost unique to the older diabetic. This type of coma may be the initial presenting feature and may be especially insidious in its symptomatic onset. Three underlying elements are found in the usual case: (1) mild renal insufficiency with impaired clearance of glucose and urea, facilitating the development of extreme hyperglycemia and azotemia; (2) the chronic administration of certain drugs, including corticosteroids, phenothiazines, thiazide diuretics, furosemide, diphenylhydantoin, or sedatives; and (3) the presence of either a chronic brain syndrome or a physical disability that impairs recognition of or response to the extreme thirst that accompanies the dehydration and advancing hyperosmolar state. The syndrome is characterized by progressive confusion and obtundation advancing to coma, vomiting, seizures, hypotension, extreme dehydration, extreme hyperglycemia (plasma glucose rarely <1,000 mg/dl and often >2,000 mg/dl), azotemia, and extreme hyperosmolarity (often >360 mOsm/dl). Potential complications of the extreme dehydration and hypotension include cerebrovascular accident, myocardial infarction, or peripheral vascular occlusion. Mortality is in the range of 30 to 40 percent. Management must be aggressive, employing vigorous rehydration with normal or half-normal saline within cardiovascular tolerance, insulin, and other supportive measures. Although it has been stated that there is extreme sensitivity to insulin in this setting, the use of low-dose insulin regimens such as those employed in ketoacidosis appears to be safe and effective.

CHRONIC COMPLICATIONS

The older diabetic is subject to the same complications as the individual who develops the disease earlier in life, namely, retinopathy and other ocular problems, nephropathy, and peripheral and autonomic neuropathy. Unique to the older diabetic, however, is the fact that such complications are commonly manifest at the time of diagnosis and indeed may be responsible for the presenting symptoms. While this may sometimes indicate diabetes that has existed undiagnosed for years, in most cases this is certainly not true and a clear explanation for this clinical observation is lacking.

There is increasing investigative and clinical evidence that diabetic cataracts, retinopathy, neuropathy, and nephropathy can in many cases be related to the degree and duration of sustained hyperglycemia, and this has led to greater concern for tighter plasma glucose control, even in older diabetics. Treatment should be aimed at minimizing the number and duration of excursions of the plasma glucose above 180 mg/dl; that such a goal may be unattainable in some elderly diabetics should not deter the physician from striving for tight control in every situation in which it can safely be achieved.

Finally, although the incidence of atherosclerosis and its complications is increased in all diabetics, this problem assumes major proportions in the older diabetic population and thus deserves special mention, as does the so-called diabetic foot, which results from a combination of neuropathic, vascular, and septic factors.

Ophthalmologic Complications
Although there remains disagreement as to whether cataracts develop with greater frequency in diabetics, most diabetologists believe that they do, and virtually all agree that cataracts mature more rapidly in the presence of diabetes. In addition, the elderly diabetic may develop all aspects of classic diabetic retinopathy, including microaneurysms, exudates, macular edema, retinal hemorrhages, neovascularization, vitreous hemorrhage, and retinal detachment. The cataracts and retinal disease of diabetes make it the leading cause of new cases of blindness in the United States. In addition, diabetics may be more prone to ocular infection and are subject to glaucoma and all the other ophthalmologic problems of the general population.

The 1976 National Institutes of Health cooperative study on the treatment of diabetic retinopathy made it clear that aggressive early intervention with laser photocoagulation can significantly reduce the risk of total loss of vision.[2] The availability of vitrectomy and improved surgical techniques for cataracts requires that physicians observe diabetic patients carefully for eye disease and coordinate timely intervention. Every diabetic over the age of 60 should receive careful

---

2. Diabetic Retinopathy Study Research Group, National Institutes of Health. Preliminary report on effects of photocoagulation therapy. *Am. J. Ophthalmol.* 81:383–396, 1976.

ophthalmologic evaluation biannually or more frequently if indicated.

Neuropathy

Common presentations of neuropathy in the older diabetic include the various mononeuropathies, symmetric polyneuropathy of the lower extremities with pain and hypoesthesia, isolated motor loss such as oculomotor palsy, and unilateral amyotrophy affecting the pelvic girdle musculature or quadriceps femoris. Important and diagnostically confusing manifestations of autonomic neuropathy include postural hypotension, impotence, bladder atony, esophageal dysfunction, gastroparesis, diarrhea, gustatory sweating, or cardiac rhythm disturbance. Isolated motor neuropathies and the painful phase of sensory neuropathies usually spontaneously resolve in weeks to months; in situations of severe or protracted pain, diphenylhydantoin, carbamazepine, or amitriptyline alone or fluphenazine/amitriptyline combinations are sometimes useful. The newer agent metoclopramide offers promise in the treatment of gastroparesis and certain other autonomic problems. Physical and occupational therapy may be beneficial. The patient with sensory neuropathy is, of course, at extreme risk for unnoticed and potentially catastrophic injury to hypoesthetic areas, especially the feet. Tight plasma glucose control appears to be of both preventive and therapeutic value in diabetic neuropathy.

Nephropathy

Renal insufficiency in the older diabetic can rarely occur as a result of isolated diabetic glomerulosclerosis; more commonly it results from diabetic injury superimposed on the arteriolar nephrosclerosis of antecedent or concurrent arteriosclerosis or hypertension or on the changes of chronic pyelonephritis or interstitial nephritis. Hydronephrosis due to a neurogenic bladder may also be a contributing cause. Once chronic renal failure has developed, management becomes highly specific and should be directed by an accomplished internist or nephrologist. Hemodialysis may prove particularly difficult in the older diabetic with a tendency to postural hypotension and congestive heart failure. The proper role of chronic ambulatory peritoneal dialysis and of renal transplantation in this age group remains to be elucidated; both have enjoyed recent success in younger diabetics. Adjustment of insulin or sulfonylurea dosage may be extremely difficult in the presence of significant renal insufficiency.

Urinary tract infection is more common in diabetics than in non-diabetics, especially when neuropathy impairs bladder emptying. Such infections are commonly asymptomatic and so must be looked for frequently and treated appropriately.

The risk of acute renal failure from radiologic contrast agents is vastly increased in the older diabetic. Intravenous pyelography and vascular contrast procedures should be avoided whenever possible; when undertaken they should be performed only after generous intravenous hydration. Careful attention to urinary output and renal function in the 48 hours following the procedure is mandatory.

Cardiovascular Disease
Since the introduction of insulin with the attendant increase in longevity, atherosclerosis has emerged as the most common and most severe complication of diabetes, and ischemic heart disease as the leading cause of death in type II diabetes. This increased incidence of atherosclerosis and ischemic heart disease is particularly striking among diabetic women.

There are no unique histologic features in the atherosclerosis of the diabetic; it would appear that diabetes essentially accelerates the atherogenic process. Although diabetics are more prone to hypertension, which may adversely influence atherosclerosis, this factor alone does not provide adequate explanation. Among the many atherogenic factors that may be abnormal in the diabetic are lipoprotein fractions (increased LDL and VLDL, decreased HDL, increased triglycerides), platelet dynamics, soluble clotting factors, prostacyclin-thromboxane balance, and arterial smooth muscle cell proliferation and metabolism. The fact that many of these abnormalities may be caused at least in part by hyperinsulinemia may explain the particularly striking increase in atherosclerotic problems among obese type II diabetics. Clinically, the accelerated atherosclerosis of diabetes results in an increased incidence of cerebrovascular accident, myocardial infarction, and peripheral vascular occlusion.

Diabetics have a vastly increased incidence of coronary heart disease, and myocardial infarction is a more frequent cause of death in diabetics than in the general population. Acute myocardial infarction in the diabetic is more likely to be complicated by congestive failure, myocardial rupture, or cardiogenic shock. Both early and late mortality following infarction are increased approximately threefold, and recurrent infarction is more common. Silent infarction is strikingly more common in the diabetic, apparently due to the interruption of afferent pain impulses by autonomic neuropathy. Independent of myocardial infarction or obvious coronary disease, most type II diabetics show abnormal systolic time intervals, increased left ventricular end-diastolic pressure, and decreased ejection fraction, and overt congestive heart failure in the absence of symptomatic ischemic heart disease is common. Whether these functional impairments reflect myocardial microangiopathy or a diabetic cardiomyopathy, or indeed whether these entities exist at all, is disputed; the pathologic observation of increased interstitial fibrosis in diabetic hearts uninvolved by gross coronary disease, however, is not disputed.

Indications for carotid surgery, myocardial revascularization, and peripheral vascular surgery are essentially the same as in the nondiabetic, and with proper attention to perioperative management and the prevention of infection these procedures can be undertaken in the diabetic with similar risks and expectations.

The Diabetic Foot

Diabetes is the leading cause of nontraumatic amputation of the lower extremity. Amputation is usually necessitated by the combination of neuropathic, ischemic, and septic processes resulting in the so-called diabetic foot. The problem commonly begins when impaired sensation leads to unrecognized minor trauma, which in turn becomes the site of infection. Ill-fitting footwear, burns, penetrating injuries, self-inflicted injury during self-care of the feet, pressure ulcerations, and ulceration over various points on clawed toes (themselves the result of neuropathy) may be implicated. The diabetes itself, as well as the ischemia of small- or large-vessel disease, impairs healing and allows progression to deeper infection, often osteomyelitis or eventually gangrene.

Proper management begins with prevention through proper education of the patient and insistence on attention to proper footwear and hygiene. The feet should be examined at each visit to the physician. Antibiotic therapy and aggressive local measures should be instituted early, with consultation by a competent surgeon or podiatrist when appropriate. Trophic neuropathic ulcers and the resultant septic lesions must be carefully distinguished from the ulcers of vascular disease, since proper management is distinctly different. When circulation is adequate and lesser measures have failed, early and aggressive local surgery may prevent later more radical amputation.

SUGGESTED READING

1. Andres, R. Aging and diabetes. *Med. Clin. North Am.* 55:835–846, 1971.
2. Christlieb, A.R. Diabetes and hypertensive vascular disease: Mechanism and treatment. *Am. J. Cardiol.* 32:592–606, 1973.
3. Davidson, M.B. The effect of aging on carbohydrate metabolism: A review of the English literature and a practical approach to the diagnosis of diabetes mellitus in the elderly. *Metabolism* 28:688–705, 1979.
4. Diabetic Retinopathy Study Research Group, National Institutes of Health. Preliminary report on the effects of photocoagulation therapy. *Am. J. Ophthalmol.* 81:383–396, 1976.
5. Fein, F.S. Heart disease in diabetes. *Cardiovasc. Rev. Rep.* 3:877–896, 1982.
6. Kreisberg, R.A. Diabetic ketoacidosis: New concepts and trends in pathogenesis and treatment. *Ann. Intern. Med.* 88:681–695, 1978.
7. Levin, M.E., Boniuk, I., Anderson, B., Avioli, L.V. Prevention and treatment of diabetic complications. *Arch. Intern. Med.* 140:691–696, 1980.
8. National Diabetes Data Group. Classification and diagnosis of diabetes mellitus and other categories of glucose intolerance. *Diabetes* 28:1039–1057, 1979.
9. Olefsky, J.M., Kolterman, O.G. Mechanism of insulin resistance in obesity and non-insulin-dependent (type II) diabetes. *Am. J. Med.* 70:151–168, 1981.
10. Steiner, G. Diabetes and atherosclerosis: An overview. *Diabetes* 30(Suppl 2):1–7, 1981.
11. Stillman, T.G., Feldman, J.M. The pharmacology of sulfonylureas. *Am. J. Med.* 70:361–372, 1981.

Menopause and Beyond

ROBERT H. FLETCHER, M.D., M.SC.

Editor's note: Estrogens are prescribed to prevent the conditions that follow ovarian failure—osteoporosis, cardiovascular disease, and genital and urinary atrophy—as well as to relieve perimenopausal symptoms. The frequencies of endometrial cancer, gallstones, and breast cancer have all been thought to be increased by the use of exogenous estrogens, although the current evidence does not support the suspicions for some of these. There is now sufficient evidence to estimate the magnitude of benefit and risk accompanying the use of estrogens, and armed with these estimates, the physician can then decide whether postmenopausal and perimenopausal estrogen therapy is appropriate for individual patients.

All women who survive to mid-life pass through the menopause. The ordinary course of events is for menses to begin to diminish in frequency and amount, then to cease altogether around the age of 50. Preceding menopause, bleeding may be irregular or heavy or may occur between periods. Bleeding rarely resumes after a pause of several months in otherwise normal women. In the United States roughly 30 percent of women have hysterectomies prior to natural menopause. For them, the nonmenstrual symptoms and sequelae of menopause are believed to be the same, or perhaps more pronounced.

SYMPTOMS OF MENOPAUSE

Among the many symptoms that have been attributed to the menopause are depression, excitability, nervousness, irritability, insomnia, and fatigue. These "menopausal symptoms" are frequently listed in textbooks of gynecology, reflecting the impressions of specialists who care for women during the perimenopausal years. It may be, however, that women with unusual and persistent symptoms, who are likely to be referred to physicians who are textbook authors, contribute to these impressions of the menopause out of proportion to their numbers. Furthermore, many of these symptoms are prevalent in people who are not experiencing the menopause. It still is unclear what the symptoms of menopause are in unselected women, over and above what they might have experienced if the menopause had not occurred.

Only a minority of women, about one-third, associate any symptoms other than change in menses with their menopause. A much smaller number visit a physician because of a symptom they attribute to the menopause. Of those women who do have symptoms, nearly all describe hot flashes. Women rarely associate other symptoms— irritability, nervousness, weakness, tiredness, headaches—with their menopause; in one study, each of these was mentioned by less than 1 percent of women.[1] In general, nonspecific symptoms do not seem to occur more commonly during this time than they might otherwise. In one community survey, 948 women over the age of 20 were asked about twenty symptoms.[2] Some of those symptoms progressively increased in prevalence with increasing age, some decreased, and some did not change with age. None of the twenty symptoms occurred with unusual frequency, in relation to the trend it was following, in the age range in which menopause ordinarily occurs (45 to 54 years).

Hot Flashes

It is clear that hot flashes (the British say hot *flushes*) are a specific symptom of the menopause in some women, and for a few they can cause considerable morbidity. Because few women and no men have experienced hot flashes themselves, many do not really understand what they are like. A typical severe hot flash, as described by Glaevech in 1889, "starts with a kind of aura, with a discomfort in the lower abdomen or epigastrium, often with a chill, followed quickly by an intense hot feeling ascending towards the head. The affected skin, mainly the face, becomes red. This is accompanied by anxiety and unease in the precordium. After a short interval, a variable amount of sweat breaks out. A feeling of exhaustion ends the attack."[3]

1. C. Wood. Menopausal myths. *Med. J. Aust.* 1:496–499, 1979.
2. Ibid.
3. Hot flushes (editorial). *Lancet* 2:965–966, 1981.

Treatment

Ever since they became available in this century, estrogen preparations have been used to relieve the symptoms of menopause, particularly hot flashes. It has been reasonably presumed that symptoms were the result of estrogen deficiency and thus could be improved by exogenous estrogens. Besides this physiologic argument, there have been emotional ones as well; as one author asserted, "Whatever a female's destiny, whether death before birth, at the time of delivery or up to age 100, it is inextricably intertwined with estrogen . . . It is the essential fuel for all stages of her life."[4] Whatever the reasons, exogenous estrogens are frequently given to women in the menopause and beyond. Depending on the region of the country and socioeconomic class, between 10 and 40 percent of women in the United States receive exogenous estrogens.

When estrogen is given, it is usually in the form of conjugated estrogens (Premarin), 0.625 or 1.25 mg/day. Some gynecologists have recommended 10 days off the pill or cyclic progestogen per month, on the theoretical grounds that continuous unopposed estrogen is less physiologic than cyclic estrogen. In general, studies of risks and benefits for patients taking estrogens have not revealed different effects at different dose levels.

When estrogens are given to women experiencing symptoms during the menopause, many respond. However, relief of symptoms may result in large measure from any well-intended medication, given with conviction—that is, there may be a placebo effect. Since taking estrogens involves some expense, inconvenience, and risk, it is important to know whether estrogens relieve symptoms over and above what might be expected from a placebo.

There have been few clinical trials of estrogens for menopausal symptoms. One was particularly well done: a randomized, double-blind, controlled trial with crossover for 30 women complaining of menopausal symptoms.[5] During three months of treatment, both estrogen-treated and placebo-treated (control) patients improved. The patients on "active" drugs experienced the greater improvement and were relieved of virtually all their symptoms. After crossover, the patients originally given a placebo improved even more, while those

---

4. R.A. Wilson, T.A. Wilson., The basic philosophy of estrogen maintenance. *J. Am. Geriatr. Soc.* 20:521–523, 1972.
5. J. Coope, J.M. Thomson, L. Poller. Effects of 'natural estrogen' replacement therapy on menopausal symptoms and blood clotting. *Br. Med. J.* 2:139–143, 1975.

changed from estrogen to placebo experienced a return of symptoms, virtually back to pretreatment levels. These differences were large and statistically significant, despite the small size of the study. From this study, supported by the conclusions of less sound trials as well, it seems clear that estrogens do relieve the symptoms of menopause, specifically hot flashes, and that this effect is over and above the response to placebos.

Besides estrogens, other drugs have been touted for treating menopausal symptoms, including antianxiety and parasympatholytic drugs. There is evidence that an anticholinergic/tranquilizer combination relieves symptoms in menopausal women, but the effect appears to be nonspecific.[6] Recently it has been supposed that if endogenous opioids are involved in hot flashes, naloxone might reduce the number of hot flashes, but the evidence is too preliminary to draw any reasonably firm conclusions.

BENEFITS OF ESTROGEN USE AFTER THE MENOPAUSE

Two chronic diseases of later life, osteoporosis and cardiovascular disease, are believed to be partly consequences of estrogen deficiency following the menopause. Because of this belief, estrogens are frequently given well beyond the time hot flashes are a problem, and also to women who do not have hot flashes at all, in the hope of preventing disease later in life.

Osteoporosis
Failure of endogenous estrogen production is believed to be a contributing cause of osteoporosis. Women are more prone to osteoporosis, and consequently to hip and spine fractures, than are men of similar age, and early (surgical) menopause is associated with more severe complications of osteoporosis later in life.

It seems clear that giving exogenous estrogens does in fact prevent both osteoporosis and fractures. It has been shown that the usual 1 to 3 percent per year decline in bone mineral content after the menopause can be reduced by daily estrogen administration, at least for several years after the menopause. However, retarding bone mineral loss is clinically important only to the extent that fractures are prevented as well. Available studies show that about one-third to two-

---

6. T.B. Lebherz, L. French. Nonhormonal treatment of the menopausal syndrome. *Obstet. Gynecol.* 33:795–799, 1969.

thirds of fractures can be prevented by regular use of exogenous estrogens. Protection increases with the duration of treatment but becomes substantial and statistically significant only after six years. One study found a greater reduction in fractures if estrogens were begun within five years of the menopause.[7] Another study found most of the protective effect among oophorectomized women; little protective effect could be demonstrated among women with natural menopause.[8] No study demonstrated differences in effect among the various forms and doses of estrogen; most women were taking conjugated estrogens in one of the common daily doses (0.625 mg or 1.25 mg).

Cardiovascular Disease

The incidence of cardiovascular disease is lower in women than in men. Before the menopause, women's rates are only about a quarter of those of men of similar age, but they triple after menopause, independent of age-related increases. Following the menopause, the difference between age-adjusted rates for men and women progressively diminishes, and the rates are roughly the same by age 65.

It is therefore reasonable to ask whether administration of exogenous estrogens would protect against cardiovascular disease in women after the menopause—or in men for that matter. Unfortunately, the answer seems to be no. In a large clinical trial of estrogens for the prevention of second myocardial infarctions in men, there was an excess of deaths in the treated group.[9] It is clear that women taking oral contraceptives, particularly older women who smoke, have an increased risk of coronary disease. As for postmenopausal women, the available data suggest that exogenous estrogens confer neither risk for nor protection against coronary disease.

Atrophic Vulvovaginitis

Since genital tissues are estrogen-dependent, all women experience some degree of vulvar atrophy after the menopause. The time of onset and severity of this effect are extremely variable. In some women atrophy results in vaginal dryness and secondary infections, and hence

7. T.A. Hutchinson, S.M. Polansky, A.R. Feinstein. Post-menopausal oestrogens protect against fractures of hip and distal radius. *Lancet* 2:705–709, 1979.
8. A. Paganini-Hill, R.K. Ross, V.R. Gerkins, et al. Menopausal estrogen therapy and hip fractures. *Ann. Intern. Med.* 95:28–31, 1981.
9. The Coronary Drug Project Research Group. The Coronary Project. Findings leading to discontinuation of the 2.5-mg/day estrogen group. *J.A.M.A.* 226:652–657, 1973.

unpleasant symptoms. It is generally believed that exogenous estrogens maintain genital tissues, and so prevent or reverse atrophic vulvovaginitis. One randomized controlled trial involving a small number of women supports this possibility.[10] Topical estrogens have been used for this purpose, but it is clear that estrogens are absorbed through the vaginal mucosa so that there is no particular advantage to topical treatment—and the disadvantage of inconvenience as well.

Genitourinary Atrophy
It has been said that the urethra and bladder, embryologically related to the genital tract and thereby estrogen-dependent, also involute when estrogen is withdrawn, resulting in symptoms such as urinary frequency, urgency, and dysuria. There is no rigorous evidence that these symptoms are in fact more frequent in postmenopausal women, are related to estrogen withdrawal, or respond to treatment with exogenous estrogens.

RISK OF ESTROGEN USE

In recent years it has become apparent that the use of estrogens involves some risks as well as benefits. In particular, three conditions have been under suspicion: cancer of the endometrium, gallstones, and cancer of the breast. The extent and strength of the evidence that associates these three conditions with exogenous estrogens are quite different.

Endometrial Cancer
More than a dozen studies have addressed the question of whether exogenous estrogens increase the risk of endometrial cancer. All have found risk; they disagree over the degree of the risk, but not its existence. Reported relative risks have ranged from 1.4 to 11.3; most studies have reported a fourfold to sevenfold increase in risk.

Although the use of exogenous estrogens seems to increase the risk of developing endometrial cancer, cancers in estrogen users are, on the average, found at earlier stages and so generally have a better prognosis and offer a better opportunity for effective treatment. However, this relationship might not be one of cause and effect, since women given estrogen are under the care of a physician and may thereby stand a better chance of early detection. Some experts have

---

10. Coope et al. Effects of 'natural estrogen' replacement therapy. *Br. Med. J.* 2:139–143, 1975.

recommended that women taking exogenous estrogens have endometrial biopsies at six-month intervals for the early detection of endometrial cancer to minimize the danger associated with the increased risk of this type of cancer. While this advice is logical enough, it lacks practicality. The inconvenience and expense of this approach, at the rate estrogens are currently prescribed, would be staggering.

Could we choose a regimen that would confer the benefits of estrogens while avoiding the risks? Relative risk does appear to increase with increasing duration of use. There is some suggestion of risk after just a few years' use, but risk is certainly present after about five years. No consistent relationship has been found between type of drug or dose and risk. Similarly, the relationships of the various schedules by which estrogens are given—intermittent, cyclic, continuous, and with intermittent progestogens—have not been studied.

Gallbladder Disease
Estrogens are suspected of causing gallbladder disease. They increase the cholesterol concentration in bile. The evidence for the increase is largely circumstantial, though, since women suffer from gallbladder disease more than men. However, oral contraceptive use in premenopausal women seems approximately to double their risk of gallbladder disease.

There is little direct evidence for or against the risk of gallbladder disease after estrogens. One study, involving surveillance of a large number of drug exposures and potential complications among hospitalized patients, found an estimated relative risk of 2.5.[11] However, this small observed risk could have been a result of chance because the data were extensively searched for associations. It is also possible that estrogen users are no more likely to *have* gallbladder disease but are simply more likely to have it *detected* because, by virtue of their taking estrogens, they are more likely to be receiving medical care in general. Therefore, we can continue to consider gallbladder disease a possible complication of estrogen use, but the evidence is by no means conclusive.

Breast Cancer
Because breast tissue is estrogen-responsive, and the growth of some breast cancers is estrogen-dependent, exogenous estrogens are

---

11. The Boston Collaborative Drug Surveillance Program. Surgically confirmed gallbladder disease, venous thromboembolism, and breast tumors in relation to postmenopausal estrogen therapy. *N. Engl. J. Med.* 290:15–19, 1974.

suspected of being a risk factor for breast cancer. So far, the evidence from clinical studies is inconsistent. Some suggest small risk, about twofold, particularly in some subgroups of women; others do not confirm these estimates of risk. For the present, we simply do not have enough information to settle the question. Presumably the relative risk must be, at most, small. However, because of the relatively high incidence and severity of breast cancer and the prevalence of estrogen taking, the question cannot be dismissed lightly.

Uterine Bleeding
Finally, use of exogenous estrogen is associated with an increased frequency of uterine bleeding, estimated to be about 0.3 per month. This condition would be a source of additional morbidity, and of cost relating to diagnostic evaluation of postmenopausal bleeding, and could even result in the rare major complication or death from dilatation and curettage.

BENEFIT VERSUS RISK

It is apparent that estrogens can alleviate some of the annoying symptoms of menopause (hot flashes, atrophic vulvovaginitis) and prevent important sequelae of the menopause (osteoporosis and consequent fractures). It is also apparent that the use of estrogens involves some risk as well. Where does the proper trade-off between risk and benefit lie?

From the point of view of individual women no general recommendation can be made—the decision depends on how each woman wishes to weigh the particular set of risks and benefits associated with estrogen use (summarized in Table 1). That risk is best conceptualized as the incidence of events (good and bad) among those taking estrogens, taking into account the incidence in those not exposed (attributable risk). The attributable risks for endometrial cancer and fractures are of roughly similar magnitude—about 0.3 to 3.0 per thousand per year for hip fracture, depending on age, and 5 to 25 per thousand per year for endometrial carcinoma in women with an intact uterus. The decision for or against estrogens would then be heavily influenced by the respective importance an individual attaches to fractures and endometrial cancer.

Two commonly occurring situations should strongly influence the decision to give estrogens. First, when estrogens are given only for the relief of hot flashes, the duration of their use can be limited. Hot

TABLE 1

The Benefits and Risk of Estrogens

Benefits	Risks	Insufficient Evidence

Prevention of:
  Hot flashes
  Osteoporosis/fractures
  Atrophic vulvovaginitis
	Endometrial cancer
	Uterine bleeding
		Cardiovascular disease
		Urinary atrophy
		Cholelithiasis
		Breast cancer

flashes rarely last more than five years, and the increased risk of endometrial cancer is relatively minor up to about five years. In this situation, benefit can be had with little risk. Second, many women have had a hysterectomy by the time of the menopause, so for them there is no risk of endometrial carcinoma. They are in a position to experience the major benefits of estrogen use and only the small and poorly substantiated risks.

Thus, individual circumstances strongly affect risks and benefits. For this reason several authoritative bodies, reviewing the data on estrogen use during the menopause and beyond, have chosen not to issue a recommendation that would apply to all women, or a policy that might be followed by the nation as a whole. The decision rests, as perhaps it should, with patients and their physicians making value judgments, informed by existing estimates of the probabilities involved.

SUGGESTED READING

1. Coope, J., Thomson, J.M., Poller, L. Effects of natural estrogen replacement therapy on menopausal symptoms and blood clotting. *Br. Med. J.* 2:139–142, 1975.
2. Hulka, B.S. Effect of exogenous estrogen on postmenopausal women: The epidemiologic evidence. *Obstet. Gynecol. Survey* 35(Suppl.):389–399, 1980.
3. Hulka, B.S., Grimson, R.C., Greenberg, B.G. et al. Alternative controls in a case-control study of endometrial cancer and exogenous estrogen. *Am. J. Epidemiol.* 112:376–387, 1980.
4. Weinstein, M.C. Estrogen use in post-menopausal women—costs, risks and benefits. *N. Engl. J. Med.* 303:308–326, 1980.
5. Weiss, N.S., Ure, C.L., Ballard, J.H., et al. Decreased risk of fractures of the hip and lower forearm with post-menopausal use of estrogen. *N. Engl. J. Med.* 303:1195–1198, 1980.

7

INFECTIONS

Urinary Tract Infections in the Elderly

TIMOTHY W. LANE, M.D.

Editor's note: Urinary tract infection is one of the most common bacterial infections of the elderly. The majority of such infections are asymptomatic and relatively benign. There is no evidence that antibiotic therapy is of any lasting benefit in asymptomatic bacteriuria, and antibiotics, which are more toxic in the elderly, must be used judiciously. Anatomic abnormalities and chronic bacterial prostatitis are common in elderly men with relapsing and recurrent urinary infections. Chronic catheterization is invariably accompanied by infection; preventive measures are inefficacious.

In the past two decades, urinary tract infections have been recognized as one of the most common bacterial infections in the geriatric population. Research in this area has been limited, and controversy exists in both diagnosis and therapy. Understanding the epidemiology and examining the current problems in diagnosis and management of this frequent problem should be important to anyone who cares for the elderly.

EPIDEMIOLOGY

Bacteriuria is remarkably common in the elderly. Its prevalence in those over age 65 is dependent on age, gender, and living environment (i.e., ambulatory outpatient versus an institutional setting). For the elderly living at home, prevalence rates of bacteriuria range from 5 to 15 percent for men, compared to 0.1% for younger men. The range for women is 15 to 30 percent compared to 3 to 5 percent for younger women. The percentage with bacteriuria rises sequentially as debility progresses and placement in a chronic care facility occurs, with the highest prevalence occurring in hospitals (Table 1). Increas-

287

TABLE 1

Prevalence of Bacteriuria ($\geq 10^5$ bacteria/ml) in Elderly Populations

	Percentage of Bacteriuric Individuals	
Setting	Men	Women
Home	5–15	15–30
Nursing Home	15–25	20–35
Hospital	30–35	30–50

TABLE 2

Age as a Determinant of Bacteriuria

	Percentage of Bacteriuric Individuals	
Age	Men	Women
65–70	5	15–20
70–80	10–15	20–30
>80	20–25	25–40

ing age exerts an independent effect on the prevalence of bacteriuria, with rates rising markedly in each decade beyond 60 years of age and particularly in the eighth decade of life (Table 2).

While the prevalence rates of bacteriuria remain fairly constant, many urinary infections spontaneously resolve and other persons become newly infected. For example, in Sourander's large-scale study of bacteriuria in an elderly (> 65 years of age), ambulatory Finnish population, the same prevalence of bacteriuria was observed over a five-year follow-up period, but 85 percent of men and over 50 percent of women initially bacteriuric no longer were five years later.[1] Thus the majority of infected patients at the conclusion of the study were initially uninfected. There is no substantial evidence to indicate that antimicrobial therapy accounted for the resolution of bacteriuria in those patients who became uninfected.

DIAGNOSIS

In all age groups, the diagnosis of urinary tract infections, whether symptomatic or not, has traditionally relied on the finding of 10^5 or

---

1. L.B. Sourander, A. Kasanen. A 5 year follow-up of bacteriuria in the aged. *Gerontol. Clin.* 14:274–281, 1972.

more bacteria per milliliter of urine in quantitative cultures of mid-stream voided urine specimens. The accuracy of this method was established initially in young women with pyelonephritis by comparing voided specimens with quantitative cultures of suprapubic urine aspirates. A single-voided urine with 10^5 or more bacteria per milliliter in young women has an 80 percent probability of predicting infection as compared to bladder aspirates. Two consecutively voided urines with 10^5 or more bacteria of the same species per milliliter have a 95 percent probability of indicating true infection.

Problems in using this criterion for the diagnosis of urinary infection in the elderly, however, were pointed out in a systematic study of 100 noncatheterized and asymptomatic elderly women on admission to a geriatric hospital.[2] Contamination with periurethral bacteria can be a particular problem: 30 percent of the voided "clean-catch" specimens were found to have 10^5 or more bacteria per milliliter, but only 13 percent of the suprapubic cultures had 10^5 or more bacteria per milliliter. In addition, 3 percent of suprapubic specimens were infected with fewer than 10^5 bacteria per milliliter, supporting the common clinical observation that urinary tract infection can occur when fewer than 100,000 organisms per milliliter are present. Over-all, the false-positive rate of a single-voided urine culture in this elderly population was 57 percent (17/30) and the positive predictive value only 43 percent; a lower false-positive rate of 15 to 20 percent for a single-voided urine culture can probably be achieved by careful supervision of the patient when the specimen is obtained.

Water loading to provoke diuresis has been studied in asymptomatic elderly patients whose initial voided cultures are sterile or contain fewer than 10^4 bacteria per milliliter. Diuresis has been shown to induce significant ($>10^5$ bacteria/ml) bacteriuria in approximately 20 percent of these subjects. By inference, it is concluded that an upper tract or renal focus of infection exists whose recognition depends on a "washing out" of the bacteria into the bladder. This phenomenon has not been studied extensively, and its clinical importance is unclear. Nevertheless, it compounds the difficulties in determining the true prevalence of urinary tract infection by usual bacteriologic methods.

The first approach to diagnosis should be careful instruction and

2. B. Moore-Smith. Suprapubic aspiration in the diagnosis of urinary infection in the elderly. *Mod. Geriatr.* 1:124–127, 1971.

assistance in the collecting of a midstream-voided urine specimen. Only if the results of the culture are confusing should suprapubic aspiration be considered. Aseptic in-and-out bladder catheterization for urine culture is a less invasive alternative that appears to be as sensitive and specific as a suprapubic aspiration.

The urinalysis is less helpful than a urine culture. Pyuria (>5 white blood cells per high-power field) is a relatively insensitive indicator of asymptomatic infection, or so-called bacteriuria, in the elderly, being present only 50 to 70 percent of the time.

Urinary frequency and dysuria are common complaints in non-infected elderly women and are not reliably predictive of infection; these symptoms may be caused by neurogenic changes in bladder function or atrophic urethritis from declining estrogen synthesis. In fact, the majority of urinary tract infections are asymptomatic.

BACTERIAL ETIOLOGY

The aerobic gram-negative bacilli that are part of the normal gastrointestinal flora are the most common bacteria causing urinary infections in all age groups. *Escherichia coli* accounts for 75 to 85 percent of infections in the elderly. The remainder are caused by *Klebsiella-Enterobacter*, *Proteus*, enterococcus, and *Pseudomonas* species. Non–*E. coli* bacteria are more likely to be responsible for infections following hospitalization or urologic manipulation. Chronic bladder catheterization almost invariably is accompanied by bacteriuria, and multi-antibiotic-resistant strains of *Pseudomonas*, *Serratia*, and indole-positive *Proteus* are frequently the infectious organisms, especially if the patient has been institutionalized. *Proteus* species are often associated with renal calculi because of the organism's ability to split urea and enhance deposition of struvite stones with an alkaline urine pH.

PATHOGENESIS

The striking increased prevalence of urinary tract infection in the elderly appears to be multifactorial and related in part to several degenerative changes of aging. Progressive prostatic hypertrophy and subsequent urologic procedures in elderly men account in part for the increase, but possibly just as important is the diminution in the natural bactericidal activity of prostatic secretions found in patients who have chronic infection. The role of periurethral colonization with enteric bacteria and adherence of urinary pathogens to uroepithelial cells, etiologically related to chronic recurrent bladder infections in young women, has not been studied in the geriatric population but may well be important. Some investigators have found an increased risk of infection when there is greater than 50 ml of residual urine, and since the aging bladder is less efficient in emptying completely, the risk of a significant residual is greater. The association of dementia with an even greater prevalence of bacteriuria supports the notion that perineal fecal contamination and poor hygiene are involved in pathogenesis.

LONG-TERM EFFECTS OF BACTERIURIA

The long-term consequences of asymptomatic urinary infection in the elderly are believed to be generally benign. Some investigators have found an association between bacteriuria and decreased glomerular filtration rate, but many others have been unable to corroborate this finding. A more consistent abnormality is the loss of maximal tubular concentrating ability with renal infection. Progressive renal damage does not appear to result unless obstructive lesions are present.

Recent epidemiologic surveys in populations of women and elderly subjects have demonstrated an increased mortality rate in those with bacteriuria compared to the rate in noninfected individuals. Since the most prevalent causes of death in elderly bacteriuric groups are related to dementia and other degenerative disorders of the central nervous system, bacteriuria may merely be a marker for these neurologic diseases that are accompanied by fecal incontinence and poor periurethral hygiene. Further research is required before bacteriuria can be directly incriminated as a significant cause of mortality.

ANTIMICROBIAL THERAPY AND MANAGEMENT OF SYMPTOMATIC URINARY INFECTION

The choice of appropriate therapy depends on the severity of infection and the environment in which infection occurs; achieving adequate urine levels of antibiotics is essential for successful treatment of infection. Minor symptomatic infections related to cystitis can be treated with oral agents. Ampicillin and sulfisoxazole are reasonably safe and inexpensive choices. Trimethoprim-sulfamethoxazole, nitrofurantoin, nalidixic acid, and oral cephalosporins are more expensive alternatives. Forced oral fluids have traditionally been advised, but their true value has never been tested. Therapy is usually prescribed for 7 to 10 days. Shorter treatment periods, including single-dose regimens, have recently been shown to be equally effective in younger women with cystitis localized to the lower urinary tract by the absence of antibody coating of the bacteria. Single-dose therapy and anatomic localization of infection have not been adequately examined in elderly populations, but there is no reason to assume that single-dose therapy would not be effective.

Recurrence of bacteriuria, defined as infection with a different bacterial strain or species, occurs in as many as 40 to 50 percent of women within a year of a conventional 7- to 10-day treatment course. Most often recurrences are asymptomatic, but some women will have frequent symptomatic recurrences. If three or more symptomatic episodes occur within a year, then long-term prophylactic antibiotic therapy (usually several months to a year) can be justified on a cost-benefit basis. Trimethoprim-sulfamethoxazole, one regular-strength tablet (80 mg/400 mg) daily, and nitrofurantoin, 100 mg daily, are two effective prophylactic agents.

Relapse of bacteriuria, defined as infection with the identical bacterial strain, ordinarily occurs within a few days to weeks after a conventional period of treatment. This usually indicates a persisting upper tract or renal focus of infection, chronic prostatitis, structural abnormalities, or infected renal calculi. If relapse occurs, and especially if it is symptomatic, intravenous pyelography may be indicated to look for correctable obstructive lesions. Longer courses of full-dose therapy of six weeks or more should be considered if a symptomatic relapse is caused by an upper tract focus of infection.

Acute pyelonephritis is one of the few serious consequences of urinary infection. Although the incidence of pyelonephritis in the elderly is not exactly known, it is common enough to account for the majority of episodes of gram-negative-rod bacteremia in hospitalized patients. The usual symptoms of high fever, flank pain, and dysuria seen in younger adults are not as uniformly present in the elderly. Constitutional symptoms, obtundation, and gastrointestinal symptoms may be diagnostically misleading to the unaware. Bacteremia is present in more than 50 percent of the elderly with pyelonephritis and necessitates prompt and vigorous parenteral antibiotic therapy. Until culture and antibiotic susceptibility results are available, a combination of ampicillin or a cephalosporin and an aminoglycoside is a reasonable empirical regimen. An aminoglycoside is especially indicated if the patient has chronic bladder catheterization or has been cared for in a nursing home. These situations indicate the increased likelihood of resistant organisms like *Pseudomonas* or *Serratia*.

Toxic effects of antibiotics are more common in the elderly, in particular aminoglycoside nephrotoxicity. Aminoglycosides must be judiciously dosed in the elderly because they are eliminated by glomerular filtration, which progressively declines with age, and serum creatinine measurements often are within the range of normal and do not reflect the decline in glomerular function. Dosing aminoglycosides and other toxic antibiotics cleared by renal routes requires careful estimates of glomerular filtration rate.[3] Because aminoglycosides and many of the other antibiotics used for treating urinary tract infection are concentrated in the urine, maximal doses with increased toxicity are not necessary; a 1 mg/kg dose of either tobramycin or gentamicin every 8 hours when creatinine clearance is 50 cc/min of urine or greater is usually adequate aminoglycoside therapy.

BLADDER CATHETERS AND INFECTION

The incidence of catheter-associated urinary tract infections exceeds 500,000 per year in the United States, accounting for nearly half of all nosocomial or hospital-acquired infections. Incontinent nursing home patients with dementia who are relegated to chronic catheterization inevitably develop infection.

Frequent diapering, bladder training, and intermittent, supervised catheterization are safer alternatives to chronic catheterization. Economic considerations and the labor-intensive nature of these techniques may explain why they have not been widely adopted. Catheter-related infections are difficult to prevent, and they are impossible to avoid if catheterization exceeds two weeks. A sterile closed drainage system will delay acquisition of infection over several days but not over longer periods. Many measures have been advocated and practiced for prevention of such infections, including oral "prophylactic" antibiotics, daily application of antiseptic ointments to the catheter-meatal junction, bladder irrigation with antibiotics, and, more recently, addition of hydrogen peroxide to the catheter collection bag. None of these methods has been found to be of benefit when submitted to carefully designed studies.

---

3. $CrCl = \dfrac{(140 - age) \times kg \, (\times \, 0.85 \text{ for women})}{S_{Cr} \times 72}$

BACTERIAL PROSTATITIS

Relapses of infection may occur in elderly men as a result of anatomic abnormalities, renal calculi, and chronic bacterial infection of the prostate. Chronic prostatic infection is usually silent; the major recognized manifestations are recurrent symptomatic urinary tract infections or prompt relapse of bacteriuria after a conventional course of antibiotics. The aerobic gram-negative rods, *E. coli, Proteus,* and *Klebsiella,* are the usual infecting organisms.

Bacterial prostatitis has been an elusive entity because of the difficulty in establishing the diagnosis; several years may elapse between clinically recognized infections. Digital examination of the prostate is of little diagnostic aid because the "boggy" prostate is a normal finding in elderly men. If chronic prostatic infection is suspected from a pattern of frequent relapse, a complicated method of culturing prostatic secretions called the four-glass test is required. This method requires the comparison of quantitative cultures of (1) a first-voided urine specimen, (2) a midstream-voided urine, (3) postmassage prostatic secretions, and (4) first-voided urine postmassage. Generally a tenfold increase in bacterial counts should be present in prostatic fluid to confirm the diagnosis. A quantitative culture of ejaculated semen that yields a tenfold increase in bacteria over first-voided and midstream-voided urine cultures may be less cumbersome and as sensitive as the four-glass technique. Sterile bladder urine is a prerequisite for either method, and a three- to five-day course of oral antibiotic therapy is necessary if bacteriuria is present. Such short-term treatment will not eradicate prostatic bacteria.

Therapy of chronic bacterial prostatitis is frustrating because of high failure rates, and treatment should be attempted only for frequent symptomatic relapses of urinary tract infection. Poor prostatic penetration of most antibiotics, including the tetracyclines, and prostatic calculi that serve as a protected nidus for bacteria explain the high failure rate of therapy. Therapeutic regimens that have cured about a third of these infections include a double-strength tablet of trimethoprim-sulfamethoxazole twice daily, or oral carbenicillin, one tablet four times daily; either agent should be administered for twelve weeks. The two-thirds of patients who fail to benefit from long-term therapy and still have symptomatic relapses are candidates for chronic suppressive antibiotics. The same regimens that are recommended for prophylaxis in women with recurrent cystitis are also effective in chronic prostatitis. Transurethral prostatectomy is of limited benefit since complete removal of infected tissue is difficult. Total prostatectomy is usually unacceptable to both patient and physician because of subsequent incontinence and impotence.

EPIDIDYMITIS

Chronic tuberculous and acute gonococcal epididymitis are less common since the introduction of effective antimicrobials. Acute infectious epididymitis still occurs but is more common in young than elderly men. The bacterial etiology is distinctly different in these two age groups and carries important implications for appropriate therapy. *Chlamydia trachomatis* and occasionally gonorrhea are the most likely causes in those 35 years of age and younger. In contrast, acute epididymitis in older men is caused by *E. coli, Klebsiella,* and occasionally *Pseudomonas.* While tetracycline would be the antibiotic of choice in younger men, gentamicin or tobramycin is the most rational empirical choice for elderly men. Cultures of midstream-voided urine are useful in determining the responsible bacteria in the older age group.

SUGGESTED READING

1. Dontas, A.S., Kasviki-Charvati, P., Papanayiotou, P.C., et al. Bacteriuria and survival in old age. *N. Engl. J. Med.* 304:939–943, 1981.
2. Garibaldi, R.A., Brodine, S., Matsumiya, S. Infections among patients in nursing homes: Policies, prevalence, and problems. *N. Engl. J. Med.* 305:731–735, 1981.
3. Gleckman, R., Blagg, N., Hibert, D., et al. Acute pyelonephritis in the elderly. *South. J. Med.* 75:551–554, 1982.
4. Kaye, D. Urinary tract infections in the elderly. *Bull. N.Y. Acad. Med.* 56:209–220, 1980.
5. Meares, E.M., Jr. Prostatitis. *Ann. Rev. Med.* 30:279–288, 1979.
6. Papanayiotou, P., Dontas, A.S. Water-loading test in bacteriuria. *N. Engl. J. Med.* 287:531–548, 1972.
7. Sourander, L.B., Kasanen, A. A 5 year follow-up of bacteriuria in the aged. *Gerontol. Clin..* 14:274–281, 1972.

Pneumonia and Influenza in the Elderly

TIMOTHY W. LANE, M.D.

Editor's note: The variety of bacterial pathogens that commonly cause pneumonia increase with aging, as do the morbidity and mortality of respiratory infections in general. Judicious initial choice of antibiotics depends on some easily obtained clinical information described in this chapter. Vaccination against influenza and pneumococci is routinely recommended for elderly patients, but unfortunately the supporting data are far from definitive, leaving ample opportunity for clinical judgment.

PNEUMONIA

Osler's designation of pneumonia as "the Captain of the men of death" still applies to the elderly. Pneumonia and influenza are the leading infectious cause and overall the fourth most common cause of death in the geriatric population of the United States. Of the estimated three million cases of pneumonia and 60,000 to 70,000 deaths that occur annually, approximately two-thirds are found in the elderly. Pneumococcal pneumonia remains the predominant type, although it is no longer the cause of the vast majority of community-acquired pneumonias it once was. Improved microbiologic diagnosis, the recognition of "new" organisms, and the emergence of micro-organisms that were previously considered nonpathogens in the debilitated and immunocompromised patient have increased the variety of organisms commonly encountered, making the diagnosis and management of pneumonia in the elderly an even greater challenge.

Pathogenesis of Pneumonia in the Elderly
The age-specific attack rates of pneumonia are highest for those over 60 years of age. The precise reasons for this heightened risk of pneu-

monia are conjectural, but several phenomena appear to be important.

First, tracheal aspiration of pharyngeal secretions is the likely route of infection for the majority of pneumonias. The common bacterial etiologies of community-acquired pneumonia, *Streptococcus pneumoniae, Hemophilus influenzae,* and *Staphylococcus aureus,* are present in the oral flora of 2–10 percent of the elderly population and when aspirated may initiate lower respiratory infection. Aspiration of potential pathogens occurs during sleep, and to a greater degree when patients have altered levels of consciousness and swallowing abnormalities secondary to stroke or dementia, or when they are using psychotropic and sedating drugs.

Once aspiration occurs, local host defenses (i.e., the ciliated epithelial cells that line the bronchial airways) must clear the aspirated secretions. Aging, chronic pulmonary diseases, and cigarette smoking impair the function of this usually efficient defense. In addition, pulmonary mechanics decline in the elderly and in those with underlying respiratory disorders and thus may contribute to the development of pneumonia.

The phagocytic and bactericidal properties of pulmonary alveolar macrophages are important defenses. Their function is known to be compromised by steroids and other immunosuppressive drugs; the effect of aging on their function in nonimmunosuppressed patients has not been examined. Cell-mediated immunity of the T-lymphocytes is known to wane with age, but its role in the pathogenesis of usual bacterial pneumonia is not thought to be of primary importance.

The greater risk of gram-negative bacillary pneumonias in the elderly may be related to pharyngeal colonization with these organisms. About 5 to 8 percent of healthy young adults are colonized by gram-negative rods, but organisms like *Klebsiella, Enterobacter, Escherichia coli, Proteus,* and *Pseudomonas* are more commonly isolated from the pharynx of those over 65 years old. The prevalence of gram-negative colonization increases from 10 to 20 percent of the elderly living independently, to 40 percent of debilitated nursing home residents, and to 60 percent of those in acute care hospitals.

Clinical Features and Etiology of Pneumonias in the Elderly
The etiology of pneumonia in the elderly differs from that in younger patients. An important characteristic that helps the clinician predict the likely etiologies is the location of acquisition: whether the disease

was community-acquired, or nursing-home-acquired or nosocomial in origin.

Community-Acquired Pneumonia   Bacterial pneumonias that are community-acquired typically occur in the winter months and are characterized by the abrupt onset of fever, cough productive of purulent sputum, dyspnea, and frequently pleuritic pain. Prospective studies of elderly patients presenting with these symptoms have demonstrated that *S. pneumoniae* (the pneumococcus) is still the most commonly recognized single pathogen, although its estimated prevalence has declined from 80 to 90 percent to 50 to 60 percent in more recent surveys. The annual incidence of pneumococcal pneumonia is estimated to be three to four times higher for the elderly. The fatality rate is also higher in the elderly: 20 percent versus 5 percent for all cases. Pneumococcal bacteremia occurs in approximately one-fifth of patients, and when it does the case fatality rate doubles.

The role of *H. influenzae* in adult pneumonia has been recognized only in the past decade; it now appears to account for about 10 percent of community-acquired pneumonias. It is clinically and radiographically indistinguishable from the other common bacterial causes, but the patient is more likely to be a smoker, an alcoholic, or to have chronic lung disease. Because *H. influenzae* has unique antimicrobial susceptibilities (notably resistance to penicillin and some cephalosporin antibiotics), its early recognition is important.

Staphylococcal pneumonia causes up to 5 percent of pneumonias in the elderly and is a particularly feared complication of influenza infection, with case fatality rates as high as 75 percent. It is often more fulminant in onset and may result in cavity formation.

The term *aspiration pneumonia* connotes a mixed bacterial process that is caused by aerobic and anaerobic oral flora. Lung abscess and empyema are occasional sequelae. Transtracheal and percutaneous lung puncture aspirates have identified *Fusobacterium, Bacteroides,* and anaerobic streptococcal species as the usual anaerobic pathogens. Aspiration pneumonia and lung abscess are not particularly common in the elderly but should be suspected in patients with swallowing dysfunction, or when pneumonia is accompanied by fetid breath, poor dentition, or alcoholism.

Nosocomial Pneumonia   Two-thirds of nosocomial (hospital-acquired) pneumonias are caused by gram-negative bacilli and have extraordinary fatality rates of 40 to 60 percent. In prospective surveys, gram-negative bacilli have been implicated as the cause of 5 to 10 percent of community-acquired and 20 to 30 percent of nursing-home-acquired pneumonias. Accuracy of diagnosis by sputum culture can be problematic because of the frequent pharyngeal colonization with enteric gram-negative rods that can cause "false-positive" sputum cultures.

Atypical Pneumonias About a quarter of community-acquired pneumonias in the elderly have eluded etiologic classification. Most of the unclassified pneumonias have been called "atypical" because of marked systemic symptoms in the absence of purulent sputum production and positive cultures. *Mycoplasma pneumoniae* and viruses, frequent causes of atypical pneumonia in adolescents and young adults, are uncommon in the elderly. Since the Legionnaires' disease outbreak in Philadelphia in 1976, there is mounting evidence that *Legionella* species may be responsible for many of these previously undiagnosed atypical pneumonias. Recent studies in this country and England have demonstrated that up to 15 percent of community-acquired pneumonias are caused by *Legionella*. Clues to the diagnosis are an unusual summertime peak incidence and the extrapulmonary complications of toxic encephalopathy and severe diarrhea, but absence of these findings does not exclude the diagnosis of *Legionella*.

Diagnosis

The etiologic diagnosis of pneumonia initially relies on an examination of a Gram's stain and culture of expectorated sputum. These methods of diagnosis are not without controversy because of the subjectivity of Gram-stain interpretation and contamination and overgrowth of cultures by oral flora. For example, sputum cultures yield pneumococci only about 50 percent of the time in cases documented by bacteremia. Despite these difficulties, a carefully supervised collection of expectorated sputum for Gram's staining and culture is often helpful in arriving at a putative diagnosis. An adequate sputum specimen usually has 25 or more polymorphonuclear leukocytes and fewer than 10 squamous epithelial cells per $10 \times$ field. Transtracheal aspiration (TTA) of sputum, introduced to avoid the contamination of sputum with oral flora, is said to be a somewhat more sensitive and specific method, but the occasional life-threatening complications of bleeding and cardiac arrest in the presence of hypoxia have rightfully tempered enthusiasm for its routine use, especially in uncooperative or uremic patients. Selective application in the obtunded or severely debilitated patient who has ineffective cough, however, is appropriate.

Since 15 to 25 percent of patients with pneumococcal pneumonia are bacteremic, blood cultures should routinely be obtained before instituting therapy in all pneumonias. The prior "empirical" use of oral antibiotics (relatively common in nursing home patients) reduces the yield of sputum and blood cultures.

Improved diagnostic methods are clearly needed. Several experimental methods of detecting bacterial antigens in sputum and urine, such as counterimmunoelectrophoresis (CIE) and enzyme-linked immunosorbent assay (ELISA), hold promise for the future. Detection of *Legionella* antigen in the urine by ELISA has preliminarily been shown to be a sensitive method for diagnosing Legionnaires' disease; currently the diagnosis of Legionnaires' disease usually depends on a fourfold rise in antibodies over a four- to six-week period. Cultures and smears of sputum for *Legionella* are relatively insensitive, and immunofluorescent staining and cultures of lung tissue are sensitive but obviously require biopsy. Therapy must often be initiated and continued on an empirical basis.

Therapy and Management
Cephalosporin antibiotics are one of the most commonly prescribed classes of antimicrobials for therapy of community-acquired pneumonia. Although they are not recommended as presumptive therapy by most infectious disease experts or in authoritative reviews of pneumonia, their use persists because of their extensive commercial promotion and clinicians' uncertainty of initial etiologic diagnosis. They are, however, rarely the most rational or cost-effective choices.

When sputum smears reveal numerous granulocytes and predominant gram-positive diplococci in a patient with an acute, typical pneumonia, pneumococcal pneumonia is likely, and penicillin is the antibiotic of choice. Higher-dose penicillin, 8 million to 12 million units daily, is also an effective regimen for community-acquired aspiration pneumonia caused by mixed oropharyngeal flora.

Hemophilus influenzae pneumonia presents unique problems for the selection of appropriate therapy. Until recently ampicillin was the preferred drug, but the emergence of beta-lactamase production in 15 to 30 percent of strains necessitates selection of agents that resist this enzyme's action. Antibiotic choices for serious hemophilus infections now include chloramphenicol, the second-generation cephalosporin cefamandole, or trimethoprim-sulfamethoxazole. The newer third-generation cephalosporins moxalactam, cefotaxime, and cephoperazone are active against *Hemophilus*, including beta-lactamase-producing strains, but initial diagnosis must be secure since moxalactam does not have reliable antipneumococcal activity. A beta-lactamase-resistant antibiotic, such as nafcillin or oxacillin, is essential therapy for staphylococcal pneumonia, whether nosocomial or community-acquired.

There is general agreement, although no rigorous proof, that combinations of antimicrobials are the most efficacious regimen for gram-negative bacillary pneumonia, the goal of combination therapy being to achieve synergistic activity against these virulent organisms. A cephalosporin and an aminoglycoside are recommended for treatment of *Klebsiella* pneumonia; the newer "anti-*Pseudomonas*" penicillins (e.g., mezlocillin and piperacillin) have activity against most *Klebsiella* strains and are reasonable substitutes for cephalosporins. *Pseudomonas* and other gram-negative bacillary pneumonias that occur in nursing-home or hospitalized patients are most effectively treated initially with an anti-*Pseudomonas* penicillin and an aminoglycoside. Local susceptibility patterns may require alteration of the foregoing recommendations and should be used to ultimately guide antibiotic selection.

Erythromycin has emerged as the antibiotic of choice for Legionnaires' disease because of its excellent in vitro activity against *Legionella* and an observed decrease in case fatality rates with its clinical use. Parenteral erythromycin followed by an oral preparation is usually given for three weeks; shorter courses of therapy have been followed by relapses in 10 to 15 percent of patients. In severe or rapidly progressive cases, rifampin, 600 mg daily, is empirically added to erythromycin therapy because of its potent in vitro anti-*Legionella* activity.

Prevention: The Pneumococcal Vaccine
The long history of the development of a pneumococcal vaccine began in 1945 when a trivalent vaccine that was shown to be effective in military recruits was licensed in this country. The nearly simultaneous introduction of penicillin limited its use, however, and eventually led to its withdrawal. In 1977 a new pneumococcal vaccine was introduced; it contains capsular polysaccharide antigens of 14 serotypes that are responsible for 80 percent of bacteremic pneumococcal infections and about 60 percent of the pneumococcal serotypes causing pneumonia in the elderly.

The efficacy of this pneumococcal vaccine was widely anticipated in the elderly and in those with underlying cardiopulmonary disorders, but two studies conducted among older adults in a prepaid health plan[1] and a chronic care facility[2] showed no reduction in pneumococcal pneumonias in the vaccinated groups. The reasons for failure in these trials are not clear, but relatively low attack rates of pneumococcal pneumonia in both vaccinated persons and controls could have obscured a protective effect. It is estimated, in fact, that as many as 100,000 subjects would have to be enrolled to demonstrate efficacy.

The protective effect of vaccine in randomized controlled studies in younger subjects has been correlated with good antibody response, and similar antibody responses have been documented in the elderly. By inference, therefore, vaccination may well be worthwhile in the elderly. Because pneumococcal vaccine is relatively safe and inexpensive (the cost is about $5.00), it is reasonable to vaccinate certain elderly patients, especially those with high-risk underlying conditions such as asplenia, cardiopulmonary diseases, cirrhosis, and chronic renal failure. Those with multiple myeloma and other dysgamma-globulinemias are also at risk for pneumococcal infections, but immunologic responsiveness to vaccination is so impaired in these patients that protection cannot be expected.

Pneumococcal and influenza vaccines can be conveniently administered simultaneously at different sites without an appreciable increase in adverse effects or loss of immunogenicity. About 30–40 percent of pneumococcal vaccine recipients experience transient local erythema and edema at the inoculation site, and 1–2 percent have a 24-hour low-grade fever. The optimal interval between vaccinations is unknown, but because of an increase in adverse reactions with repeated vaccination, currently pneumococcal vaccine should not be administered more frequently than every five years.

INFLUENZA

The three influenza viruses that infect man are designated A, B, and C. Influenza A and B are responsible for outbreaks, and influenza C causes minor childhood infections. Influenza viruses are specifically designated by the following shorthand nomenclature: type/location of first isolation/year isolated/ and, for influenza A, surface protein

1. D.W. Bentley. Pneumococcal vaccine in the institutionalized elderly: Review of past and recent studies. *Rev. Infect. Dis.* 3(Suppl.):561–570, 1981.
2. Ibid.

hemagglutinin and neuraminidase type. Two recent strains, for example, are A/Bangkok/1979(H_3N_2) and B/Singapore/1979.

Epidemiology and Transmission

Influenza is transmitted by large and small particles aerosolized by sneezing and coughing. Although attack rates for influenza are greatest for the young, the elderly suffer disproportionate morbidity and mortality. Virtually all cases of influenza occur in the wintertime, and outbreaks persist over six to eight weeks. Influenza activity cannot be predicted, so its activity must be monitored by the observation of deaths attributed to pneumonia and influenza and by sentinel viral isolation laboratories in major metropolitan areas in the United States. Local and state health departments and the Centers for Disease Control publish very current periodic epidemiologic reports on influenza activity that should be consulted by clinicians during the winter months for the likelihood of influenza virus as the cause of "flu-like" upper respiratory infections.

Clinical Presentation

Classic clinical influenza infections are characterized by the abrupt onset of fever of 102–104°F, chills, myalgia, malaise, nonproductive cough, sore throat, headache, and nasal congestion. Nausea and vomiting occur in about a quarter of cases. Patients complain mostly, however, of systemic symptoms. Clinical findings besides fever include nonexudative pharyngitis, occasional cervical adenopathy, and muscle tenderness. Influenza B is considered to be less virulent but may be indistinguishable clinically from influenza A infection. Subclinical cases are as common as symptomatic clinical cases during an outbreak.

In young and healthy hosts, influenza is usually a three- to five-day self-limited illness; about a third of patients will experience malaise, fatigue, and a persistent cough for an additional two to three weeks, probably related to necrosis and inflammation of virally infected nasal and bronchial epithelial cells.

Because viral shedding begins during the incubation period and continues for four to five days, nursing home residents and the hospitalized elderly with influenza should be isolated during this period to prevent nosocomial spread.

Diagnosis

During an epidemic of influenza, a clinical diagnosis of a typical case is usually sufficiently sensitive. In a nonepidemic situation, most cases of respiratory illness that are called "flu" are more likely to be caused by other viruses such as parainfluenza and respiratory syncytial virus. Because in most situations specific therapy is not indicated, the current laborious methods of definitive diagnosis are unnecessary. When exact diagnosis is required for management or epidemiologic surveillance, the only accurate methods of diagnostic confirmation are viral isolation from nasal and throat swabs or conversion of antibody titers. Tissue cultures for influenza become positive within two to five days of incubation; serologic confirmation depends on a fourfold rise in specific antibodies and requires three to four weeks, thereby diminishing its clinical utility.

In the future, experimental methods of rapid direct viral detection in respiratory secretions offer the possibility of definitive diagnosis within hours. Rapid and accurate diagnosis is desirable because the prognosis of influenza in the elderly, especially in the presence of underlying disease, is worse than with other viral respiratory infections, and specific treatment with amantadine may avert complications.

Treatment

Supportive management of uncomplicated influenza has become medical folklore: adequate fluids, bed rest, and minor analgesics like aspirin or acetaminophen. Judicious use of phenylephrine drops or spray for nasal congestion and codeine for persistent cough can ameliorate symptoms. "Prophylactic" antibiotics have no role.

Amantadine has antiviral activity against influenza A and has been shown to shorten the febrile period and occasionally to reduce other symptoms. It is effective only for influenza A and must be administered within 48 hours of the onset of symptoms to have therapeutic efficacy. Usual oral dosages have been 200 mg/day for four to seven days, but dosage should be reduced by half in patients with creatinine clearances of 30–50 cc/min, often a "normal" level of renal function for those 70 years of age or older. Amantadine has been recommended for those at risk of complications, particularly the elderly, and those with chronic illnesses. Prospective clinical trials, however, have been limited to young healthy subjects with influenza, so the usefulness of amantadine in the elderly needs confirmation. In the interim, its careful use is justified, particularly if chronic cardiopulmonary disorders are present.

Five to fifteen percent of elderly patients given amantadine develop nausea, dizziness, and difficulty with mental concentration. These adverse effects are reversible upon discontinuing the drug and possibly by dosage reduction. Because of the difficulties in early diagnosis, fear of central nervous system side effects, and the lack of prospective trials in the elderly, amantadine has so far achieved limited use.

Complications

Bacterial infections are frequent sequelae of influenza, most likely because of alterations in host defenses caused by viral infection and necrosis of the bronchial mucociliary cells. Tracheobronchitis and sinusitis are well-known complications of influenza, but primary viral and secondary bacterial pneumonias contribute the most to morbidity and mortality. Both viral and bacterial pneumonias develop four to six days after the onset of typical influenza. Roentgenographic pneumonia is seen in about 3–5 percent of influenza cases. Recrudescence of fever and respiratory symptoms (the so-called biphasic illness) heralds pneumonia. The development of purulent sputum can be a helpful clue to a secondary bacterial infection. The most common bacterial causes, in descending order of frequency, are pneumococcus, *S. aureus,* and *H. influenzae.* Enteric gram-negative bacillary and meningococcal pneumonias have occasionally been described. Risk factors for these infectious sequelae of influenza, in addition to age greater than 65 years, include chronic renal, metabolic (including diabetes), hematologic, immunodeficiency, and cardiopulmonary disorders.

Prevention

Chemoprophylaxis Amantadine, when used as prophylaxis against influenza A, reduces infection rates by 50–70 percent. Its prophylactic use during epidemics should be especially considered for patients with underlying diseases and those in chronic care institutions who have not received the appropriate vaccine.

The dosage of amantadine for prophylaxis is the same as that recommended for therapy; it must be administered over the usual six- to eight-week period of an outbreak to be effective. An optional and more attractive approach is to administer amantadine and updated influenza vaccine simultaneously; vaccine immunogenicity is not impaired, and amantadine can be discontinued after two weeks, when 80 percent of those vaccinated will have developed protective levels of antibodies.

Vaccination Prospective field trials in young adults have shown a 50–80 percent reduction in influenza infection after vaccination, but such studies have not been carried out in the elderly. Several retrospective studies in elderly, high-risk groups have demonstrated 30–60 percent reduction in infection. Annual influenza vaccination is recommended for those 65 years of age and older regardless of chronic underlying conditions, because the majority of excess morbidity and mortality occurs in this group. Despite a targeted vaccination policy, only about 25 percent of high-risk individuals actually receive vaccine in any given year.

Yearly immunization is necessary because of the short-lived protective immunity gained from killed virus vaccines and because of constant minor and occasional major antigenic changes in viral strains that necessitate periodic vaccine reformulation. The antigenic changes of influenza viruses often cannot be anticipated rapidly enough to produce and widely distribute updated vaccine, which accounts for the limited ability to control influenza. Currently, a single injection of inactivated whole virus vaccine containing the A and B strains that circulated in the preceding years is recommended. There is some reduction in immunogenicity in those with underlying renal and metabolic disorders, and the vaccine should be given during drug-free intervals to patients receiving immunosuppressive chemotherapy.

Adverse reactions to vaccination are generally mild; about a third of vaccinated persons experience local discomfort, and 1–2 percent have a 24- to 48-hour syndrome of malaise and low-grade fevers. Rarely a history of serious allergy to egg protein will be elicited, and in this situation the vaccine should not be given because it contains residual egg antigens. The Guillain-Barré syndrome was associated with the mass swine influenza vaccination program in 1976. Nationwide surveillance has shown no such risk with subsequent vaccine formulations, and this episode should not be a reason for the patient to avoid or for the physician to withhold vaccination.

SUGGESTED READING

Bacterial Pneumonias
1. Boerner, D.F., Zwadyk, P. The value of the sputum Gram's stain in community-acquired pneumonia. *J.A.M.A.* 247:642–645, 1982.
2. Garb, J.L., Brown, R.B., Garb, J.R., et al. Differences in etiology of pneumonias in nursing home and community patients. *J.A.M.A.* 240:2169–2172, 1978.
3. Horton, J.M., Pankey, G.A. Pneumonia in the elderly: A growing problem demanding special handling. *Postgrad. Med.* 71:114–123, 1982.
4. Schwartz, J.S. Pneumococcal vaccine: Clinical efficacy and effectiveness. *Ann. Intern. Med.* 96:208–220, 1982.
5. Valenti, W.M., Trudell, R.G., Bentley, D.W. Factors predisposing to oropharyngeal colonization with gram-negative bacilli in the aged. *N. Engl. J. Med.* 298:1108–1111, 1978.

6. Wallace, R.J., Musher, D.M., Martin, R.R. *Hemophilus influenzae* pneumonia in adults. *Am. J. Med.* 64:87–93, 1978.
7. Yu, V.L., Kroboth, F.J., Shonnard, J., et al. Legionnaires' disease: New clinical perspective from a prospective pneumonia study. *Am. J. Med.* 73:357–361, 1982.

Influenza

1. Barker, W.H., Mullooly, J.P. Influenza vaccination of elderly persons: Reduction in pneumonia and influenza hospitalizations and deaths. *J.A.M.A.* 244:2547–2549, 1980.
2. Douglas, R.G., Jr., Betts, R.F. Influenza virus. In Mandell, G.L., Douglas, R.G., Jr., Gennett, J.E. (Eds.), *Principles and Practice of Infectious Diseases.* New York: John Wiley and Sons, 1979.
3. Hirsch, M.S., Swartz, M.N. Antiviral agents (first of two parts). *N. Engl. J. Med.* 302:903–907, 1980.
4. Horadan, V.W., Sharp, J.G., Smilack, J.D., et al. Pharmacokinetics of amantadine hydrochloride in subjects with normal and impaired renal function. *Ann. Intern. Med.* 94 (pt. I):454–458, 1981.
5. Recommendations of the Immunization Practices Advisory Committee: Influenza vaccines 1982–1983. *Morbidity and Mortality Weekly Report* 31:349–352, 1982.

8

HEMATOLOGIC
DISORDERS

Anemia in the Elderly

WILLIAM B. HERRING, M.D.

Editor's note: Marginal hemoglobin values occur commonly enough in the elderly that physicians might disregard borderline abnormalities that may be an early indication of a serious disease. In particular, the diagnosis of "anemia of chronic inflammation," most frequent in the elderly, must be made cautiously after excluding other causes. While the evaluation of true anemia in the elderly is no different from that in younger adults, serious and often treatable causes are more likely to be found.

The frequency and complexity of anemia increase with advancing age, in keeping with the accelerating rate of clinical expressions of dysfunction in other organ systems. Anemia is a more ominous sign of disease in the elderly than in younger persons, for it is more often a harbinger of malignancy. Often multifactorial in origin, it is commonly more difficult to diagnose and manage in the elderly and is a greater threat to well-being because of the fragility of other organ systems that are affected by it.

HEMOGLOBIN LEVELS

Establishing the Normal Range

In the elderly, as in other age groups, establishing the presence of anemia when hemoglobin (Hb) concentrations are borderline is often problematic. Many studies have been carried out in an attempt to establish normal ranges for blood values in the aging person. Table 1 shows the mean Hb values by decade from several of these studies. The last column shows estimated ranges, based on these studies, within which 95 percent of Hb values for elderly persons would be expected to fall. Common deficiencies among these studies are small

311

TABLE 1

Mean Hemoglobin Concentrations (g/dl) by Decade in Elderly Men and Women

Study[a]	Sex	Decade				Mean (all)	±2 S.D.[b]
		7th	8th	9th	10th		
1	M	13.4	12.9	12.2	—	12.9	9.9–15.9
	F	—	—	—	—	—	
2	M	—	—	—	—	15.3	13.1–17.5
	F	—	—	—	—	14.0	11.6–16.4
3	M	14.2	13.5	13.2	—	13.6	13.3–14.0
	F	13.1	13.2	12.9	—	13.1	12.9–13.4
4	M	14.5	13.6	13.8	14.4	14.3	11.4–17.1
	F	13.7	13.5	12.7	12.9	13.5	10.8–16.2
5	M	—	15.0	14.8	—	—	
	F	—	14.4	14.2	—	—	
6	M	14.8	14.7	13.9	—	—	
	F	13.7	13.6	13.3	—	—	
7	M	13.9	13.4	12.4	11.2	—	
	F	12.9	13.0	13.0	11.4	—	
Composite Means (non-weighted)	M	14.1	13.8	13.3	12.8	14.0	11.0–16.1
	F	13.3	13.5	13.2	12.1	13.5	11.7–15.3

[a]Sources of these data will be supplied on request.
[b]Ranges encompass 95 percent of the values.
Dashes in columns indicate testing was not done for that category. Blank spaces indicate value could not be calculated for lack of certain information.

numbers of subjects, selection of groups that are poorly representative of the general elderly population, and inadequate precautions to exclude a significant proportion of subjects who might, in fact, be anemic. In two studies, senility, vascular disease, and degenerative arthritis were common and considered nondisqualifying. Although these disorders are not generally associated with anemia, it is debatable whether persons so afflicted may be assumed to be hematologically normal.

In spite of these limitations, nearly all studies of Hb concentrations show a slight but gradual decline with advancing age (Table 1). Women have consistently lower values than men, by about 0.5 to 1.0 g/dl, but there is a trend toward narrowing of the difference with advancing age. In men the mean values decline steadily and after the eighth decade are below the standard normal range for all males (14 to 18 g/dl). In women the mean values remain within the standard normal range for all females (12 to 16 g/dl).

Cellularity of the marrow diminishes from 80 to 100 percent to about 50 percent during the first 30 years of life, remains stable until the seventh decade, and then declines further to about 30 percent during the next decade. Although there are no reliable estimates of functional marrow volume, shrinkage of the erythron is a likely phenomenon and is consistent with the principle that "age begets atrophy," demonstrated by the losses in mass that occur in other systems (e.g., skeleton, muscles, kidneys, brain). Since the kinetics of erythropoiesis appear to be uniform throughout life, one concludes that the Hb *mass* decreases. Whether or not the Hb *concentration* decreases depends on the plasma volume and other factors. Thus, although a decline in Hb production occurs with aging, this knowledge is unlikely to be helpful in assessing individual values.

Contributing to the uncertainty of the relationship between aging and Hb levels is the wide disparity between the biologic and chronologic ages of individuals. The latter may be an inadequate reference standard. Pending the availability of a reliable "senility index," or of age-adjusted normal values based on studies of large numbers of well persons, however, I believe the more rigorous standard normal values should be used for elderly patients, even though some excess of diagnostic studies may result.

Evaluating a Borderline Hb Level

When the Hb value is equivocal, its significance may be tested by a series of basic observations. The measurement of Hb concentration in virtually all hospitals and most office practices today is automated and is measured by the cyanmethemoglobin method. If not, the Hb concentration should be checked by this method. A carefully taken history and meticulous physical examination, searching especially for evidence of bleeding, gastrointestinal or renal disease, and chronic inflammatory conditions, may be productive. The automated cell counter will usually give a directly measured mean red cell volume (MCV) along with the Hb concentration. This value should be noted (the other indices are of little worth). A well-stained blood smear made from a drop of nonanticoagulated blood should be examined for variations in the size and shape of red blood cells (RBCs), abnormal forms, inclusions, and evidence of fragmentation. Maturation defects, if present, and approximate proportions of the various populations of leukocytes should be observed. An estimate of the num-

TABLE 2
Assessment of Marginal Hemoglobin Values

1. History	4. Blood smear
2. Physical examination	5. Platelet count
3. Mean red cell volume	6. Reticulocyte count

bers and average size of platelets may provide clues to the presence and cause of anemia, but if there is doubt that the concentration of platelets is normal, a direct platelet count should be performed, since the "indirect" method is unreliable. An absolute reticulocyte count, which reflects the rate of production of RBCs by the bone marrow, completes this series of basic observations (Table 2).

If all of these parameters are normal, the borderline Hb value is probably normal for that patient and further investigation is usually not warranted. If doubt persists, a biochemical profile and chest x-ray may be indicated. Bone marrow biopsy should not be used as a screening test for anemia; it is rarely helpful in such cases. After the examinations described above are completed with negative results, a marginal Hb determination should be repeated at monthly intervals until it is clear it represents the normal value for that patient. If the borderline value is due to anemia, usually a downward trend will become apparent eventually.

DIAGNOSIS OF ANEMIA IN THE ELDERLY

Once the presence of anemia is established, a systematic approach to diagnosis should be pursued. Diagnosis is facilitated by dividing anemias into morphologic categories on the basis of the MCV (i.e., microcytic, normocytic, or macrocytic), although there is some overlap early in the course of evolution of anemia. Those anemias that are encountered most commonly in the elderly in each category are briefly considered in the following sections.

Microcytic Anemias
The most common cause of microcytic anemia in the elderly, as in other age groups, is iron deficiency. In adults of all ages, iron-deficiency anemia is virtually always due to recurrent or chronic blood loss. Thus, an unremitting search for a source of bleeding is indicated. When anemia is microcytic and bleeding is obvious, confirmation of

iron deficiency is superfluous; correction of the cause of bleeding and treatment with iron are sufficient. When the source of bleeding is inapparent, iron stores should be assessed. Serum ferritin measurement is the preferred method even though, because of labile acute phase reactivity of this protein, the level may be increased when inflammation is present, leading to falsely high estimates of iron stores. Serum iron and transferrin levels measure only the iron transport pool and are a reliable index of stores only if iron metabolism is unperturbed by the absence of inflammation and renal failure. Estimation of stainable marrow iron by Prussian blue staining of marrow specimens is often helpful and should be done if marrow biopsy is performed for other indications.

In elderly adults of both sexes, inflamed diverticula, colonic polyps, peptic ulcer disease, and hiatal hernia are common sources of recurrent bleeding and iron-deficiency anemia. Significant bleeding from hemorrhoids may be overlooked. Carcinoma of the colon must not be missed, since it is curable when resectable but invariably attended by much suffering and short survival after it has spread. Mainly for this reason, proctoscopic and barium enema examinations are indicated when iron-deficiency anemia is found, unless another cause is obvious. In postmenopausal women vaginal bleeding, often due to endometrial carcinoma, should be suspected.

The use of aspirin and other antiinflammatory drugs for rheumatic complaints, common in the elderly, is a frequent cause of gastrointestinal blood loss and may lead to iron deficiency. It is prudent to establish a baseline Hb concentration and to monitor it periodically in patients taking these medications.

The term *nutritional anemia* is often used to include iron-deficiency anemia. The smaller iron stores of women, related to their smaller body mass and therefore lower food (iron) intake and their vulnerability to iron deficiency due to menstruation, pregnancy, and lactation, are cited as predisposing factors. However, it has not been shown in adults of either sex that iron-deficiency anemia may occur solely as a result of inadequate dietary intake of iron. Labeling iron-deficiency anemia a form of nutritional anemia, therefore, seems undesirable since it could lead to an inadequate workup for bleeding. Further evidence against a role for dietary iron lack as a contributor to iron deficiency in the elderly is the fact that iron stores, as measured by serum ferritin levels, increase steadily throughout life in men and postmenopausal women.

When treating iron deficiency, one should eliminate the cause of bleeding if possible. To replenish the depleted iron pools, a single tablet of ferrous sulfate taken at bedtime is sufficient, unless bleeding persists; this treatment should be continued for six months to a year, or until the serum ferritin level is satisfactory. This regimen is more convenient, less expensive, equally effective, and more likely to be complied with than the usual three-times-a-day regimen, since the side effects that occur with the latter are avoided.

Although severe thalassemia is unlikely to be found in elderly patients, mild forms of alpha-thalassemia are said to occur in nearly a third of American blacks. This diagnosis should be considered in elderly patients with mild microcytic anemia in the absence of bleeding and when iron stores are normal. The presence of target cells and basophilic RBC inclusions (aggregates of excess beta chains) in the blood film are supportive evidence. Although Hb analysis, as usually reported, is normal (i.e., normal *percentages* of Hbs A, A_2, and F), analysis of globin chain synthetic rates shows impaired alpha-chain synthesis. Family studies may help to confirm the diagnosis.

Sideroblastic anemia is a rare but usually severe and slowly progressive disorder that occurs mainly in older persons. There may be several RBC populations: one is severely microcytic with many bizarre forms, another may be macrocytic, and a third is morphologically normal. Whether the MCV is low, normal, or high depends on the proportions of these forms. The marrow is intensely cellular and heavily iron-loaded. The hallmark of this disorder is the presence on marrow smears of large numbers of ringed sideroblasts, in which the mitochondria are laden with iron. The severity of the anemia is proportional to the ring count, that is, the percentage of erythroblasts containing abnormal aggregates of stainable iron (Fig. 1). Maturation in the erythroid series shows megaloblastoid features, probably accounting for the macrocytic RBC population.

The basic defect in sideroblastic anemia is unknown, although several enzyme deficiencies in the heme synthetic pathway have been identified. A fundamental disorder of iron metabolism, in addition to the stimulus to iron absorption of ineffective erythropoiesis, seems likely because of the ringed-sideroblast phenomenon.

Treatment of sideroblastic anemia is supportive. Iron unloading, by venesection if the anemia is mild or by iron chelators in the usual case, may be helpful, but the abnormalities will not completely reverse. Unfortunately many of these patients will have had empirical

FIGURE 1

Comparison of ring counts with hematocrits in nine patients with acquired sideroblastic anemia. Solid black circles represent control subjects.

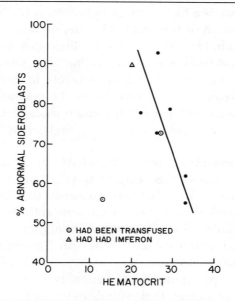

iron therapy, sometimes for years. Supplemental ascorbic acid should be avoided since it enhances iron toxicity. Some patients respond partially to vitamin B_6 and folic acid, but transfusion is the main treatment. Acute myeloid leukemia develops in about 10 percent of patients with sideroblastic anemia.

Macrocytic Anemias

When anemia is associated with significant numbers of oval macrocytes on blood smear, megaloblastic maturation is suspected. Usually neutropenia and thrombocytopenia are also present. In elderly non-alcoholic patients this condition is most often due to pernicious anemia, although loss of intrinsic factor from total gastric resection or malabsorption of the vitamin B_{12}–intrinsic factor complex due to severe ileal disease may also cause vitamin B_{12} deficiency. Serum vitamin B_{12} levels under 100 pg/ml are sufficient for diagnosis in the proper clinical setting, but since lifelong treatment is required, it is prudent to confirm megaloblastic maturation by bone marrow biopsy and to confirm the absence of intrinsic factor by the Schilling test (<1% urinary excretion of a test dose of $^{60}Co-B_{12}/24$ hr). Monthly injections of 50 to 100 μg of vitamin B_{12} are appropriate treatment for vitamin B_{12}–deficient subjects.

When alcoholism is a factor, megaloblastosis is likely to be responsive to administration of folic acid. The diet of alcoholics is deficient in folates, but alcohol also impairs folate absorption and inhibits conversion of folic acid to its active form, folinic acid. Occasionally folate deficiency is a result of a sustained severely inadequate diet. An increased folate requirement, as in chronic hemolytic anemia or malignancies associated with greatly increased rates of DNA synthesis, usually combined with inadequate dietary intake, may lead to megaloblastosis.

Serum folate determinations are unreliable in the diagnosis of folate deficiency because of the rapid turnover of serum folate. When laboratory confirmation is deemed necessary the RBC folate level should be measured, since it more accurately reflects available folate and is a more stable value. Generally, when vitamin B_{12} deficiency has been excluded, empirical treatment with 1 mg of folic acid daily, given orally, is acceptable, together with correction of the cause of the deficiency. Supplemental folate generally need not be continued after restoration of hematologic values to normal.

Nonmegaloblastic macrocytic anemia is associated with round, rather than oval, macrocytes on blood smear and usually normal granulopoiesis and thrombopoiesis. The MCV is only slightly increased. If the macrocytes are polychromatophilic, reticulocytosis may account for the macrocytosis. This situation may occur a few days following blood loss or when a responsive anemia has been only partially treated. If the macrocytes are normochromic they may be the progeny of precursors that have skipped divisions, as in aplastic anemia. The anemia of myxedema is often macrocytic. Alcoholics and heavy smokers may show macrocytosis that is unresponsive to folate; they are not always anemic. The treatment of these conditions depends on recognition and correction of the causes.

Normocytic Anemias

Normocytic anemias may be divided into those due to recent blood loss, those in which the rate of production of RBCs by the marrow is inadequate, and those in which there is accelerated destruction of RBCs.

While acute blood loss may be occult, it is usually easily recognized.

In elderly persons especially, however, dangerous hypovolemia may occur before there has been sufficient hemodilution to drop the Hb concentration. The decision to replace lost blood should be made earlier in older patients and should be based on careful monitoring of symptoms, vital signs, and mental status, and whether coexisting vascular disease is present.

The hypoproliferative anemias comprise the largest group of normocytic anemias in the elderly. There are four main categories; most common is the "anemia of chronic disorders." This term is in danger of losing its utility if invoked, as it often is, to explain anemia associated with virtually any chronic disease. Although this type of anemia is characterized by changes in iron metabolism and some shortening of RBC survival, the mechanism of decreased production (manifest by a low absolute reticulocyte count) remains unknown. Until the cause is clarified, this diagnosis should be reserved for the anemia accompanying those conditions in which there is evidence of inflammation. The "anemia of inflammation" might, in fact, be a better term.

The anemia of chronic renal failure deserves to be separated from the anemia of chronic disorders because a significant contributing factor is erythropoietin deficiency resulting from renal damage. The adverse effects of uremia on RBC production and survival remain obscure but are surely important. About 33 percent of patients with rheumatoid arthritis and anemia and 19 percent of patients with the anemia of chronic renal failure have microcytic RBCs, with MCVs as low as 63 femtoliters, in the absence of evidence of iron deficiency or other causes of microcytosis. The mechanisms of microcytosis are unknown. It is important to recognize these subpopulations in order to avoid unwarranted diagnostic procedures and ineffective or possibly injurious iron therapy.

Myelophthisic anemia is most common in elderly persons, since the predisposing conditions that displace erythroid marrow are most common in this age group. They include the hematologic malignancies (multiple myeloma, lymphomas, acute and chronic leukemias) and others with a predilection for metastasis to the skeleton (carcinomas of the prostate, lung, and breast). Least common among the hypoproliferative anemias are aplastic anemia and erythroid aplasia. While the causal agent is a drug or toxin in many cases, at least half are idiopathic. Recent work indicates that the disease is often mediated by immune mechanisms in a hostile "hematopoietic microenvironment." These observations afford new opportunities for rational treatment with greater hope of success. Bone marrow transplantation, to be considered early in young persons with aplastic anemia, is seldom an option for the elderly patient, however.

Treatment of the hypoproliferative anemias is dictated mainly by the nature of the associated conditions; control of the latter will usually result in improvement of anemia. Drugs used to treat the primary condition, especially anticancer agents, may themselves cause anemia and must be used judiciously. Unfortunately, transfusion must often be employed as the main treatment, which creates new opportunities for complications and adds greatly to the costs of care. Generally, one or two units of packed RBCs given just often enough to control symptoms represents the most efficient use of this precious resource.

Hemolytic anemias are divided into two groups; in one the basic defect is intrinsic to the RBC (intracellular), and in the other the cause of hemolysis is extrinsic (extracellular). Mainly, the former are hereditary and the latter are acquired. Severe anemias of hereditary origin are unlikely to be seen in elderly persons, but mild (heterozygous) forms are occasionally found. These conditions include membrane defects (e.g., hereditary spherocytosis) and metabolic derangements (e.g., glucose-6-phosphate dehydrogenase deficiency). Acquired causes of hemolysis encountered in the elderly include hypersplenism, due to splenic enlargement from any cause, and autoimmunity. Autoimmune hemolytic anemia may be idiopathic or incited by drugs, infections, or predisposing malignancies, especially chronic lymphocytic leukemia and lymphomas.

Splenectomy is a major form of treatment of the hemolytic anemias, but it should not be used indiscriminately, especially in the elderly. Unfortunately, there are no good techniques for quantifying the contributions of the spleen to the anemia or for predicting the benefits of splenectomy. The decision regarding splenectomy is further complicated by new evidence that hyposplenism may be a significant disease state at any age. Often in fragile elderly patients a degree of splenic hyperfunctioning is preferable to the risks of surgery and absence of the spleen, but the risks of continued hemolysis, transfusion, and steroid therapy must be given appropriate weight.

SUGGESTED READING

1. Freedman, M.C., Marcus, D.L. Anemia and the elderly: Is it physiology or pathology? *Am. J. Med. Sci.* 280:81–85, 1980.

2. Htoo, M.S.H., Kofkoff, R.L., Freedman, M.L. Erythrocyte parameters in the elderly: An argument against new geriatric normal values. *J. Am. Geriatr. Soc.* 27:547–551, 1979.
3. Williams, W.J. Hematology in the aged. In Williams, W.J., et al. (Eds.), *Hematology*, 2nd ed. New York: McGraw-Hill, 1977.

9

PREVENTIVE CARE

Screening for Cancer in the Elderly

WILLIAM B. HERRING, M.D.

Editor's note: Any primary physician responsible for patients over 55 years old must be familiar with the age-specific recommendations for cancer screening. Though the frequency and cost-effectiveness of the screening procedures summarized are not, in general, securely established by large, well-designed studies, they represent the current state of the art. Deviations from the American Cancer Society standards should be made only with clear understanding of these recommendations.

The incidence of cancer increases markedly with aging. Mortality due to cancer of the five most commonly affected sites is six times higher in men and four times higher in women over 55 years of age than under. Twenty-one percent of all deaths are due to cancer, the second leading cause of death in nearly all age groups. Although much progress has been made in recent years in the treatment of some cancers, even at advanced stages, morbidity and mortality due to cancer remain unacceptably high. The elderly are further victimized, for they often tolerate cancer and its treatment less well than do younger patients, for reasons that are unclear. Also, treatment must often be compromised in the elderly because of intercurrent diseases and a poor performance status.

Cancer control depends on prevention and on the effectiveness of treatment. Known preventive measures, such as avoidance of smoking, are few and difficult to implement. Survival, a commonly used index of the success of treatment, is strongly related to the stage of cancer at the time of diagnosis. Unfortunately most patients come to the physician when their cancers are too advanced for optimal treatment, due to the insidious nature of some cancers or to indifference, ignorance, or denial born of fear. Education of the public is vitally important to advancements in prevention and treatment.

Since early detection enables more successful treatment and improved survival, it is reasoned that screening (to detect cancer in asymptomatic persons) will lead to optimal results, for cancer could then be detected in its earliest stages. The principle of screening has become widely accepted, although its methods are uncertain and its effectiveness, at least for certain cancers, remains to be established. Still, the philosophy of screening appeals so strongly to reason, and screening is currently so vigorously promoted, that a policy is clearly needed. Although there are significant obstacles to implementation, including cost, logistics, and compliance, the guidelines published by the American Cancer Society (ACS) in 1980 are the best available. It is emphasized that these are guidelines only, designed to help the clinician deliver optimal medical care to his elderly patients who are *asymptomatic* in the parts being screened, and that his clinical judgment may dictate departures from these recommendations in individual cases. These guidelines are not designed for screening large populations, such as residents of nursing homes, although they might be adapted for this purpose.

Those guidelines that apply to the most frequent cancers in the elderly are reviewed in the following sections.

CANCER OF THE LUNG

In 1982 there were approximately 129,000 new cases and 111,000 deaths due to cancer of the lung; of these, about 84 percent occurred in persons over 55 years of age. Cancer of the lung is by far the most common cause of death due to cancer in elderly men. In women over 55, its frequency as a cause of cancer death is exceeded only by breast and colon cancer and is rapidly rising. At current rates it will become the leading cause of death due to cancer in women by 1985.

Several studies of screening for lung cancer using periodic chest x-ray and sputum cytology studies, including three well-designed and controlled studies now in progress, have thus far failed to show any reduction of mortality due to screening. The only benefit that might accrue from detection at earlier stages is that less extensive initial treatment might be required. Although the ACS endorses regular chest films and sputum cytologies in high-risk patients, it does not presently offer guidelines nor advocate screening for lung cancer.

CANCER OF THE COLON AND RECTUM

Colorectal carcinoma is second only to cancer of the lung as a cause of cancer death among Americans. In 1982 there were about 123,000 new cases and 57,000 deaths from colorectal cancer; 90 percent were in persons over 55 years old. In women over age 75, it is the leading cause of cancer death by a wide margin.

In addition to aging, there are several other risk factors for colorectal cancer, including concurrent ulcerative or granulomatous colitis, a history of colorectal adenomas or prior cancer of the large bowel, and cancer of the uterus, ovary, or breast. Also, there are a number of familial syndromes characterized by polyposis of the colon that are strongly associated with malignancy of the large bowel. Recently diet has received much attention; a high intake of fat and cholesterol, leading to increased synthesis of bile acids, and a low content of fiber are thought by some to be significant causative factors.

There is convincing evidence that adenomatous polyps of the colon may become cancers after an interval of about five years, the risk increasing with both the size and number of polyps present. Thus the finding of one or more polyps places the patient in a high-risk category and dictates closer surveillance than would be indicated in their absence. Polyps should be removed, at colonoscopy if possible.

The evidence that screening reduces mortality from colorectal cancer is strong, although controlled studies are presently lacking. In a large study of asymptomatic persons at the University of Minnesota Hospital, 78 percent of the cancers detected by the Hemoccult test were staged as either Dukes A or B,[1] whereas about 50 percent of colon cancers found in symptomatic persons are at stage Dukes C (lymph nodes involved). Although the five-year survival rate among these patients is not yet available, several other studies suggest a five-year survival rate of more than 80 percent when the patient is asymptomatic, as opposed to less than 50 percent when the patient presents with symptoms.

Screening techniques for colorectal cancer vary widely in feasibility, cost, and patient acceptance. Digital rectal examination detects a significant number of cancers, but despite the advantages of simplicity and low cost it has limitations that are obvious. Proctosigmoidoscopy,

---

1. V.A. Gilbertson, R. McHugh, L. Schuman, and S.E. Williams. The early detection of colorectal cancers: A preliminary report of the results of the occult blood study. *Cancer* 45:2899–2901, 1980.

especially with the new flexible endoscopes, improves the detection rate to about 60 percent but will miss lesions beyond the sigmoid colon. Colonoscopy is the most sensitive procedure but is limited by availability, patient acceptance, and cost. The sensitivity of full-column barium enema for small lesions is low; air-contrast barium enema is better but is still less sensitive than colonoscopy. The costs, discomfort to the patient, and limited availability to large numbers of asymptomatic persons render barium enema and endoscopy impractical as screening procedures.

The most satisfactory single method of screening for colorectal cancer is the Hemoccult II slide test for occult blood in the stool; its advantages are simplicity, good patient compliance, low cost, and reliability when correctly performed. In a large study at the Strang Clinic in New York City, half of those asymptomatic screened subjects who had at least one positive Hemoccult slide were found to have polyps larger than 5 mm in diameter (38 percent) or cancers (12 percent); the remainder had diverticula, polyps less than 5 mm in diameter, or no pathology, for a false-positive rate of 0.5 percent.[2] A high percentage of cancers detected by the Hemoccult test are localized and thus curable. Comparison of results with those of sigmoidoscopy, however, suggests a substantial false-negative rate; nearly as many adenomas are missed as are found and about 20 percent of cancers escape detection.

The Hemoccult test depends on the phenolic oxidation of guaiac by the peroxidase-like action of hemoglobin. It can detect about 2 ml of blood per 100 g of stool. Peroxidase-containing foods (fruits and raw vegetables, especially radishes) and hemoglobin (red meat) in the diet may give false-positive results. Large amounts of vitamin C, a reducing agent, may interfere with a positive result. The slides are stable for at least four to five days after the specimen is applied and thus can be returned to the physician by mail, but rehydration is required to dissolve crystallized hemoglobin in the dried specimen and restore sensitivity. Unfortunately, rehydration also increases the false-positive rate, since interfering peroxidases are also returned to solution.

The ACS currently recommends the following procedures to screen for colorectal cancer: (1) a yearly digital rectal examination for every-

---

2. S.J. Winawer, M. Andrews, B. Flehinger, et al. Progress report on controlled trial of fecal occult blood testing for the detection of colorectal neoplasia. *Cancer* 45:2959–2964, 1980.

one over 40 years of age, (2) yearly stool guaiac slide tests on three consecutive days for all those over 50, and (3) sigmoidoscopy for everyone over 50 every three to five years after two negative examinations separated by a year.

CANCER OF THE BREAST

In 1982 there were an estimated 112,000 new cases and 37,000 deaths due to cancer of the female breast, currently the most common site for cancer in women (26 percent). Seventy-four percent of these deaths were in women over 55 years of age. Although the death rate due to breast cancer has not changed significantly in the last 50 years, this is one of the few major cancers in which there is convincing evidence that early detection (prior to lymph node involvement) saves lives. Women now receiving treatment for breast cancer without node involvement have an 85 percent chance of surviving five years, whereas only 53 percent survive five years when more advanced disease is present at diagnosis.

The most important modalities of screening for breast cancer are breast self-examination, regular physical examination of the breasts, and mammography. The ACS recommends that all women be taught the technique of breast self-examination and that it be performed monthly after 20 years of age. Women between 20 and 40 should have a breast examination by a physician every three years; after age 40 this should be done annually. Women should have a baseline mammogram at age 35 to 40, and women over 50 should have mammography performed annually. The appropriate frequency of mammography in women between 40 and 50 years of age has not been decided, but all women over 35 who have a history of breast cancer, or whose mothers or sisters have such a history, should have mammograms at least annually. Routine mammography is not recommended for women under 35 due to the risk of radiation-induced cancer, but in older women the benefits far outweigh the risks. While there is an estimated excess incidence of 6 cases per million women per year per rad of radiation exposure after ten years, mammography performed with modern techniques can detect over 90 percent of breast cancers, whereas only about two-thirds may be discovered by physical examination alone. The value of mammography is further shown by the fact that women whose breast cancers were detectable only by mammography had a 78 percent ten-year survival, whereas this figure decreased to 58 percent when the tumor was palpable.

GYNECOLOGIC CANCER

Cancer of the Cervix

Although there has been a steady decline in the incidence of invasive cancer of the uterine cervix during the past 25 years, an estimated 16,000 new cases occurred in 1982. Risk factors include coitus at an early age, multiple sexual partners (prostitutes have a threefold increase in incidence), multiparity, and a history of venereal disease.

Invasive carcinoma of the cervix evolves in most if not all cases from carcinoma in situ, which appears to be preceded by cervical dysplasia. The duration of carcinoma in situ is long, averaging at least eight years; dysplasia precedes carcinoma in situ by five to ten years. Appropriate treatment of cervical dysplasia and carcinoma in situ can prevent invasive carcinoma in virtually all cases. The widespread use of the Papanicolaou (Pap) smear for cervical cytology since its introduction for screening in the 1950s undoubtedly accounts for the decline of invasive cancer, although this question has never been the subject of a randomized controlled study. Cancer of the cervix is rare after age 65 in women who have previously had negative cervical cytology.

These features of cervical cancer are reflected in the recommendations of the ACS for screening. When sexual activity begins or at age 20 all women should have two consecutive yearly Pap tests, followed by a Pap test every three years until age 65, after which regular screening for *cervical* cancer appears unnecessary. Indeed, Pap tests every five years may be sufficient to control cervical cancer; this interval is recommended in Canada, Great Britain, and Finland and by the American College of Preventive Medicine. However, the optimal frequency of Pap tests is still being vigorously debated, and annual smears are recommended by some investigators.[3]

Since there is a significant incidence of false-negative smears, proper technique is important. At each examination two smears should be made, one from the endocervical canal and one from the squamocolumnar junction, if visible, or the cervical os. Prompt fixation and interpretation by qualified cytopathologists are essential.

Cancer of the Endometrium

Endometrial carcinoma is the most common gynecologic cancer, accounting for 39,000 new cases and 3,000 deaths in 1982. Its peak

---

3. W.T. Creasman, W.C. Fowler, and H.D. Homesley. Screening for cervical cancer, 1982—an update. *N.C. Med. J.* 43:771–773, 1982.

incidence is in the seventh decade. The proportion of uterine cancer arising in the endometrium has increased in the last 20 years as the population of aging women has increased and the frequency of cervical carcinoma has declined. Risk factors for endometrial cancer include a history of infertility, failure of ovulation, prolonged estrogen therapy, late menopause, obesity, diabetes, and hypertension.

There are no simple and reliable screening procedures for endometrial cancer. The most successful means of controlling endometrial cancer with the techniques now available is the prompt reporting and appropriate investigation of abnormal uterine bleeding. The Pap test, highly effective in screening for cancer of the cervix, will detect only about 40 percent of endometrial cancers. Current recommendations of the ACS are limited to endometrial biopsy at menopause in women at high risk. Pelvic examination, recommended every three years between ages 20 and 40 and annually after age 40, may detect some endometrial cancers if associated with uterine enlargement or local extension, and annual Pap tests, although unnecessary for adequate screening for cervical cancer, may modestly enhance the sensitivity of the pelvic examination. Fortunately, most endometrial cancer is diagnosed in stage I or stage II when the five-year survival rate, after hysterectomy and radiotherapy, exceeds 80 percent. Over 90 percent of recurrences occur within three years.

Cancer of the Ovary

Cancer of the ovary is the fourth-ranking cause of cancer death in American women. In 1982 there were 18,000 new cases and 11,400 deaths due to this tumor. Ninety percent of the tumors are of epithelial origin and occur mainly in women from 40 to 70 years old. The presenting symptoms are most often pain and abdominal distension, since the cancer is usually advanced at the time of diagnosis, accounting for the high death rate.

The only practical method of screening for cancer of the ovary is periodic pelvic and rectal examinations with careful attention to the uterine adnexae. Ovaries larger than 5 cm in diameter in premenopausal women and ovaries that are palpable in postmenopausal women should be regarded with suspicion. The ACS recommends annual pelvic examinations for women over 40 years of age.

CANCER OF THE PROSTATE

Cancer of the prostate accounted for 73,000 new cases and over 23,000 deaths in 1982. It is the third leading cause of cancer death in men, and in those over 75 it is second only to lung cancer. While prostatic cancer often follows an indolent course, only 10 percent are detected when localized; thus 90 percent of men who have prostatic cancer are destined to die of or with it.

While the benefits of screening are unproved, localized cancer of the prostate is amenable to surgery or radiotherapy. Except for the transient benefits from hormonal manipulation, the treatment of advanced disease is unsatisfactory. It seems probable that early detection would improve the cure rate; thus elderly men should be offered the likely benefits of screening.

Unfortunately, there is no highly satisfactory screening test. In a comparison of 10 tests in 300 men with prostatic cancer, the digital rectal examination was best.[4] It detected 69 percent of cancers with an efficiency (correct classification) of 85 percent. The acid phosphatase measured by enzyme activity was next, but all other tests gave poorer results and their technical difficulties and costs were significant. They included other methods for measuring acid phosphatase, urine and prostatic fluid cytologies, ratios of lactic dehydrogenase isoenzyme V to isoenzyme I, and leukocyte-adherence inhibition tests. This study was performed by urologists; digital rectal examination may be less sensitive when done by others.

The ACS recommends a digital rectal examination annually for men over 40 years of age. Presently, careful palpation of the entire gland for nodularity, symmetry, and texture, not omitting the seminal vesicles, followed by appropriate investigation of any abnormalities, remains the best approach to the control of cancer of the prostate.

SKIN CANCER

About 400,000 nonmelanoma skin cancers occur annually in the United States, mostly in older men. Over 90 percent are curable. They tend to occur in sun-exposed areas—that is, the face, lips, and dorsum of hands. Prolonged sun exposure and fair skin are risk factors; acquired immune deficiency, perhaps an accompaniment of aging, possibly makes a permissive contribution. Careful inspection of the skin, especially the exposed areas, is adequate for screening.

---

4. P. Guinan, N. Gilhan, S.R. Nagabadi, et al. What is the best test to detect prostate cancer? *CA* 31:141–145, 1981.

CANCER OF THE ORAL CAVITY

About 27,000 new cases and 9,000 deaths due to cancer of the oral cavity and pharynx occurred in 1982. Approximately 70 percent were in men. The use of alcohol or tobacco is a risk factor. Many of these cancers arise from leukoplakia. Thorough inspection of the buccal mucosa, tongue, and appurtenant structures should be done at the time of physical examination.

RECOMMENDATIONS

While the value of screening for cancer in the elderly is hardly controversial in principle, the impact of screening on the morbidity and mortality rates of most cancers is unclear, and cost/benefit ratios are not established. There are special problems with screening the elderly. Compliance is likely to be low, limiting the success of screening efforts, since many older people have lost their independence and must rely on others for seeing to their health care needs. Episodic medical problems or chronic diseases are almost universal and preoccupy both patient and physician. Nearly all elderly persons have accepted a changing bodily image that includes not only physical but

TABLE 1
Screening for Cancer in the Elderly

Test	Sex	Age	Frequency
Physical examination (including digital rectal)	M, F	Over 40	Every year
Stool guaiac slide test	M, F	Over 50	Every year
Pelvic examination	F	Over 40	Every year
Pap test	F	To age 65	Yearly ×2; if negative then every 3–5 years
Sigmoidoscopy	M, F	Over 50	Yearly ×2; if negative then every 3–5 years
Breast self-examination	F	Over 20	Every month
Physical examination of breasts	F	Over 40	Every year
Mammography	F	35–40	Baseline
		Under 50	As indicated
		Over 50	Every year
Endometrial tissue sampling	F	At menopause	At menopause in women at high risk

mental deterioration. Thus the prospect and even the symptoms of cancer may be seen as natural and inevitable processes, leading to delay in diagnosis and generally poorer results of treatment.

Education of the public and active participation in screening by primary care physicians is vital to the success of cancer control programs. Studies of areawide screening have shown that intensive public education can improve compliance with screening programs from about 15 percent to 40 to 80 percent. Studies of screening in primary care practices and efforts to improve screening procedures for groups of elderly persons, such as those in group residences and nursing homes, are needed. Until proved screening practices based on such studies are available, it is prudent to follow guidelines, such as those listed in Table 1, for early detection of cancer in the elderly.

SUGGESTED READING

1. *Cancer Facts and Figures 1982*. American Cancer Society, 1982.
2. Creasman, W.T., Fowler, W.C., Homesley, H.D. Screening for cervical cancer, 1982—an update. *N.C. Med. J.* 43:771–773, 1982.
3. DeVita, V.T., Jr., Hellman, S., Rosenberg, S.A. (Eds.), *Cancer: Principles and Practice of Oncology*. Philadelphia: J.B. Lippincott, 1982.
4. Guidelines for the cancer-related checkup: Recommendations and rationale. *Am. Cancer Soc.* 30:194–240, 1980.
5. Guinan, P., Gilhan, N., Nagabadi, S.R., et al. What is the best test to detect prostate cancer? *CA* 31:141–145, 1981.
6. Scanlon, E.F., Taylor, W.J., Brown, H.G., et al. Mammography 1982: A statement of the American Cancer Society. *CA* 32:226–230, 1982.
7. Silverberg, E. Cancer statistics, 1982. *CA* 32:15–31, 1982.
8. Weisburger, J.H., Wynder, E.L., Horn, C.L. Nutritional factors and etiologic mechanisms in the causation of gastrointestinal cancers. *Cancer* 1982;50:2541–2549, 1982.
9. Winawer, S.J., Fleisher, M., Baldwin, M., et al. Current status of fecal occult blood testing in screening for colo-rectal cancer. *CA* 32:100–112, 1982.

Nutritional Requirements of the Elderly

TERRY L. BAZZARRE, PH.D.

Editor's note: Older adults, especially those in institutions, are frequently malnourished and get inadequate amounts of exercise. Calcium, vitamin A, vitamin C, iron, protein, and calories are commonly present in deficient amounts. Changes in the elderly in taste, vision, smell, and dentition, as well as the presence of chronic diseases, make attention to nutrition even more important.

By the year 2020, it is estimated that almost one of every five Americans will be over age 65; and of all Americans older than 65, more than half will be over age 75. Since the nutritional requirements of most adults are thought to change significantly near the eighth decade of life, large numbers of people will have special, largely poorly understood, nutritional needs.

At the turn of the century about six nutrients were known to be constituents of foods. Currently, we know of more than 60 nutrients present in the foods we consume; however, the actual requirements for most of these nutrients are not well defined. Most of the research on nutrient requirements has been based on young adult populations, growing children, and women during pregnancy. Thus, little work is available on adults over age 50 that would provide insight into the nutritional problems of the elderly. The Food and Nutrition Board of the National Academy of Sciences is one of several groups of researchers that periodically publishes information about nutritional needs (The U.S. Recommended Dietary Allowances). The most recent edition (1980) includes, for the first time, recommendations for the energy needs of people over age 50.

Physicians and other health professionals need to be aware of three major limitations of the Recommended Dietary Allowances (RDA) in evaluating the nutritional needs of older adults. The first limitation

335

is that the RDAs were developed as guidelines for groups of people rather than for individuals. The second limitation concerns the danger of generalizing; given the paucity of available information on nutrition and the elderly, health professionals need to recognize that the food (and drug) metabolism of an 85-year-old woman is likely to be quite different from that of a 50-year-old woman. Finally, the RDAs do not take into account the effects of disease or infection on nutrient requirements. This final limitation is of considerable concern because the major chronic disease entities (cardiovascular heart disease, high blood pressure, adult-onset diabetes mellitus, osteoporosis, and obesity) all require that dietary modifications be included in both treatment and prevention.

STUDIES OF NUTRITIONAL STATUS OF THE ELDERLY

A majority of the reports of food intake among the elderly are based on an institutionalized population or participants of a congregate meal program for the elderly. Because only about 5 percent of the population over age 65 live in an institutionalized setting and because the majority of surveys reported in the literature used relatively small sample sizes, the generalizability of the available data is limited. Moreover, very few of the dietary surveys have included laboratory testing of clinical measures of nutritional deficiencies.

On the basis of the food survey data that are available, however, there are some trends that suggest that a large percentage of older Americans have inadequate diets. Caloric intake was less than the standard in the majority of surveys reported, including all national surveys (e.g., Ten-State Nutrition Survey, 1968–70; Nutrition Canada National Survey, 1970–72; U.S.D.A. Household Food Consumption Survey, 1965). These data are surprising, given the incidence of obesity reported among older adults in the Ten State Nutrition Survey, which ranges from up to 20 percent of males to about 50 percent of females. The RDAs for energy may be too high for older adults, or conversely, the level of physical activity among aging adults may be insufficient to prevent excessive adiposity.

In addition to an inadequate intake of calories, several major surveys, including my own,[1] observed dietary inadequacy of calcium, especially among females, and dietary inadequacy of vitamin A, es-

---

1. T.L. Bazzarre, J.A. Yuhas. Measures of food intake among rural elderly. *J. Nutr. Elderly.* In press.

pecially among males. Iron and vitamin C intake may be inadequate. Ascorbic acid concentrations were low in almost one of every ten black females from low-income states and were deficient in almost one of every ten Spanish-American males. Low or deficient hemoglobin levels were common among both males and females. Over 50 percent of black males from low-income states had low hemoglobin levels, while almost 15 percent had deficient levels.

The mean intake of dietary protein among older Americans appears to be, in general, adequate on the basis of most surveys. Individuals over 70 years of age appear to need more than 1 gram of high-biologic-value protein per kilogram of body weight in order to maintain nitrogen balance (assuming they meet the RDA for energy); younger adults, by comparison, require 0.8 g/kg of body weight. About 15 to 20 percent of older black and Spanish-American adults were found to have low serum albumin levels, however, possibly indicating protein malnutrition.

ASSESSMENT OF NUTRITIONAL STATUS AND NEEDS

When reviewing the nutritional requirements of older adults, it is important that the assessment include: (1) evaluation of food intake; (2) the collection of appropriate body measures; (3) laboratory testing; (4) physical examination for gross signs of deficiency; and (5) a review of the individual's personal and medical history, including income, transportation, and other factors that affect food purchasing. A few of the salient aspects of these five categories of evaluation and some of the physiologic changes occurring during the aging process that are considered in nutritional assessment will be discussed.

Changes in Body Composition

Body composition studies in both animals and humans note a decrease in lean body mass, a decrease in bone density, and an increase in adiposity with aging. Between 25 and 70 years of age, man's lean body mass decreases from 47 percent to 36 percent; skeletal tissue decreases from 6% of total body mass to about 4%; and body fat as a percentage of total body mass increases from 20 to 36 percent. The changes in body composition such as percentage of body fat appear to be more prominent in women than in men. For example, body fat in males increases from 15 to 30 percent, whereas in females body fat increases from about 25 percent to about 50 percent between the ages of 25 and 70.

Since women have a longer average life span than men, these alterations indirectly suggest that obesity as a mortality risk factor is perhaps of lesser concern in older adults than in younger adults. In addition, it is not clear if adiposity during adult life is a reflection of the aging process or of the lack of regular physical activity. The percentage of body fat for athletes is lower: male athletes 60 years of age have 10 to 15 percent body fat, and one group of older female athletes had 20 percent body fat.

The changes in body composition that occur during aging are accompanied by a decrease in the basal metabolic rate and impaired thermoregulatory capacity. The combination of these changes affects appetite and nutritional requirements as well. Nutritional implications include:

- decreased energy requirements
- increased protein requirements
- increased calcium requirements
- altered appetite regulation
- increased need for physical activity

Taste and Smell Sensitivity
Changes in taste and smell sensitivity are some of the most important changes affecting appetite. By 45 years of age there is a significant reduction in the number of olfactory neurons lining the nasal passages and in the number of taste buds; the rate of cell death is slower for taste buds than for olfactory neurons. Smoking and some drugs also may add to the impairment of taste and smell sensitivity. Initially, a decrease in taste buds leads to an increased taste recognition threshold. Thus, an individual will use more sugar to achieve a satisfying "sweet" sensation, and more salt in order to achieve a satisfying "salty" sensation. Obesity and poorly controlled diabetes or high blood pressure may, therefore, be results of taste and smell changes during the middle and later phases of adult life.

Eventually the number of taste buds is reduced to the extent that almost all taste sensitivity is lost, and the elderly may be less interested in food. Decreased consumption of food eventually leads to anorexia, weight loss, and malnutrition, which in turn lead to impaired health and perhaps ultimately to premature death. The elderly may also complain that the food served to them, particularly in institutional settings, tastes bad. The problem may not be a result of poor cooking practices but may simply represent an inability to taste food. Alterations in vision may also contribute to decreased appetite, difficulties in food preparation, and finally poor food intake.

Dental Health

Changes in dental health among the elderly include fewer teeth, decreased salivary flow, and poor periodontal condition. A decrease in food choices (especially fibrous foods such as fruits and vegetables), a decreased interest in eating, and decreased food digestibility are likely to occur following a loss of dental health. Many drugs commonly used by the elderly result in reduced salivary flow.

Gastrointestinal Function

Among the problems of gastrointestinal function reported in the literature are diminished hydrochloric acid secretion by the gastric mucosa, impairing protein digestibility,and reduced intestinal absorption of protein, which is perhaps responsible for the observation that the elderly may need about 20 percent more protein per kilogram of body weight in order to maintain nitrogen balance than younger adults.

Poor gastrointestinal absorption of glucose, lactose, and xylose could mean that these sugars are less available as energy substrate and could contribute to increased energy and protein needs. Lactose intolerance, very common among the elderly, leads to decreased consumption of dietary calcium. The combination of decreased dietary calcium and decreased physical activity is likely to contribute to the development of osteoporosis.

Other gastrointestinal problems among the elderly include decreased bile secretion, which may contribute to hypercholesterolemia and therefore to increased risks of coronary disease; fecal incontinence or constipation, which may lead to a fear of eating and anorexia; and urinary incontinence, which may lead to an inadequate fluid intake and subsequent dehydration.

CHRONIC DISEASES AND NUTRITION

There is considerable controversy about whether or not a prudent diet reduces the risk of developing chronic diseases. Unfortunately, no longitudinal studies are yet available that clearly demonstrate that dietary modifications do prevent illness. There is, however, a consensus among most health professionals that if an individual has one or more risk factors, he or she should adhere to appropriate dietary guidelines, and it may be wise in general for all older adults to avoid excesses in their dietary habits.

The *Dietary Guidelines for Americans*[2] is a practical starting point in promoting sound food preparation and consumption patterns that can help maintain the good health of older Americans. These commonsense guidelines include the following:

- maintain ideal weight
- eat a variety of foods
- avoid too much dietary fat, saturated fat, and cholesterol
- eat food with adequate starch and fiber
- avoid too much sugar
- avoid too much sodium
- if you drink alcohol, do so in moderation

Obesity

Chronic diseases like heart disease, high blood pressure, adult-onset diabetes, and osteoporosis are more common among older adults than in any other age segment of the general population. Obesity may play a salient role in the development, poor control, or complications of all these disease entities. Since recidivism rates for weight reduction programs are well over 90 percent by many estimates, perhaps programs aimed at the prevention of obesity rather than its treatment would be more successful. Prevention and treatment programs should incorporate regular physical activity as an integral component of dietary and other life-style changes. Physical activity like walking can result in small but significant improvements in cardiovascular function and reductions in body fat. Physical activity programs should be of a continuous nature using large muscle groups (aerobic exercise). In order to gain the physiologic benefits from exercise, individuals should "work" about 30 to 45 minutes per day three to four times per week.

Drug-Nutrient Interaction

Most of the elderly take medications daily, and drugs can affect appetite and nutrient metabolism. Anorexia may result from altered taste sensitivity, nausea, or from suppression of appetite. Over-the-counter medications, commonly used by the elderly, may contain large amounts of sodium, which is dangerous for those patients with heart disease or high blood pressure.

---

2. U.S. Department of Agriculture and U.S. Department of Health and Human Resources, February 1980.

NUTRITION PROBLEMS OF THE ELDERLY LIVING IN HEALTH CARE FACILITIES

The range and severity of dietary problems among elderly persons living in either acute-care or long-term nursing facilities require consideration. The incidence of protein-calorie malnutrition for all patients ranges from 20 to 60 percent. Patients in a hypermetabolic state (e.g., patients who have an acute infection or are recovering from severe tissue injury due to surgery) may require up to 3,000 to 6,000 calories per day. Evidence of protein-calorie malnutrition is frequently supported by other clinical findings such as a decrease in immunoglobulins, lymphocyte count, body weight, lean body mass, serum albumin, and serum transferrin. A number of criteria have been developed to identify individuals who are at risk of suffering protein-calorie malnutrition; these include the following:

- body weight less than 70% of ideal body weight
- total lymphocyte count less than 1,000/mm^3
- serum albumin less than 3.0 g/100 ml
- serum transferrin less than 98
- negative delayed hypersensitivity by skin tests (e.g., PPD)

If three or more of the above criteria are present, the person should receive some form of hyperalimentation.

On the basis of biochemical analyses, 39 percent of ambulatory patients in a nursing home setting were deficient in one or more of these vitamins: pyridoxine, nicotinate, vitamin B_{12}, and folate. Deficiencies of vitamins A, D, E, and K have also been observed in nursing home populations. Poor food consumption is the probable explanation for most of these nutrition problems.

SUGGESTED READING

1. Albanese, A.A. *Current Topics in Nutrition and Disease*, vol 3. New York: Alan R. Liss, 1980.
2. Bazzarre, T.L., Yuhas, J.A. Measures of food intake among rural elderly. *J. Nutr. Elderly*. In press.
3. Natow, A.B., Heslin, J. *Geriatric Nutrition*. Boston: CBI Publishing, 1980.
4. O'Hanlon, P., Kohrs, M.B. Dietary studies of older Americans. *Am. J. Clin. Nutr.* 31:1257–1269, 1978.
5. Weg, R.B. Nutrition and the later years. Ethel Percy Andrus Gerontology Center, University of Southern California, 1978.
6. Winick, M. (Ed.). *Nutrition and Aging*. New York: John Wiley and Sons, 1976.

Preoperative Evaluation of the Elderly

M. ANDREW GREGANTI, M.D.

Editor's note: The efficient preoperative evaluation of the elderly requires a search for abnormalities of intravascular volume, cardiac status, pulmonary status, and renal status. If no abnormalities are detected and emergency surgery is not planned, the preoperative risk is only slightly greater than that of a young patient. Quantitation of relative influences on operative risk of the major abnormalities that are found is limited by the inadequacy of current risk-evaluation scales. The clinical approach should not focus as much on risk analysis, however, as on the optimal preoperative management of individual risk factors.

The preoperative evaluation of the elderly is a routine task for present-day internists. It has not always been that way, however, and for good reason. Before 1960 perioperative mortality in patients over 80 was 20 percent, and surgical procedures in the elderly were approached with a great deal of apprehension. The situation was summarized best by Dr. Alton Ochsner, who noted in a 1967 address: "In 1927, as a young Professor of Surgery at Tulane Medical School, I taught and practiced that an elective operation for inguinal hernia in a patient older than 50 years was not justified." Fortunately, growth of knowledge about the surgical, anesthetic, and medical management of operations in the elderly since the days described by Dr. Ochsner has paralleled the increase in the geriatric population, resulting in much greater surgical experience with the special problems of this age group. In the last two decades, major improvements in the perioperative management of geriatric patients have allowed older and sicker patients to undergo surgical procedures successfully. Internists are now playing a major role in the preoperative evaluation and management of these patients.

342

CASE STUDY

You are asked to evaluate and medically manage Mr. A., an 85-year-old man with recurrent biliary colic who is admitted for an elective cholecystectomy. Over the past three months he has had three episodes of right upper quadrant, postprandial pain. Fever and chills occurred during the third episode. An oral cholecystogram confirmed multiple radiopaque stones.

The patient's general health has been good until his present problem. His only other significant medical problem is hypertension, which has been easily controlled with hydrochlorothiazide, 50 mg daily. He has not had symptoms of congestive heart failure or angina pectoris. Although he has smoked one pack of cigarettes daily for fifty years, he has no dyspnea on exertion or cough.

The patient's blood pressure is 140/90 mm Hg; his pulse is 88, regular. There is mild hypertensive retinopathy. Chest examination is notable only for a generalized decrease in vesicular breath sounds. Cardiac and abdominal examinations are normal. There is no peripheral edema.

Laboratory data include a normal complete blood count (CBC), blood chemistries profile, urinalysis, and coagulation profile. His electrocardiogram is normal; a chest film reveals flattened diaphragms but is normal otherwise. His pulmonary function tests are compatible with a mild obstructive pattern.

After interviewing and examining Mr. A., you conclude that he is healthy for his age, excluding probable asymptomatic obstructive lung disease. Before making your final assessment and recommendations, you consider the following questions:
1. Does the perioperative mortality rate of patients like Mr. A differ significantly from that of similarly healthy younger patients?
2. If Mr. A. does develop fatal perioperative complications, what complications are most likely?
3. What particular characteristics of Mr. A. predispose him to these specific perioperative complications?
4. What can be done to evaluate, quantitate, and manage Mr. A.'s perioperative risk?

PERIOPERATIVE MORTALITY IN THE HEALTHY ELDERLY

Accurate age-related perioperative mortality statistics are difficult to determine from the available literature. A significant number of the most quoted studies have failed to stratify patients on the basis of age, have not defined preoperative medical status precisely, and have combined statistics for emergency and elective procedures. Elective operations on healthy patients have received comparatively little attention; in fact, urgent or emergency procedures dominate many surgical series, which often originate from university medical centers where patients commonly present during a complicated phase of their disease. As a result, it is usually impossible to assign a well-documented mortality risk to either the "healthy young" or the "healthy elderly."

Despite these limitations, sufficient reliable data are available to confirm the general impression that recent surgical, medical, and anesthetic advances have made perioperative death a rare event in "healthy" patients of any age. Statistics on the eight most common surgical procedures done on healthy patients, ages 25 to 44, confirm that the mortality rate for cholecystectomy, appendectomy, hysterectomy, and inguinal hernia repair was less than 0.1 percent in the early 1970s. The mortality rate for the same procedures in healthy elderly patients is probably only slightly higher provided that surgery is not required on an emergency basis and does not result in a complication. Substantiation of this statement is difficult, however, since it is based primarily on anecdotal impressions of experienced clinicians. The most recent published series, including patients with varying degrees of medical illness, quote overall mortality rates of 4 to 5 percent in elderly patients. The true risk probably lies somewhere between the lower figure (0.1 percent) and the upper figure (5 percent).

Several key observations, common to most series examining operative mortality rates, warrant emphasizing. (1) Most deaths occur postoperatively, not intraoperatively. In fact, many elderly patients do relatively well for 72 hours postoperatively, only to develop complications later. The importance of maintaining careful observation until the patient is well into the recuperative phase has been noted in multiple studies. (2) Emergency procedures are not well tolerated by the elderly and are associated with 4 to 5 times the mortality rate of elective procedures. Among other reasons, the lack of sufficient time to prepare the patient adequately preoperatively causes the noted increased risk. (3) If one potentially fatal perioperative complication develops, the likelihood of the occurrence of others increases significantly.

The causes of increased perioperative mortality in the elderly are brought into clearer perspective by examination of the causes of perioperative mortality in patients of all ages (Table 1). Although

TABLE 1
Percentage of Postoperative Deaths in Series of
Consecutive Surgical Admissions

Etiology	Carp (1950)	Ryan (1960)	Randle (1968)	Lewin (1971)
Pneumonia	33	31	27	18
Cardiac arrest	20	6	12	26
Pulmonary embolus	8	6	6	13
Peritonitis	17	31	28	
Sepsis	4			16
Renal failure	5	10		8
Inoperable cancer	4	6	18	
Hypovolemic shock		10		5
Stroke				
Miscellaneous	9		9	14

Adapted from Feigal, D.W., Blaisdell, F.W., The estimation of surgical risk. *Med. Clin. North Am.* 63:1131–1143, 1979.

TABLE 2
Postoperative Morbidity and Mortality in 147 Patients
Over 90 Years of Age

Condition	Percentage of Patients	
	Morbidity	Mortality
Myocardial infarction	3.4	2.0
Cardiac failure	4.8	—
Pulmonary embolus	2.0	0.7
Bronchopneumonia	7.5	6.1
Cerebrovascular accident	1.4	—
Transient dementia	2.7	—
Septicemia	5.4	2.7
Renal failure	0.7	—
Gastrointestinal bleeding	1.4	0.7
Urinary infection	8.8	—
Paralytic ileus	2.0	—
Decubitus ulcer	4.8	—
Wound infection	1.4	—
Electrolyte imbalance	1.4	—
Total	47.7	12.2

Adapted from Miller, R., Marlar, K., Silvay, G., Anesthesia for patients aged over ninety years. *N.Y. State J. Med.* 77:1421–1425, 1977.

there is some slight variation in the results of the studies listed, the degree of agreement among the series is impressive: pulmonary, cardiac, and infectious complications are the major causes of perioperative death. It is noteworthy that surgical series of mortality in the elderly have depicted similar findings (Table 2): bronchopneumonia, septicemia, and myocardial infarction are the major causes of mortality (and morbidity) in both "healthy" and chronically ill geriatric patients. Why, then, is an elderly patient who is "healthy" more likely to develop these particular complications? The answer, it seems, lies in understanding the physiologic changes that occur in major organ function as a concomitant of aging.

PHYSIOLOGIC CHARACTERISTICS OF THE "ELDERLY NORMAL": RELATIONSHIP TO PERIOPERATIVE COMPLICATIONS

Many elderly patients are physiologically young for their age; indeed, no "disease" results from the passage of time only. Differences in the physiology of the elderly should, therefore, be viewed as quantitative, not qualitative. Nevertheless, in general, "elderly normal" patients do have a decreased ability to compensate for unusual physiologic stresses; old age has been appropriately described as "a continuation of life with decreasing capacities for adaptation." In large part, the limited ability to adapt explains the observations of operative morbidity and mortality in healthy geriatric patients: they do as well as young patients if their physiologic balance is not maximally stressed by an emergency procedure or surgical complications.

Subclinical changes in pulmonary function partially explain the geriatric patient's increased risk of bronchopneumonia and other pulmonary complications. Decreases in vital capacity, tidal volume, minute volume, and maximal breathing capacity have been well documented. Residual volume, dead space, residual volume to total lung capacity ratio, and closing volume all increase. Although the quantitative changes involved are subclinical in most circumstances, they may become clinically significant in the setting of anesthesia and surgery. Alveolar closure with associated ventilation-perfusion abnormalities and decreased clearance of secretions are the pathophysiologic mechanisms that underlie the resulting pulmonary infections; these complications are even more likely in the setting of superimposed chronic lung disease, as in the patient described earlier in the case study.

Age causes a diminished cardiac function with a decrease in cardiac index at rest and in the expected increment in cardiac output under stress—a general state of limited cardiac reserve referred to as "presbycardia" by some authorities. Predictably, complications that require adjustments in cardiac output, such as fever and volume depletion, are tolerated poorly. As in the case of pulmonary disease, the effects of anesthesia exacerbate the basic physiologic impairments to produce clinically overt problems—for example, a decreased cardiac output state in volume-depleted patients. Poor coronary perfusion may lead to infarction, especially in elderly patients with clinical or subclinical coronary artery disease. Volume overload may stress the compensatory mechanisms of the elderly myocardium and acutely precipitate left ventricular failure.

On the other hand, age-related decreases in renal concentrating ability, renal blood flow, and glomerular filtration rate necessitate a relatively volume-expanded state to assure adequate excretion of urinary solutes. When volume deficits occur, prerenal azotemia commonly develops and, if untreated by volume expansion, progresses to acute renal failure.

In general, impairments of drug absorption, metabolism, and excretion increase with age. Failure to make appropriate adjustments in drug and anesthetic dosing results in delirium, oversedation, hypotension, or other problems that increase the risk of pulmonary, cardiac, and renal complications.

EVALUATION AND MANAGEMENT OF THE ELDERLY SURGICAL PATIENT

To maximize the chances for optimal patient outcome, four areas of perioperative evaluation and management deserve special attention: intravascular volume status, cardiac status, pulmonary status, and renal status.

Intravascular Volume
The increased sensitivity of the elderly to both volume depletion and volume overload necessitates an accurate perioperative assessment of intravascular volume status. Unfortunately, this task is fraught with diagnostic pitfalls, many of which result in major perioperative com-

plications. Nevertheless, as in many other clinical situations, the key to making the diagnosis of abnormal fluid balance is thinking of the diagnosis.

Volume depletion in the acute surgical patient occurs in a variety of settings, most of which are easily recognized. Acutely ill patients with fever, decreased oral intake, persistent diarrhea, or other sources of fluid loss usually manifest easily detectable signs of decreased intravascular volume (e.g., orthostatic hypotension, dry mucous membranes, and decreased skin turgor). Aggressive fluid replacement preoperatively prevents intraoperative hypotension secondary to the vasodilatory effects of anesthesia.

In contrast, volume depletion in the elective surgical patient commonly presents in a more subtle manner. Typically, the patient complains only of mild weakness and malaise and has a slightly increased serum blood urea nitrogen (BUN) to creatinine ratio or a mild contraction alkalosis. The volume deficit frequently remains undetected until hypotension develops intraoperatively, particularly in patients whose sympathetic reflexes are blocked by spinal anesthesia, with resultant myocardial ischemia or infarction. Although this scenario may also complicate the chronic use of diuretics, it more commonly develops in the setting of preoperative diuretic therapy instituted within one week of elective surgery. In such cases, fluid has been selectively depleted from the intravascular compartment, and there has been insufficient time for equilibration with the extravascular compartment.

Because of the potential complications of instituting diuretics preoperatively, the specific indications for these agents should be considered carefully. In general, patients with mild hypertension (diastolic pressure 90 to 100 mm Hg) do not require preoperative antihypertensive treatment, since this level of blood pressure elevation has not been shown to increase perioperative morbidity and mortality. In contrast, preoperative diastolic pressures of greater than 110 mm Hg do significantly increase surgical risk. Whether pressures in the 100–110 mm Hg diastolic range increase risk remains in debate; a conservative management plan would be to postpone elective surgical procedures for at least two weeks while instituting antihypertensive therapy, which usually includes a diuretic. The two weeks' delay allows sufficient time to control the patient's hypertension and prevents preoperative intravascular volume depletion. Obviously, a more aggressive approach is required in patients who need emergency surgery; nevertheless, diuretics should be used judiciously, and hypertension control should primarily depend on short-acting vasodilators like nitroprusside.

In contrast to volume depletion, preoperative volume overload is usually easier to detect. The patient with pulmonary rales, S3 gallop, and peripheral edema rarely presents diagnostic problems. As in the case of preoperative antihypertensive therapy, diuretic therapy of elective surgical patients should allow time for volume equilibration prior to anesthesia.

Volume overload presents greater problems intraoperatively and postoperatively in patients whose preoperative volume status was clinically normal. In most cases these patients have subclinical cardiac abnormalities that become clinically overt when the administration of large volumes of intravenous fluid and/or blood products precipitates acute congestive heart failure. Although this complication is easily treated in most cases, the best treatment is prevention, with routine judicious fluid management in the elderly patient.

Cardiac Status

Despite the major technical advances during the past two decades in the detection of cardiac abnormalities, the key to successful preoperative cardiac evaluation continues to be a detailed history and physical examination. The major focus should be to determine whether the patient has symptoms and signs of congestive heart failure, coronary artery disease, or both. A recent study of cardiac risk factors demonstrated that the presence of congestive heart failure, evidenced by an S3 gallop or jugular venous distention, had the greatest "weight" in predicting cardiac morbidity (perioperative myocardial infarction, ventricular tachycardia, or pulmonary edema) and mortality.[1] The occurrence of myocardial infarction within six months of the date of surgery had the second greatest weight.

Other risk factors also warrant particular attention. Based on data from the same study, the presence of more than 5 ventricular premature contractions per minute documented at any time before surgery or any nonsinus rhythm on the routine preoperative electrocardiogram significantly increased the chances of perioperative morbidity and mortality. Interestingly, age greater than 70 was associated with a significant relative risk. This observation probably

---

1. L. Goldman, D.L. Caldera, S.R. Nussbaum, et al. Multifactorial index of cardiac risk in noncardiac surgical procedures. *N. Engl. J. Med.* 297:845–850, 1977.

reflects the prevalence of subclinical heart disease or limited cardiac reserve that becomes clinically significant when stressed by a surgical procedure.

Optimal preoperative management entails minimization of cardiac risk by treating those abnormalities that are reversible, in part or totally. Controlling congestive heart failure with digitalization and diuresis, treating abnormalities of cardiac rhythm, and delaying elective surgery in patients who have had a myocardial infarction within the previous six months are all of critical importance.

Since perioperative morbidity and mortality in the elderly most often occur in the postoperative phase, careful observation and management should continue well into the recuperative period. This should include scrutiny for perioperative myocardial infarction, particularly in those patients who develop intraoperative hypotension, who undergo emergency surgery, or who have documented significant coronary artery disease. Other factors that increase the risk of myocardial infarction include vascular procedures, upper abdominal procedures, procedures of long duration, and significant preoperative hypertension (diastolic pressure >110 mm Hg). Even with careful clinical observation, cardiac complications may be difficult to recognize since the classic symptoms are usually obscured by incisional pain, sedation, and analgesia. The usual perioperative presentation includes sudden hypotension, new onset congestive heart failure, or signs of decreased cardiac output, with the peak of recognition of these problems at day 3 to day 6 postoperatively. Patients who are at high risk, therefore, should have a routine postoperative electrocardiogram even in the absence of suspicious signs.

Pulmonary Status
The proper evaluation of pulmonary status is a greatly debated step in preoperative evaluation. The case study presented is typical of many elderly patients who present with a history of smoking and minimal symptoms or signs of respiratory compromise.

Contrary to popular belief, pulmonary function tests (PFTs) do not necessarily offer the most accurate assessment of perioperative pulmonary risk. In fact, few studies provide convincing evidence that PFTs are superior to the routine history and physical examination in patients who are undergoing procedures not involving lung resection. Patients with chronic cough and greater than 1 ounce of sputum production per day are at major risk, since their compromised ability to clear secretions will be even further impaired by anesthesia. Similarly, the presence of a history of combined cardiac and pulmonary disease is a particularly serious risk factor, as is a history of dyspnea on mild exertion.

Physical examination provides other useful indicators of risk. Simply observing the strength of the patient's cough can predict whether the effects of anesthesia and postoperative sedation will significantly impair the ability to clear secretions by coughing. In general, patients with significant prolongation of expiratory time (greater than 3 to 4 seconds) have ineffective coughs and, as a result, have a greater risk of major postoperative pulmonary complications.

Pulmonary function tests, in particular the $PaCO_2$ and the midmaximal expiratory flow rate (MMEFR), may provide further assistance. An elevated preoperative $PaCO_2$ is a foreboding sign, since postoperative ventilatory insufficiency will invariably occur. A depressed MMEFR of less than 0.6 L/sec correlates with a severe impairment of the ability to generate an effective cough. None of the many other tests of pulmonary function has been shown to add significant predictive capacity to the history and physical examination in patients who are not undergoing lung resection.

The routine preoperative chest radiograph offers little useful information when the history and physical examination fail to reveal cardiopulmonary problems. Nevertheless, the routine chest film has become a standard of clinical practice—albeit one with a poor cost/benefit ratio. Most proponents argue that the study serves as a helpful baseline should pulmonary or cardiac complications arise.

The specific site of the surgical incision determines pulmonary risk; incisions transecting the primary or accessory respiratory muscles have the greatest deleterious effect (i.e., intrathoracic procedures, upper abdominal procedures, and intraabdominal vascular procedures requiring long incisions). For example, the pulmonary risk of the patient in the case study would be less for a lower abdominal procedure than for cholecystectomy.

Management of the patient who has significant pulmonary risk should focus on improving the patient's abilities to clear airway secretions. Preoperative instruction in the use of the incentive spirometer is particularly important. Treatment of bacterial bronchitis with antibiotics preoperatively will decrease the risk of pulmonary infection postoperatively. Other useful approaches include (1) using an optimal bronchodilator regimen, (2) minimizing anesthesia time,

(3) early postoperative mobilization, and (4) minimizing postoperative narcotic analgesia with its potential for impaired ventilation and poor clearance of secretions.

Renal Status

The first step in evaluating renal status is estimation of the patient's intravascular volume and then treatment of intravascular volume depletion. If intravascular volume is carefully maintained at adequate levels, elderly patients with and without renal dysfunction do well. A mortality rate of more than 50 percent when postoperative renal failure occurs makes prevention far preferable to treatment.

METHODS OF PREDICTING PERIOPERATIVE COMPLICATIONS

Although evaluation of the organ systems usually involved in perioperative complications provides helpful data for risk assessment, a practical numerical estimate of overall operative risk is not always possible. In most cases, the evaluator is faced with stating a highly subjective impression in general terms, such as "acceptable," "poor," and "unacceptable." Such descriptive terminology provides a global risk assessment but does not accurately quantitate the risk of morbidity and mortality. Unfortunately, a better method is not available; however, other methods that are being used deserve a brief discussion.

The American Society of Anesthesiologists' (ASA) Physical Status Classification is probably the oldest and the most commonly utilized risk evaluation scale. Based on the history, physical examination, and laboratory data, a patient is placed into one of five classes, ranging from class 1 (a normal, healthy patient) to class 5 (a moribund patient who is not expected to survive 24 hours with or without an operation). A letter E is appended to the class number in emergency cases. Although this scheme seems simplistic and permits subjective biases of individual anesthesiologists, several studies have shown a direct correlation between class number and 48-hour and six-week operative mortality. In addition, the same studies have documented a clear increase in the risk of perioperative death in emergency cases, no matter what the numerical scale class or the patient's age. Unfortunately, the scale fails to define the specific causes of morbidity and mortality to facilitate intervention, nor does it allow a distinct separation between acceptable and unacceptable risk.

A scale developed by Dr. Lee Goldman and colleagues has been used to evaluate cardiac risk more objectively.[2] By studying the perioperative cardiac morbidity and mortality of approximately 1,000 patients, Dr. Goldman used multifactorial analysis to define the nine factors with the greatest influence on cardiac risk. By assigning each factor a specific number of points, each patient could be given an overall total point score. Using total point scores, Goldman defined four classes, each correlating with a specific risk of life-threatening cardiac complication or cardiac death. There are two major advantages of this scale over the ASA scale: the risk of a specific type of morbidity and mortality is defined based on specific preoperative medical problems, and patients in class 4 (having 26 or more total points) have a tremendous increase in risk compared to patients in class 3. The degree of the increase allows a distinct separation of acceptable (class 3) and unacceptable (class 4) surgical risk. Since patients in class 4 have clinically obvious severe cardiac disease and would be defined as "unacceptable" by more global risk scales, it is questionable whether the Goldman scheme offers any practical advantage in the evaluation of the elderly.

Finally, the use of routine preoperative screening tests to assist in defining operative risk deserves some discussion. The popularity of these tests has increased with the rapid expansion of medical technology and with the tendency to deemphasize the value of the routine history and physical examination. The most commonly ordered screening studies include complete blood count, blood chemistries profile, urinalysis, coagulation profile, electrocardiogram, and chest radiograph. Despite cogent arguments that can be made in support of each of these studies, there is no well-documented evidence that routine screening adds any information useful in predicting the perioperative risk of young or elderly patients who are found to be healthy after the routine history and physical examination. Perhaps the best rationale for using the tests is that they provide an accurate assessment of the patient's baseline major organ function.

SUGGESTED READING

1. Burnett, W., McCaffrey, J. Surgical procedures in the elderly. *Surg. Gynecol. Obstet.* 134:221–226, 1972.
2. Cain, H.D., Stevens, P.M., Adaniya, R. Preoperative pulmonary function and complications after cardiovascular surgery. *Chest* 76:130–135, 1979.

---

2. Ibid.

3. Cole, W.H. Medical differences between the young and the aged. *J. Am. Geriatr. Soc.* 18:589–614, 1970.
4. Djokovic, J.L., Hedley-Whyte, J. Prediction of outcome of surgery and anesthesia in patients over 80. *J.A.M.A.* 242:2301–2306, 1979.
5. Ellison, N. Problems in geriatric anesthesia. *Surg. Clin. North Am.* 55:929–945, 1975.
6. Goldman, L., Caldera, D.L., Nussbaum, S.R., et al. Multifactorial index of cardiac risk in noncardiac surgical procedures. *N. Engl. J. Med.* 297:845–850, 1977.
7. Miller, R., Marlar, K., Silvay, G. Anesthesia for patients aged over ninety years. *N.Y. State J. Med.* 77:1421–1425, 1977.

Index